DOCTORS, NURSES, AND MEDICAL PRACTITIONERS
A BIO-BIBLIOGRAPHICAL SOURCEBOOK

EDITED BY LOIS N. MAGNER

Greenwood Press
Westport, Connecticut • London

Library of Congress Cataloging-in-Publication Data

Doctors, nurses, and medical practitioners : a bio-bibliographical
  sourcebook / edited by Lois N. Magner.
     p. cm.
  Includes bibliographical references and index.
  ISBN 0–313–29452–6 (alk. paper)
    1. Medicine—Bio-bibliography—Dictionaries. I. Magner, Lois N.,
  1943– .
  R153.D63   1997
  610'.92'2—dc21
  [B]   97–2232

British Library Cataloguing in Publication Data is available.

Library of Congress Catalog Card Number: 97–2232
ISBN: 0–313–29452–6

First published in 1997

Greenwood Press, 88 Post Road West, Westport, CT 06881
An imprint of Greenwood Publishing Group, Inc.

Printed in the United States of America

The paper used in this book complies with the
Permanent Paper Standard issued by the National
Information Standards Organization (Z39.48–1984).

10 9 8 7 6 5 4 3 2 1

Copyright Acknowledgments

The editor and publisher gratefully acknowledge permission for the following material:

Extracts from Jacqueline Corn, *Protecting the Health of Workers: The American Conference of
Governmental Industrial Hygienists 1938–1988* (Cincinnati, OH: ACGIH, 1989), pp. 157–158. Reprinted with permission of ACGIH.

Every reasonable effort has been made to trace the owners of copyright materials in the book, but
in some instances this has proven impossible. The editor and publisher will be glad to receive
information leading to more complete acknowledgments in subsequent printings of the book and in
the meantime extend their apologies for any omissions.

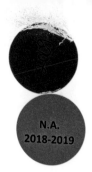
To Ki-Han and Oliver, as always

CONTENTS

INTRODUCTION

LOIS N. MAGNER

Medical biography has been of considerable interest to the medical community since ancient times, but most representatives of this genre have been celebrations of the great doctors in their role as biomedical scientists. Some medical biographies celebrated the lives of rather special figures of the history of medicine, such as master surgeons, physicians as men of letters and men of action, doctors whose names were immortalized in medical eponyms, or even the *Musical Sons of Aesculapius*. Interest in medical biography has certainly not diminished since these pioneering works were assembled. However, the kinds of questions of interest to historians, scholars, and general readers continue to evolve and lead to the demand for new approaches to medical biography.

The ''great doctors'' approach generally ignores and excludes the contributions of nurses, public health workers, practitioners, and educators who played a large part in the establishment of the social, cultural, and institutional foundations of health care, and it tends to exclude the contributions of women and minorities. A more nuanced account of history requires that studies of heroic figures must be balanced by paying attention to the much larger cast of supporting players: educators, activists, teachers, administrators, scientists, and practitioners. Such an approach can reveal complex networks of relationships and interactions, direct and indirect, and the elusive and often ephemeral sense of community that links medicine, science, and society.

The goal of this collection was to identify and explore the work of significant but lesser-known individuals. It is easy to compile a list of Nobel Laureates or famous European and American biomedical scientists, but very difficult to produce a representative list of individuals from all parts of the world who reflect, in their lives and achievements, the issues that have become central to social and contextual approaches to the history of health care, the special concerns of women and minorities, and international aspects of health and disease.

This book contains biographical essays on fifty-six remarkable individuals in the medical field. Many of these figures are not well known outside their own country, calling, or specialized field, but the stories told here include the famous and even the infamous. They are the people who "get things done" and work toward establishing a "more egalitarian system of health care delivery." They are significant for their ideas, diagnostic or therapeutic methods, writings, the institutions that they founded, and the impetus they imparted to their students.

By integrating biographies of doctors, nurses, and practitioners of different time periods and different cultures, this book addresses the kinds of questions currently of interest to historians, scholars, and students. Profiles of individuals from different cultures and time periods provide a valuable perspective on changing patterns of health and disease and differences in medical philosophy.

In order to assemble a collection of individuals who can best be described as extraordinary yet unsung, a preliminary list was circulated among historians of medicine, and suggestions were obtained from colleagues and contributors. Of course, given the nature of this collection, an almost infinite variety of final assemblages was possible, but we believe that this book provides an intriguing entry into a world of lesser-known but not less interesting men and women. Although most of the individuals profiled can be classified as American and European physicians, individuals from other parts of the world and other professions are included as well. Issues in biomedical science, public health, preventive medicine, education, and so forth are truly global problems. The authors of these essays have attempted to transcend traditional nationalistic and disciplinary boundaries. Unfortunately, space limitations prevented us from including many other equally remarkable individuals and forced us to keep the essays shorter than many of the contributors might have liked. But by keeping the number of entries relatively small, the treatment of each one is more detailed than possible in many other biographical dictionaries.

The subjects of these essays are too diverse to lend themselves to a rigid format, but to encourage overall consistency, contributors were asked to follow a set format. Each essay focuses on one person's life and career, and the relationship of that individual's work to the universal quest for health and healing. Authors have also provided a bibliography including, wherever possible, a guide to the archival materials available, works written by and about the individual, and recent scholarship concerning related topics to help readers seek out further information on subjects that pique their interest. Names marked with an asterisk are found elsewhere in the book.

We hope that this collection will serve many ends. As a bio-bibliography, it is intended as a reference work designed for students and scholars, but it should also provide inspirational reading for high school and college students. Although a one-volume reference book cannot be exhaustive or comprehensive in its coverage, we hope that readers will find this collection of essays accessible, thought provoking, and informative. We hope as well that these individual stories will raise questions, suggest possibilities and patterns, and provide readers with useful guidelines and strategies for seeking out additional information.

As a teacher in the history of medicine, I have found the biographical approach particularly effective in reaching students. Biographies help us to think critically and compassionately, and they establish a sense of kinship with patients and practitioners, past and present, a sense of humility, and a critical perspective with respect to today's medical problems. Biographical studies can throw light on the encounter between patient and practitioner, changing patterns of medical practice, professionalization, institutions, education, human experimentation, innovation, and resistance to change. Above all, these essays should encourage further reflections on the factors determining patterns of health and disease and a point of entry into a diverse and fascinating field of scholarship.

Many people helped this work evolve. In particular, I thank the authors of the essays for their cooperation and their enthusiasm for the project. I also express my appreciation to the always helpful, efficient, and cheerful staff of the History Department at Purdue University—especially Julie Mántica, Judy McHenry, and Peggy Quirk. Without the cooperation and assistance of the staff of the Interlibrary Loan Division of the HSSE Library, it would have been impossible to complete this project.

I am particularly indebted to John Parascandola for his invaluable advice, encouragement, and help, especially concerning subjects, contributors, and assistance in revising particular sections. I also thank Nancy Eckerman for help in tracking down elusive references. Special thanks go to Oliver J. Kim for revising and editing several of the more recalcitrant essays and for his always stylish advice.

WILLIAM BEAUMONT
(1785–1853)

William Beaumont, physician and physiologist, was born in Lebanon, Connecticut, November 21, 1785, shortly after the close of the American Revolution.
He was the third child in a family of nine who toiled steadfastly on the few
acres of their New England farm. Although Beaumont had only minimal training
in medicine and was self-taught in physiology, he earned an international reputation in medical research for his experiments on Alexis St. Martin, known
popularly as "the man with a hole in his stomach." Beaumont's work, the first
documented case of such human experimentation in the United States, is a landmark in the field of biomedical ethics (Numbers 1979: 113–135). Beaumont's
work provided empirical evidence about the exact nature of the human digestive
process that called into question prevailing theories, such as vitalism. Advocates
of vitalism believed that gastric fluid has no solvent properties when removed
from the body. Until Beaumont's work, scientists had been able to extract only
minute quantities of gastric fluid from dogs, birds, or other animals. Beaumont
proved that gastric fluid, even when removed from the body, possesses solvent
properties. Remarkably, all of Beaumont's research was conducted on the American frontier, far from the eastern educational-scientific establishment. For all of
these reasons, Sir William Osler in 1907 hailed William Beaumont as a "pioneer
physiologist" and a major figure in the development of medicine and science
in America (Beaumont 1959: vii–xxxix).

It may be assumed that Beaumont received his primary and secondary education in the local public school in Lebanon. The earliest documented event in
his life was his leaving the farm at age twenty-one to seek employment as a
schoolmaster in the village of Champlain, New York (Myer 1939: 15). Whatever
the nature of his early education, he was considered competent enough to hold
a post as schoolmaster from 1806 to 1810. Augmenting his income with a
second job, he saved enough money to secure a medical apprenticeship with
Dr. Benjamin Chandler, a distinguished physician in St. Albans, Vermont. The
year that Beaumont spent with Chandler was the only formal medical training
he ever received. In June 1812, as America was again going to war with England, Beaumont left his mentor, still owing him tuition, a debt he never paid.
Beaumont joined the army at Plattsburgh, New York, as surgeon's mate. After
his service in the War of 1812, he attempted to set up a practice in Plattsburgh.
For five years he struggled to make a living, and in 1819, when financial failure
overwhelmed him, he rejoined the army. The Medical Department was being
reorganized by a young surgeon general, Joseph Lovell, and Beaumont was
readily accepted. His first duty station was a remote army post on the north-

western frontier, Fort Mackinac, located on an island in the straits of the Great Lakes. Mackinac Island was an outpost of the American Fur Company.

On May 3, 1820, Beaumont boarded the steamer *Walk-in-the-Water* to travel to Mackinac Island in the Territory of Michigan to assume the duties of post surgeon. Still deeply in debt, he secured Lovell's permission to establish a private medical practice in the Village of Mackinac down the hill from the fort. It is indicative of Beaumont's temperament that by the following autumn he was involved in a dispute over a public vegetable garden inside the military reservation. Before the dispute was settled, Beaumont had taken the matter all the way up the chain of command to the War Department in Washington. In August 1821, at the end of his first lonely tour of duty, Beaumont traveled back to Plattsburgh to marry the innkeeper's daughter, Deborah Green Platt, described as a widow. The second year at the fort was less lonely for Beaumont; his wife gave birth to their first child, Sarah, in the spring, and Beaumont met his professional destiny when he encountered Alexis St. Martin, a young French Canadian who on June 6, 1822, was accidentally shot in the abdomen. Years later, a fur company employee remembered the scene: "One of the party was holding a shot gun which accidentally discharged, the whole charge entering St. Martin's body . . . the muzzle was not over three feet from him . . . the wadding entering, as well as pieces of his clothing, his shirt took fire; he fell, as we supposed, dead" (Beaumont 1959: ix).

Beaumont, who had been summoned from the fort hospital, pushed a portion of stomach and lung that were protruding back through the wound and applied a fermenting poultice of flour, charcoal, yeast, and hot water. Although Beaumont expected the wound to be fatal, St. Martin survived. For the next seventeen days, Beaumont changed his dressings several times a day and bled him once "to the amount of eighteen or twenty ounces." When St. Martin's fever subsided, he was still critically ill and his wound continued to exude bits of cloth and bone. Paid by the village charity funds, Beaumont continued applying poultices and brought St. Martin to the post hospital, when he seemed strong enough to be carried on a stretcher. Beaumont attempted to clear the wound of bone and debris and close it surgically. In preanesthesia days, this was a traumatic procedure. When the wound did not respond to efforts at closure, Beaumont placed a compress over the aperture and bound it tightly.

St. Martin gradually improved and expressed his intention of returning to the Canadian woods, but according to the memorial Beaumont later presented to Congress, he believed the journey would kill the young man. Because village charity had been exhausted, Beaumont hired St. Martin as a household servant. Beaumont unsuccessfully attempted to close the wound, and following the surgical procedure, he wrote in his journal: "After trying every means within my power to close the puncture of the Stomach by exciting adhesions between the lips of the wound . . . without the least appearance of success, I gave over trying, convinced that the Stomach of itself will not close a puncture in its coats by granulations" (Beaumont 1833).

In time, it became clear to Beaumont that St. Martin's gastrostomy was permanent. Although he was not a university-trained physician, Beaumont knew from his reading that he had a rare opportunity to observe digestion in a healthy human being. These observations might definitively test the many conflicting theories concerning normal human digestion. Encouraged by his correspondence with Lovell, who provided books on physiology, Beaumont began a systematic scheme of observations of St. Martin's stomach. Beaumont wrote a description of the case that Lovell submitted for publication. As a consequence of this article, Beaumont was given honorary membership in the Medical Society of the Territory of Michigan, his first accolade relative to the St. Martin case. In May 1824, Beaumont began to experiment on his patient by inserting and then withdrawing items of food from St. Martin's stomach in order to ascertain the "length of time required to digest each." For the next nine years Beaumont and St. Martin maintained their difficult relationship. Although he was paid a small wage, St. Martin frequently ran away.

As the importance of his work became more and more evident, Beaumont planned a tour of European medical centers to lecture and exhibit St. Martin's gastrostomy. He depended on the full cooperation of Surgeon General Lovell to place the resources of the army at his disposal. After the publication of his first article, Beaumont feared that St. Martin might be lured away by another scientist and sought a way to secure exclusive rights to his unique human subject. Further complications arose when Beaumont was assigned to Fort Crawford, Prairie du Chien, in the Wisconsin Territory. In 1831, St. Martin, with his wife and two children, went to Fort Crawford, where Beaumont performed an important series of experiments. Beaumont directly tested vitalist theory by withdrawing gastric fluid from St. Martin and conducting experiments on artificial digestion outside the body. The situation in the Beaumont household, especially the relationship between Mrs. St. Martin and Mrs. Beaumont, was strained. In this domestic turmoil, Beaumont observed for the first time the effects of emotional stress on his subject's digestion. When St. Martin left for Canada this time, it was with a promise to meet Beaumont in Plattsburgh to prepare for the European tour.

To assist Beaumont, Lovell granted him a year's furlough and contacted European medical schools and learned societies where Beaumont might lecture and exhibit St. Martin. During these preparations, Beaumont's orders granting the furlough were rescinded because two calamities on the frontier required his presence at Fort Crawford. The Black Hawk Indian War, followed by an outbreak of cholera, cost Beaumont a delay of another year. Not until August 1832 was Beaumont permitted to travel to the East. St. Martin was waiting for him in Plattsburgh as promised, and Beaumont drew up a contract, securing his exclusive right to experiment on St. Martin's gastrostomy. The contract was signed before the notary in Plattsburgh and an official of Clinton County Court. This was the first document of its kind in the history of human scientific experimentation; it placed St. Martin in Beaumont's custody in a relationship tantamount to indentured servitude. Lovell arranged for St. Martin to receive a sergeant's wage and a clothing allowance for five years, placing the army, for the first time, in the position of granting a direct subsidy to scientific investigation.

While Beaumont was in Washington preparing the final draft of his manuscript for publication during the winter of 1832–1833, Lovell invited Robley Dunglison, a distinguished professor of physiology at the University of Virginia, to come to Washington to meet Beaumont and St. Martin. Dunglison, who had recently published his own textbook in physiology, supported the theory of an Italian researcher, Lazzaro Spallanzani, that gastric fluid contains solvent properties. As an antivitalist, Dunglison was eager to work with Beaumont and, above all, to obtain gastric fluid from St. Martin for chemical analysis. Beaumont, however, immediately saw Dunglison as a threat to his exclusive authorship and rudely withdrew from Dunglison, leaving behind a vial of St. Martin's gastric fluid with a note begging for an analysis from the physiologist's university laboratory and a suggestion that Dunglison might plan to precede him to publication. Dunglison, who was deeply insulted, repeated his conversations with Beaumont verbatim in his personal memoir and recorded in detail his impressions of the unsophisticated frontiersman. Dunglison made a substantial contribution to Beaumont's book, and he suggested a line of experimentation comparing gastric fluid and artificially acidified solutions to demonstrate that the action of gastric fluid is not due simply to its acidity. Within days of his return to the University of Virginia, Dunglison had reported the results of his chemical analysis to Beaumont who was still in Washington with St. Martin. Dunglison found that gastric fluid contains both muriatic and acetic acids, and this analysis supported his own work as well as Beaumont's. Again, Dunglison urged Beaumont to publish promptly and not to fear piracy of his work. Beaumont replied with characteristic self-interest, "I shall hasten publication of experiments as fast as my circumstances and abilities permit, consistently [sic] with a view to future benefit and to secure credit to myself" (Myer 1939: 78–79).

Lovell arranged for Beaumont and St. Martin to travel to New York City, where Beaumont met leading physicians and physiologists. To obtain further analyses of gastric fluid, Beaumont submitted a specimen to Benjamin Silliman, a renowned professor of chemistry and natural history at Yale University. Rather than conducting the analysis in his own laboratory, Silliman suggested that Beaumont contact the well-known Swedish scientist, Jacob Berzelius, in Stockholm. This Beaumont did with the aid of the Swedish consul, but he also asked Franklin Bache of the Philadelphia College of Pharmacy to perform an analysis. He even contacted Dunglison again, begging for further analyses. Lovell made it possible for Beaumont and St. Martin to travel to Plattsburgh in July 1833 for the final round of sixty-two experiments, which took him until November. Waiting anxiously for the results of the analyses, Beaumont delayed final publication of his book and drew up a second contract with St. Martin, binding him in service for two years at a stipend of four hundred dollars, to be paid by the army.

By December, none of Beaumont's requests for analysis of gastric fluid had materialized, so he published without them. His book, 280 pages long, paid for by Beaumont himself, had been vigorously promoted prior to publication at a cost of three dollars, and it sold briskly. In title, format, and style it is reminiscent of Benjamin Franklin's book on electricity. Dedicated to Joseph Lovell, it is entitled *Experiments and Observations on the Gastric Juice and the Physiology of Digestion*, with an acknowledgment to eleven physicians and physiologists whose support and interest he valued. The introduction contains a detailed case history of St. Martin and Beaumont's routine of experimentation, emphasizing that the procedure caused no harm to the subject. In order to elucidate his opinions on the subject of digestion and comment on his experiments, Beaumont divided his observations into seven sections: 1) aliments, 2) hunger and thirst, 3) satisfaction and satiety, 4) mastication, insalivation and deglutition; 5) digestion by the gastric juice; 6) the appearance of the villous coat and the motions of the stomach; 7) chylification and the uses of the bile and pancreatic juice. After reviewing the literature pertaining to each topic, Beaumont attacked the work of leading investigators if his experiments led him to different conclusions. He extolled his own lack of sophistication and training as a liberating factor, claiming that he had no prior knowledge or adherence to any given theory that might color or distort his conclusions about human digestion (Beaumont 1959: 6–7).

The year 1833 was the summit of Beaumont's career. He had successfully maintained control of St. Martin, for the duration of the experiments at least; he had kept exclusive right to publication, allowing no one, not even Dunglison, to share the credit; he had become not merely an army doctor but a scientist, physiologist, and candidate for the pantheon of American medical pioneers. Even before his book came off the presses, Beaumont had begun his memorial to Congress requesting financial remuneration. Beaumont must have felt instinctively that his work had bridged the gaping space between the two halves of American medicine: applied medicine and medical science. Within the year, the army ordered him to report for duty as army surgeon at Jefferson Barracks, near St. Louis, Missouri. Disappointed, he protested and procrastinated, but as he boarded a steamer bound for St. Louis, he received another blow: Congress rejected his request for financial remuneration in the spring of 1834. Not until November 1835 was Beaumont allowed to travel to Washington to argue his case for a change in duty station. After meeting with Lovell, Beaumont was transferred to the St. Louis Arsenal, with permission to establish a private medical practice within the city. In May 1835, Beaumont returned to St. Louis, a place he had described in a letter to Major Kirby as "an abode of savages, alligators & Indian traders."

Beaumont never again obtained the services of St. Martin, although he never ceased trying. He published a second edition of his book with the assistance of his cousin, Samuel Beaumont of Plattsburgh. With the duties of post surgeon to perform at the arsenal and a medical practice to build in the city, Beaumont worked tirelessly during his first year in St. Louis, a thriving city of more than 16,000 inhabitants. In 1836, the city's elite physicians organized a medical society to improve the standards of practice and fight quackery. Beaumont identified himself with founders of the Medical Society of Missouri at St. Louis and received an appointment to the chair of surgery in the medical school organized by the society.

Beaumont learned of Lovell's sudden death when he wrote to the surgeon general asking if it would be proper for him, as an army surgeon, to serve as professor of surgery in the projected St. Louis University Medical Department. Lovell's successor, Thomas Lawson, who loathed Beaumont and had no interest in scientific research, ordered the physician to report to Fort Brooke, Florida, where the government was launching a military action against the Seminole Indians. Beaumont refused to move and submitted his resignation from the army. The dispute was finally resolved with the formal acceptance of Beaumont's resignation.

During this difficult period, Beaumont became embroiled in a conflict within the new medical society. The board of trustees of the St. Louis University Medical Department had waited three years for his letter concerning the appointment to the chair of surgery. As the delay lengthened, a new medical school was founded in St. Louis by Joseph Nash McDowell, Beaumont's enemy, thereby depriving the society of the distinction of establishing the first medical school west of the Mississippi River.

During the 1840s, Beaumont made a comfortable living as a private physician, but his life was disrupted by direct involvement in two major court battles. The Darnes Davis case involved a carpenter who had attacked the owner of a newspaper with an iron cane and smashed his skull. To relieve cranial pressure, Beaumont performed an emergency trephination, but the victim died. When the case came to trial in St. Louis, William Darnes, the man who had wielded the iron cane, was not the focus of the trial. Instead, the defense accused Beaumont of drilling a hole in the victim's skull to observe and experiment on the brain, as he had done with St. Martin's stomach. In 1844, already embittered by his humiliating experience in court, Beaumont was named in a medical malpractice lawsuit. Dugan, a patient whom Beaumont had seen as a consultant, sued Beaumont and a colleague for the unsatisfactory results of their treatment. Beaumont and Dr. Stephen Adreon were acquitted, but violent hostilities developed in the medical community, and Beaumont bitterly denounced his colleagues.

Although Beaumont spent his final twenty years in St. Louis trying to resume his physiological research, that never happened. His small book, published in 1833, was his only real achievement. He died on April 25, 1853, having fallen on the ice a month earlier as he was making a house call. St. Martin lived for twenty-eight years after Beaumont's death. Only briefly did he allow other doctors to study his gastrostomy during these years, but no major contribution to medical knowledge was forthcoming from their work. Beaumont is credited solely, as he dreamed he would be, with the first full description of human digestion.

BIBLIOGRAPHY

In 1915, William Beaumont's correspondence, personal library, and manuscripts were presented to Washington University School of Medicine by his granddaughter, Lily Beaumont Irwin. This collection consists of several thousand documents, beginning in 1804, and ending with family papers, which were gathered after Beaumont's death in 1853; the collection contains letters received by Beaumont, and, in almost every case, a draft of the letter he sent in reply. For almost fifty years, these materials were stored, unused and forgotten, in the medical library. Under the direction of Estelle Brodman, librarian, the papers were made available to scholars in 1964. Prior to this bequest, the Beaumont family allowed Jesse S. Myer, M.D., to use the Beaumont papers in order to write a biography, *The Life and Letters of Dr. William Beaumont*. Genevieve Miller's *William Beaumont's Formative Years* provides information about Beaumont's apprenticeship and early career.

Writings by William Beaumont

William Beaumont's Formative Years; Two Early Notebooks, 1811–1821. With Annotation and an Introductory Essay by Genevieve Miller. New York: Henry Scherman, 1946.
Experiments and Observations on the Gastric Juice and the Physiology of Digestion. (Facsimile.) New York: Dover, 1959.

Writings about William Beaumont and Related Topics

Bylebyl, Jerome J. "William Beaumont, Robley Dunglison, and the Philadelphia Physiologists." *Journal of the History of Medicine and Allied Sciences* 25 (1970): 3–21.
Myer, Jesse S. *The Life and Letters of Dr. William Beaumont*. 2d ed. St. Louis: C. V. Mosby Co., 1939.
Numbers, Ronald L. "William Beaumont and the Ethics of Human Experimentation." *Journal of the History of Biology* 12 (1979): 113–135.
Numbers, Ronald L., and William J. Orr, Jr. "William Beaumont's Reception at Home and Abroad." *ISIS* 7 (1981): 590–612.
Pitcock, Cynthia De Haven. "The Involvement of William Beaumont M.D. in a Medical Legal Controversy: The Darnes Davis Case, 1840." *Missouri Historical Review* 59 (1964): 31–45.
———. "William Beaumont, M.D. and Malpractice: The Mary Dugan Case, 1844." *Journal of the History of Medicine and Allied Sciences* 47 (2) (April 1992): 153–162.

Cynthia De Haven Pitcock

JOHN SHAW BILLINGS
(1838–1913)

John Shaw Billings, M.D., is best known for his innovative work in medical bibliography, library administration, medical statistics, and hospital planning. He was also a significant voice in the public health movement of the late nineteenth century. Billings was born in southern Indiana in Allenville, Switzerland County, where his parents were shopkeepers. Despite modest family circumstances, Billings educated himself by constant and omnivorous reading. With the help of a local clergyman, he prepared for attendance at Miami College in Oxford, Ohio. In 1857, he received his bachelor's degree from Miami College. Next he attended the Medical College of Ohio in Cincinnati founded by Daniel Drake. Drake's *Diseases of the Interior Valley of North America* (1850–1854), one of the first works to connect topography and data collection to the study of diseases in human populations, was an important influence on Billings's career in public health.

Billings's medical school thesis, "The Surgical Treatment of Epilepsy" (1861), would be forgotten except for its author's later comments on the frustration he had experienced in its preparation because of his lack of access to medical indexes and collections of medical literature. He claimed that his later work in building the Library of the Office of the Surgeon General and the production of the *Index Catalogue of the Library of the Office of the Surgeon General* was inspired by his experience in preparing his dissertation. After graduating, Billings served as a demonstrator of anatomy at the Medical College of Ohio.

He might have practiced medicine with his preceptor, George Blackman, if the American Civil War (1861–1865) had not interrupted the life of the nation. Billings went to Washington, D.C., in 1861 to take the examination for medical officers in the U.S. Army. His examiners expected him to fail since he was from Indiana, but he placed first on the list, beginning a thirty-year career with the Surgeon General's Office of the U.S. Army. During the Civil War, the young doctor was in charge of the Cliffburne Hospital in Washington, D.C. Later, he served as a surgeon in the field at the Battles of Chancellorsville and Gettysburg, and in military campaigns from the Wilderness to the Siege of Petersburg.

In 1862, Billings married Katherine Mary Stevens (1836–1912), daughter of Hestor Lockhart Stevens of Michigan, a member of the U.S. House of Representatives (1853–1857) and later a Washington lawyer. The couple had four children. Billings never practiced medicine after 1864. His duties with the Surgeon General's Office directed him to the fields of public health, hospital planning, and medical literature.

In the last months of the war (1865) Billings organized the data gathered for

The Medical and Surgical History of the War of the Rebellion (1870). European scientists considered these volumes America's first significant contribution to medicine. Billings's later work in statistics and community health derive from his participation in this project. After April 1865 the Surgeon General's Office faced the enormous task of closing the military hospitals created between 1861 and 1865. Billings supervised the dismantling of the hospitals. During this process he routed surplus medical books into the library of the Surgeon General's Office.

During the postwar years Billings also pursued microscopy and microphotography, publishing several papers reflecting this interest. His passion for the microscope is honored in the Billings Microscope Collection of the National Museum of Health and Medicine in Washington, D.C., formerly the Army Medical Museum. Postwar assignments in the Surgeon General's Office continued to draw Billings into public health. Prior to the mid-nineteenth century, the relationship between the health of the many and the health of the individual was of little interest, except in military medicine. In writing two circulars for the Surgeon General's Office, Billings worked with large amounts of data about the health of specific military communities. *A Report on Barracks and Hospitals, with Descriptions of Military Posts, Circular No. 4* (1870) and *A Report on the Hygiene of the United States Army, with Descriptions of Military Posts, Circular No. 8* (1875) established him as a hospital expert and innovator with medical statistics. Reprints of the circulars serve as a primary source of information about the U.S. Army in the American West in the late nineteenth century. From September 1869 to September 1870 Billings was assigned the task of examining the condition of the U.S. Marine Hospital Service, which was responsible for meeting the medical needs of merchant seamen. Billings recommended significant improvements in the organization that later became the U.S. Public Health Service.

In 1874, the board planning the Johns Hopkins Hospital invited Billings to submit a proposal. His successful proposal formed the basis of his fifteen-year association with Johns Hopkins (1874–1889). During this time, however, Billings continued to perform his duties with the Office of the Surgeon General. Although his original plan for the Johns Hopkins Hospital was labeled too military, he made appropriate changes, and this objection was eventually overcome. Billings also planned the Barnes Hospital (Soldiers Home in Washington, D.C.), the William Pepper Laboratory of Clinical Medicine (University of Pennsylvania), and the Peter Bent Brigham Hospital (Boston). More important than his hospital designs was the influence Billings exerted on medical education at Johns Hopkins and nationwide. Billings was among those who brought outstanding physician-scientists and clinicians, including William Henry Welch (1850–1934), William Osler (1849–1919), and the brilliant surgeon William S. Halsted (1852–1922) to Johns Hopkins.

Billings summed up his ideas for the relationship between a hospital and medical education as follows: "The Hospital should Contribute to Charity, Education and Science. First to Charity.'' This included care of the sick poor and a respectful relationship among student doctors, the medical faculty, and the patients. Billings believed that every teaching hospital needed an outpatient clinic and trained nurses. For Billings, a bachelor's degree was the prerequisite for a medical education. Medical education should consist of two years of study in the sciences, followed by two years of clinical study learning from observation, experiment, and personal investigation.

Since 1865 Billings had searched the world for medical literature to be added to the Surgeon General's Office Library. He even expected his acquaintances to donate rare items from their personal libraries. During Billings's tenure, the library of the Surgeon General's Office, which would become the National Library of Medicine, increased from several thousand volumes to over 300,000 items. Providing methods for making the information in books and periodicals accessible was as important to Billings as collecting appropriate materials. Building on the indexing work of Antonio Panizzi in the British Museum Library, Billings directed a mammoth indexing project that employed clerks and army doctors as indexers.

Acclaim for the result of this project, *The Specimen Fasciculus for the Index Catalogue of the Library of the Office of the Surgeon General* (1876), led not only to the publication of the entire *Index Catalogue*, a retrospective index, but also the *Index Medicus*, an index for current medical literature. The *MEDLINE* computer index to medical literature is a direct descendant of Billings's efforts. In 1883, the Library of the Surgeon General's Office was officially combined with the Army Medical Museum, which had grown from specimens collected during the Civil War, and moved into a new fireproof building. Billings, now officially in charge of the museum and library, fostered the growth of both collections and oversaw the construction of their new home during his ten-year directorship of the museum.

Elected vice president of the National Board of Health in 1879, Billings served in reality as its leader until 1882. The National Board of Health, born in the wake of the yellow fever epidemic of 1878, failed to overcome objections made by local governments to federal usurpation of local quarantine rights. The opposition was strongest in southern states. The National Board of Health also had to compete with the U.S. Marine Hospital Service, which was already in control of some quarantine procedures. Under Billings's leadership, the National Board of Health issued the first federal grants-in-aid to local governments and municipalities for public health and the first federal grants for medical research from a budget of $500,000, a huge appropriation in the 1880s. Billings also worked on the national census from 1880 to 1910. While working on the 1880 census, Herman Hollreith developed Billings's idea for a punch card method for tabulating census information that was based on the system used by Louis Jacquard in weaving mills. Unwisely, Billings refused to invest in Hollreith's business, which eventually became IBM.

In 1892 Billings left the army and moved to Philadelphia, where he held a professorship at the Institute of Hygiene of the University of Pennsylvania from 1891 to 1896. In 1896 he moved to New York City to consolidate its free public libraries and develop a system of branch lending libraries. He influenced the architecture of the New York Public Library, organized its staff, developed a classification system, and obtained the money from Andrew Carnegie for branch libraries. Carnegie later had Billings organize the Carnegie Institute of Washington, D.C., and made him chairman of the board.

Billings's efforts were not always successful, nor was he always rewarded by his contemporaries. He was passed over for the office of surgeon general of the U.S. Army on five occasions. The National Board of Health failed to withstand southern states' rights politics in funding battles and expired in 1883. Surgeon General John B. Hamilton of the U.S. Marine Hospital Service played on the fears of the members of the American Medical Association (AMA). Members from southern and western states feared that eastern doctors controlled the AMA. Hamilton, using the AMA, blocked Billings's bid for leadership of the Eighth International Medical Congress and became its president himself. Billings edited a medical dictionary that contains many circular definitions primarily because he refused to allow his contributors to consult previous dictionaries, hoping to produce a truly original and up-to-date work. His son, John Sedgwick Billings, M.D., believed his father might have spent more time with his family.

The recognition accorded to Billings included honorary memberships in the Royal Statistical Society of London, 1881, and the Institut Internationale de Statistique, 1883 and honorary degrees from Edinburgh, 1884; Harvard, 1886; Oxford, 1889; Munich, 1889; Dublin, 1892; Budapest, 1896; Yale, 1901; and Johns Hopkins, 1902. The National Academy of Sciences in 1883 and the American Philosophical Society in 1887 chose him as a member. He was the first American to address a session of the International Medical Congress. His many titles included those of medical inspector of the Army of the Potomac, 1864; vice president of the National Board of Health, 1879–1882; president of the American Public Health Association, 1880; deputy surgeon general, U.S. Army, 1894–1895; professor, University of Pennsylvania, 1891–1896; executive board member of the Committee of Fifty for the Investigation of the Liquor Problem, 1905; director of the New York Public Library, 1896–1913; and organizer and chairman of the board of the Carnegie Institute, 1902–1913.

Billings's successes, the result of a mixture of drudgery and vision, profoundly influenced medicine in the United States. He made the Surgeon General's Library into the world's finest national medical library and developed a useful index for its use. In medical education, Billings pointed the way for medical schools in the twentieth century. His leadership in public health is sometimes overshadowed by his work as a librarian, bibliographer, and hospital planner. Billings's paramount concern was that medicine should comport itself as a science using medical literature and statistics in conjunction with observation and experimentation.

BIBLIOGRAPHY

The largest collections of John Shaw Billings papers are in the New York Public Library and the National Library of Medicine. The National Library of Medicine has microfilm copies of key Billings papers held by the New York Public Library plus copies of items in the Philadelphia College of Physicians and the American Philosophical Society. Three book-length works on Billings are *Order Out of Chaos* by Chapman (1994), *John Shaw Billings: A Memoir* by Garrison (1915), and Lyndenburg's *John Shaw Billings: Creator of the National Medical Library, etc.* (1924). Garrison's and Lyndenburg's works do not attempt to portray Billings's life in its entirety. Chapman's book slights Billings's work as head of the Army Medical Museum, his involvement in the general milieu of science, and his deep involvement in sanitation and statistics. *Selected Papers of John Shaw Billings*, compiled by Frank Bradway Rogers (1965), concentrates on Billings's medical bibliography writings, but includes a complete and corrected bibliography of his works.

Writings by John Shaw Billings

A Report on Barracks and Hospitals; with Descriptions of Military Posts. U.S. Surgeon General's Office, Circular No. 4. Washington, D.C., 1870.
"A Bibliography of Cholera" in U.S. Congress. House. *The Cholera Epidemic of 1873 in the United States.* House Executive Document 95. 43d Cong., 2d Sess., 1875.
Billings, John Shaw. *A Report on the Hygiene of the United States Army; with Descriptions of Military Posts.* U.S. Surgeon General's Office. Circular No. 8. Washington, D.C., 1875.

Writings about John Shaw Billings and Related Topics

Chapman, Carleton B. *Order Out of Chaos: John Shaw Billings and America's Coming of Age.* Boston: Boston Medical Library, 1994.
Garrison, Fielding H. *John Shaw Billings: A Memoir.* New York: G. P. Putnam's Sons, 1915.
Lydenburg, Harry Miller. *John Shaw Billings: Creator of the National Medical Library and Its Catalogue. First Director of the New York Public Library.* Chicago: American Library Association, 1924.
Miles, Wyndam. *A History of the National Library of Medicine, the Nation's Treasury of Medical Knowledge.* Washington, D.C.: Government Printing Office, 1982.
Rogers, Frank Bradway. *Selected Papers of John Shaw Billings.* Chicago: Medical Library Association, 1965.

Nancy Eckerman

EMILY BLACKWELL
(1826–1910)

Emily Blackwell, pioneer woman physician and medical educator, was born on October 26, 1826, in Bristol, England, the sixth child of Samuel Blackwell, a sugar merchant, and his wife, Hannah, and the younger sister of Elizabeth Blackwell, who would be the first woman to receive a medical degree. Blackwell brought his family to New York City to pursue his trade in America. In 1837 the country moved into an economic depression, aggravated for Blackwell by a fire in his sugar refinery. Rather than waiting out adversity, he packed up his family again and in 1838 moved to Cincinnati, then on the edge of the western frontier. They settled into a residence on the grounds of Lane Theological Seminary, founded by Lyman Beecher. Within three months, Samuel Blackwell died of a malarial fever.

Left without resources, the Blackwells remained in Cincinnati. They quickly developed strong ties with many of the reformist families in the community, particularly with the Beechers and the Stowes. The oldest Blackwell sons took clerking jobs. Mrs. Blackwell and the oldest daughters took in boarders and established the Cincinnati English and French Academy for Young Ladies. The family's rented home was rearranged to accommodate boarders. Elizabeth worked in the school and gave piano lessons. The serious, shy, and deeply religious Blackwell daughters disliked teaching and went to great lengths to open doors to the medical profession for themselves and future generations of women.

From 1844 to 1846 Emily was able to study at St. Ann's Female Seminary in New York, where her sister Anna taught. Elizabeth was employed as a governess-teacher in Henderson, Kentucky, when a sick friend implored her to consider the revolutionary idea that women should bring their nurturing tendencies to the practice of medicine for the betterment of all women. Elizabeth set out to gain the training and accreditation needed to advance such a cause, even though no woman in modern times had attended medical school. After many serious setbacks and rejections, Elizabeth was admitted in 1847 to Geneva Medical Institute.

Emily opened her own school in Cincinnati, which she ran successfully for several years, but she began to consider Elizabeth's suggestions that she become a doctor and join her in establishing a medical clinic. In 1850, the year after Elizabeth graduated from Geneva, Emily was offered Elizabeth's former position in Henderson, Kentucky. She accepted the position in order to earn enough money to pursue a medical education, but moody by nature, she soon found herself lonely and dejected. "I ask myself," she wrote contemplatively in her diary, "whether I am off [sic] the stuff that reformers must be made of. I will strive to retain my faith in myself. If I cannot be a fine teacher, I will strive to be a noble woman.'' Her private reading and study of medical texts became her consolation, and, like her sister, Emily became more and more convinced that the gentle nature of women made them the most suitable persons to minister to the sick and suffering, especially to other women. Her spirits lifted by commitment, Emily returned to Cincinnati, where she began to study medicine more formally with Dr. N. S. Davis of Cincinnati, meeting with him on weekends for tutorials and lessons in dissections. Unfortunately, Elizabeth, who had traveled to London for clinical training, felt compelled to warn her aspiring sister that the chances for women to study medicine in Europe were no better than those in America. Indeed, in 1851, when Emily applied for admission to the Medical College of Ohio at Cincinnati, she was turned down.

John C. Vaughn, editor of the Cleveland-based antislavery newspaper, the *True Democrat*, and an advocate of women's rights, became aware of Emily's search and encouraged her to apply to the Cleveland Medical College (CMC), the medical department of Western Reserve College. Nancy Talbot Clark had matriculated at the CMC after Elizabeth Blackwell graduated from Geneva and was expected to graduate in 1852. Emily was denied admission, although she was told that a large majority of the professors and students wanted to admit her, because a minority were strongly opposed. In the next few months, Emily was rejected by Castleton Medical School and by the Ohio College of Medicine at Cincinnati. The next summer she traveled east to apply in person to Dartmouth Medical School in Hanover, New Hampshire, and the medical school at Pittsfield, Massachusetts. After visiting with Elizabeth in New York City, Emily noted in her diary that she was pleased with the prospect of working in a partnership with her sister, who as an adult ''was not nearly as particular and fidgety'' as before. Both Dartmouth and Pittsfield rejected Emily's petition. Visiting with Elizabeth again, she met Horace Greeley, well-known journalist and politician. On obtaining interviews with the attending physicians at Bellevue Hospital through Greeley's influence, Emily convinced them to allow her to visit the hospital ''like any other student.'' This, she felt, was the real beginning of her medical education.

After two months spent on the wards, Blackwell obtained favorable letters of recommendation from the Bellevue physicians. She set out for Chicago to petition Dr. Daniel Brainard, dean of Rush Medical College, who had become sympathetic to the women's cause. Without opposition from the faculty, Blackwell began attending classes on Saturday, October 30, 1852, and entered her name on the register November 2. Bravely enduring her isolation as a student, Blackwell developed a warm, tutorial relationship with Dr. Brainard. They spent long hours in his office discussing surgeries he planned to perform in the amphitheater, and she consulted with him about establishing a clinic in New York with Elizabeth. He made his private library of texts available to her. His skill and enthusiasm probably heightened Blackwell's confidence, and by midterm she had refined her professional focus. She wrote in her diary, ''I should like to be a surgeon and I would choose certain branches—make myself the most

skillful surgeon in America in that department if possible—and I think it would
be hard to keep me from succeeding. I am deeply interested in my studies and
long exceedingly for those free untrammeled opportunities of study a young
man would have.''

Emily finished the term and returned to New York, eager to continue the
planning of the clinic with Elizabeth and hopeful for the opportunity to continue
attending rounds at Bellevue. In May, Brainard visited the sisters and informed
them that the trustees of Rush had no objection to Emily's graduation. While
working on her thesis and planning for the future, she convinced herself that
she might have to go to Europe, disguised as a man, to obtain the best clinical
experience. However, in August Brainard wrote that he would be absent from
Rush the next session and that Emily probably would not have the support
necessary to continue her studies at Rush. Despite this warning, she wrote her
thesis and had herself fitted for a graduation dress. On her trip back to Chicago,
her wallet was stolen in Cleveland. At Rush the atmosphere was no longer
favorable. Members of the faculty, who had previously encouraged her, were
cool and hesitant to speak with her. At a secret meeting, her readmittance was
denied. Though no mention is made in the minutes of the Illinois State Medical
Society, medical historians attribute Emily's dismissal to censure of the school
by that society for admitting a woman. The extent of the faculty's reversal
reflected the level of influence a local medical society could bring to bear on a
medical school.

Rejected by Rush Medical College after mastering the first session of work,
Blackwell visited the medical school in Cleveland in December 1853. Having
been empowered by the faculty the previous October to admit women as students, Dean John Delamater invited Blackwell to join the session in progress.
She accepted immediately and settled into a nearby boardinghouse. Contrary to
images of harassment and ostracism surrounding the first women to enter the
study of medicine, Emily Blackwell recorded scenes of professional respect and
consideration during her brief but successful study at the Cleveland Medical
College. In February 1854, she stood for her final examination in Dr. Kirtland's
room at the college with all faculty participating. The next day Kirtland saw
Blackwell at the college and, with all professional courtesy, asked her to gather
additional data for him on her ''views with regard to the diseases of the heart
and consumption.'' She noted with some surprise, ''He and the other professors
expressed a satisfaction with my course and a kindliness toward me much beyond what I expected.''

The thesis that Blackwell formally presented to the faculty, ''A Thesis on
Certain Principles of Practical Medicine,'' was a well-organized argument on
the certain progress of medicine. The practice of medicine inevitably needed to
move, she argued, from an unreliable art form dependent on the empirical observations of individual doctors treating individual patients to an exacting science in which the action or effects of prescriptive medicines and therapeutics
would be known and standardized throughout the profession. On February 22,

1854, Emily Blackwell graduated in a simple ceremony as the only woman in a class of forty-four from the CMC.

Just over a month after her graduation, Blackwell sailed on the steamer *Arabia* out of Boston harbor, arriving in England on April 8. By July, Dr. James Y. Simpson, professor of medicine at Edinburgh University and one of the leading practitioners and thinkers in the profession, had accepted her as an assistant. This clinical experience allowed Emily Blackwell to become the first woman medical graduate to perform major surgery. Emily spent eight months working with Simpson, sometimes staying at his home to be available to assist when births were imminent. When she left, he provided a letter of praise and recommendation.

Blackwell moved from Edinburgh to London, where she declined offers from Florence Nightingale to serve in the Crimean War. Instead, she studied with Dr. William Jenner at London's Children's Hospital and St. Bartholomew's Hospital. Utilizing Simpson's unqualified recommendation, she proceeded to Paris to study with Dr. Pierre Huguier and, against Elizabeth's advice, gained access to La Maternité (the great lying-in hospital) for further study of midwifery. These experiences were followed by similar opportunities in Berlin and at Franz von Winckel's clinic in Dresden. Throughout her European clinical studies, Emily kept extensive notes on approaches and procedures in maternity cases, as well as the development of devices such as pessaries, which she forwarded to Elizabeth in New York. When she returned to New York to assist with the establishment of the Infirmary, thirty-year-old Emily Blackwell was the most highly trained woman surgeon in the world.

One of the most significant steps in the history of women in medicine occurred on May 1, 1857, when three fully trained women doctors, each with European clinical experience—Dr. Elizabeth Blackwell, Dr. Emily Blackwell, and Dr. Marie Zakrzewska*—formed a professional partnership with the formal dedication of the New York Infirmary for Women and Children. The Infirmary was staffed by the three best-qualified medical women in the world. Zakrzewska became the resident physician, and Emily Blackwell assumed administrative duties and responsibility for surgery. Elizabeth Blackwell, inclined more toward advancing the cause of women in medicine than actual practice, worked in the dispensary, maintained a private practice, and continued her leadership role, overseeing the philosophical and philanthropic survival of the institution. Patients began to arrive, and the two wards of six beds each were full within a month. Students from the Female Medical College of Pennsylvania (FMCP), founded in Philadelphia in 1850, trained at the Infirmary during the summer months between sessions and provision was made to provide rudimentary training in nursing.

Public opposition and distrust of women physicians continued for some years; the Infirmary nevertheless managed to remain open and flourished because of the tireless efforts of the three founders. However, in 1858 Elizabeth returned to England, and Zakrzewska went to Boston, where she accepted a professorship in obstetrics at the struggling New England Medical College for Women with full authority to organize and run the affiliated hospital for women. Emily remained in charge at the Infirmary. When Elizabeth returned to New York in August 1859, the Infirmary was prospering as more and more of the FMCP graduates came to the Infirmary for practical experience and helped manage the patient load. In response to the increased services provided by the Infirmary, including the introduction of a home visitor to instruct women in hygiene, the facility moved in 1860 to a house at the corner of Second Avenue and Eighth Street.

Any plans the Blackwells had for broadening their influence in England was delayed by the outbreak of the Civil War in 1861. The Infirmary's women physicians participated in the development of the Woman's Central Association for Relief, out of which grew the U.S. Sanitary Commission. The Blackwells served in the selection and training of volunteer nurses for the war effort. After the war, the Infirmary was barraged by requests from graduates of women's medical colleges for clinical training. Although the Blackwells had tolerated separate schools for women as a temporary measure, they saw that it was still difficult for women to gain admission to the established regular medical colleges. But they did not believe that any of the women's medical colleges had met the high standards that would be necessary for their graduates to attain equity in the profession.

In 1868 Elizabeth and Emily Blackwell obtained a charter and established the Woman's Medical College of the New York Infirmary. They introduced significant innovations, including entrance examinations, a three-year graded curriculum, increased clinical experience, and an outside examining board. A chair of hygiene, the first in America, was established, and Elizabeth Blackwell was its first occupant. The faculty included distinguished women physicians, such as the European-trained Mary Putnam Jacobi, M.D., and Elizabeth Cushier, M.D., a surgeon who graduated from the college in the class of 1872.

Elizabeth Blackwell left for London in 1869 to pursue her plans to assist the advancement of women in medicine in Great Britain, leaving the college and infirmary once again in the able hands of Emily Blackwell. Emily served as dean of the college and professor of diseases of women and children (later gynecology) for thirty years, until 1899, when the college merged with Cornell Medical College, which had agreed to accept women as students but not as faculty. Thousands of patients were treated every year in the Infirmary, and 364 women physicians graduated from the Woman's College of the Infirmary for Women and Children over its thirty-one years.

Emily Blackwell accepted an invitation to become a member of the New York County Medical Society in 1871, after refusing several previous offers. At about the same time she adopted a daughter, Annie. In 1882 she invited her devoted friend and former student, Dr. Cushier, to join the household. After Emily's retirement in 1900 at age seventy-four, the two women spent their time between two residences: a winter home in Montclair, New Jersey, and a summer home on the coast of York Cliffs, Maine. On September 8, 1910, just three months after the death of her sister Elizabeth, Emily Blackwell, a true woman physician, died of enterocolitis at the age of eighty-four at York Cliffs.

BIBLIOGRAPHY

Until a definitive biography acknowledges the accomplishments of Emily Blackwell, she will continue to remain in the shadow of her sister, Elizabeth (see, for examples, Blackwell, 1985/1977, and Hays, 1967). There has been no critical examination of her professional work for the three decades she oversaw and guided the Medical School of the New York Infirmary. It is likely that Emily was the more accomplished physician of the two sisters, and perhaps the more deeply dedicated. Her early struggle to find a suitable career and obtain a medical degree are captured in her diary (Emily Blackwell Papers, 1850–1910). A thorough study of pioneer women in medicine by Regina Markell Morantz-Sanchez (1985) is enlightening in regard to the establishment of the New York Infirmary by the Blackwell sisters. The Library of Congress holds the Emily Blackwell Papers, 1850–1910.

Writings by Emily Blackwell

Emily Blackwell Papers. 1850–1910. Diary. Papers of the Blackwell Family, Library of Congress.

Writings about Emily Blackwell and Related Topics

Blackwell, Elizabeth. *Pioneer Work in Opening the Medical Profession to Women: Autobiographical Sketches.* London: Longmans, Green, 1895; reprinted, with an introduction by Mary Roth Walsh, New York: Schocken Books, 1977.
Cushier, Elizabeth M. "In Memory of Dr. Emily Blackwell." *Woman's Medical Journal* 21 (April 1911): 87–89.
Hays, Elinor Rice. *Those Extraordinary Blackwells: The Story of a Journey to a Better World.* New York: Harcourt, Brace & World, 1967.
Horn, Margo. " 'Sisters Worthy of Respect': Family Dynamics and Women's Roles in the Blackwell Family." *Journal of Family History* 4 (Winter 1983): 367–382.
Markell Morantz-Sanchez, Regina. *Sympathy and Science: Women Physicians in American Medicine.* New York: Oxford University Press, 1985.

Linda Lehmann Goldstein

ERNST P. BOAS
(1891–1955)

Ernst P. Boas, cardiologist and medical and political activist, born to Marie and Franz Boas in Worcester, Massachusetts, was the scion of a distinguished lineage in which medicine figured prominently. Abraham Jacobi, often regarded as the father of pediatrics, was married to Boas's great aunt. Ernst Krackowizer, a respected New York City doctor who served as a Civil War surgeon, was Boas's maternal grandfather. (Krackowizer and Jacobi later collaborated to found the German Hospital and Dispensary in New York City, which became Lenox Hill Hospital.) Franz Boas was a seminal scholar whose iconoclastic research exploded racial and ethnic stereotypes. For thirty-seven years at Columbia University, he nurtured a generation of anthropologists. Until his death in 1942 at age eighty-four, Franz Boas remained an indefatigable activist and antifascist.

In 1914, Ernst Boas graduated first in his class from the Columbia University College of Physicians and Surgeons. After rejections from the city's leading internship programs, which he saw as a reflection of anti-Semitism in the medical profession, he interned at Mt. Sinai Hospital from 1914 to 1916. With the United States's entry into World War I, Boas became a captain in the Army Medical Corps and chief of medical services at a base hospital in France. For two years following the war, Boas practiced privately and taught physiology at the College of Physicians and Surgeons. In 1921, when he became medical director of Montefiore Hospital in the Bronx, his career took shape. At Montefiore, he developed his expertise as a cardiologist and an early proponent of geriatric medicine.

Boas challenged the prevailing medical view of chronic illness as incurable and untreatable. (This philosophic change was reflected in 1921 with the renaming of Montefiore Home for Chronic Illness as the Montefiore Hospital for Chronic Disease.) In the third decade of the twentieth century, much care for the chronically ill was custodial, in "homes for incurables," workhouses, and almshouses, with a small percentage in acute care general hospitals. Chronic illness, according to Boas, compelled hospitals to become centers for diagnosis and treatment, as well as domiciliary and custodial care (Boas 1940: 34, 93). He devoted much of his career to that end.

Boas immediately began reorganizing Montefiore around five medical divisions: neurology, tuberculosis, medicine, surgery, and laboratory. This was delicate business, as Boas confided to his father in 1921: "It is a little difficult for me because I am so young and many of the doctors present have been my teachers. Now I have to tell them how to run their sections" (Javitz 1960: 13). Although Montefiore became an acute care hospital under his successors, E. M.

Bluestone and Martin Cherkasky, Boas never abandoned his vision of specially designed institutions for the chronically ill.

In 1928, Boas returned to private practice and teaching at Columbia, activities he continued until his death in 1955. As a clinician and authority on heart disease, he earned an international reputation. He developed the cardiotachometer, which measures the heart rate electronically over extended periods of time and under different conditions (the original is on display at the Smithsonian Museum). Upon studying the link between trauma and heart attacks—an investigation initiated, according to one analyst, because of his sympathy for working people—Boas became convinced of a causal connection and testified as a legal-medical expert in compensation hearings. Boas's private practice flourished. At his death, he and Hyman Levy, his partner, boasted a long patient list that included Henry A. Wallace, Karl Menninger, Dr. Felix Adler, Sidney Hillman, and William Laurence. But Boas's involvement with his own practice did not muffle his commitment to promoting medical and social solutions to chronic maladies.

The Welfare Council of New York City conducted a study of chronic disease sufferers in 1928, the first local attempt to quantify and assess the problem. Boas headed the medical advisory committee. Based on a survey of facilities and a census of 20,700 people incapacitated by chronic problems (excluding tuberculosis, mental disease, blindness, and deafness), the 1933 report revealed a confused picture in which patients "scramble" to find "refuge" in "any institution that is willing to admit them" (Boas Papers 1934: 1). Following publication of the report, the Welfare Council established the Committee on Chronic Illness. As chairman of the committee, Boas pressed for the scientific treatment of the chronically ill.

Boas warned that without deploying more human resources and research dollars against what he later called "the unseen plague," the success of medicine would leave behind a suffering elderly population for whom physicians were unprepared. Breaking with prevailing thought that chronic disorders were inevitable by-products of stresses associated with advancing civilization, Boas asserted "Unprejudiced study demonstrates that the increasing prevalence of chronic disease is due to beneficent, rather than malign forces. We are spared attack by the infectious diseases, even in maturity, and survive to succumb at a more advanced age to one of the chronic diseases" (Boas Papers 1944: 6). Circulatory diseases, diabetes, rheumatism, cancer, and degenerative neurological diseases, "chronic in their course and lead[ing] to irreversible changes in the human organism," should receive more medical attention (Boas 1941: 11).

In three pioneering monographs—*Coronary Artery Disease, Treatment of the Patient Past Fifty*, and *The Unseen Plague—Chronic Disease*—Boas cautioned that with the aging of America, chronic illness would assume new "social significance," unquantifiable by mortality figures alone. Boas understood that in contrast to acute infectious illness, death from chronic disease typically follows years of sickness and incapacity. Comparing chronic illness to "dry-rot constantly weakening and destroying the social organism'' (Boas 1940: 4), Boas railed against medical nihilism. At best, chronic sufferers ''are scattered through the wards of a general hospital . . . apt to be regarded as interesting boarders'' (Boas Papers 1944: 21–22.) Instead, Boas believed, specialized care, bent on arresting the progress of disease, should enable many victims to ''resume [their] accustomed place[s] in society'' (Boas 1940: 22). Urging coordinated care, Boas spearheaded the move to put a fully equipped hospital for the chronically ill on Welfare (now Roosevelt) Island. After jockeying with New York City Parks commissioner Robert Moses, who wanted to set aside thirty-five acres on the island for recreational purposes, S. S. Goldwater, commissioner of the Department of Hospitals, endorsed the plan. Boas's vision and struggle resulted in Goldwater Memorial Hospital for Chronic Diseases.

While champion of medical treatment for chronic disease, Boas recognized that medicine alone would prove inadequate: ''Without adequate social service aid, most of the medical problems in the clinic are insoluble. But even the best medical care and social service cannot offset the effects of poverty, unemployment, and poor housing'' (Boas Papers 1944: 12). Like many other doctors of his generation, Boas embraced social medicine. Poverty, the maldistribution of medical resources, and financial barriers to medical care compelled physicians to assume political roles, to be alert citizens as well as first-rate clinicians; effective medical practice depended largely on public policy's addressing political and economic inequities. This model collided with mainstream medicine.

To cajole organized medicine into confronting economic issues in medical care, in 1938 Boas established the ''Progressive Group'' of doctors in the New York County Medical Society, then the largest local unit in the American Medical Association (AMA). Three years later, the group organized officially as the New York Physicians Forum for the Study of Medical Care; in 1943, with the introduction of the Wagner-Murray-Dingell bill, which called for universal and comprehensive national health care, it incorporated as a national organization, the Physicians Forum. Although eventually the Forum had thirty-eight chapters in medical societies, including the National Association of Physicians, which was made up of black doctors, under Boas's leadership the Forum remained strongest in Manhattan.

The Forum grew out of the ferment that followed the publication of the final report of the Committee on the Costs of Medical Care in 1932. Its recommendation for medical insurance galvanized organized medicine, which until 1938 fought even voluntary insurance. But the 1937 release of the Principles and Proposals of the Committee of 430 (a group of prominent physicians), endorsing a program to widen the scope of government health activities, impelled liberal doctors in New York to organize to challenge the hegemony of the AMA by attacking its flanks. The national health program formulated by the National Health Conference of 1938, where, as Boas reported to his son, papers delivered ''show clearly how at least one third of the population cannot afford medical care'' (Javitz 1960: 20), and the introduction of the Wagner bill in 1939, gave the Forum its agenda. What Boas described as "the counterblasts of the AMA" (Boas Papers 1944: 1), decrying the national health program, gave the Forum a sense of mission. "I believe," Boas told his son, "that the time has come when every physician . . . must openly take sides. . . . The lines between conservatives and liberals . . . are being more and more sharply drawn" (Javitz 1960: 21). From 1938 and beyond Boas's death, the Forum bludgeoned the New York County Medical Society with what Boas called "medical politics."

Forum members shared the conviction that laissez-faire medicine had lost its bearings; financial barriers left too many Americans medically disenfranchised. Rejecting voluntary fee-for-service insurance, advocates instead urged a tax-supported health care system. Within the Manhattan county society, contested elections, referenda, inflammatory debate, and special meetings drew the membership into discussions of medical indigency and experimental pay schemes. Attendance, previously low, soared. Beyond debating medical care and payment options, the Forum championed equal access for women and blacks to medical schools and postgraduate programs and repeatedly called on the AMA to revise its constitution to permit qualified doctors, regardless of their race, to join southern county medical societies. The Forum also led the successful drive for the inclusion of physicians in the social security program. As Boas explained, the Forum operated on the premise that "an articulate minority could exert influence" (Boas Papers 1944: 2). Although the Forum did not turn the tide, Boas saw another purpose to its counterpoint posture: "The whole point was to prove that there are many doctors who disagree with the A.M.A. and who believe that doctors must cooperate with government in working out answers to these problems" (Javitz 1960: 31).

Beginning in the late 1940s, anticommunism took on new virulence, tying domestic liberal reform to internal subversion. Amid the heightened hysteria, health reformers became targets of scurrilous attacks as the medical establishment took up the anticommunist cudgel to link compulsory health insurance with disloyalty. Under Boas, the Forum became a center of opposition to McCarthyism, resolute against the invasion of doctors' civil rights and steadfast upholders of the ideas under attack. As prominent physicians faced humiliating grillings and the Forum came under siege, Boas mounted a principled defense and counterattack. He challenged red-baiting itself as an obfuscation of the issues. In spite of the pummeling, the Forum continued to urge political roles for doctors, insisting that the status of physician confers a political responsibility; the ideal physician, it held, could not be separated from the ideal citizen. Boas saw McCarthyism in medicine as an instrument to quash dissent and stifle doctors' political participation.

Beyond challenging the medical and political orthodoxy of the early 1950s, the Forum refused to sanitize itself by becoming part of the anticommunist liberal establishment. It fought for its survival exclusively in terms of American civil liberties, refusing, as Boas wrote, "to weed out" communists (Boas Papers 1951: 2). Although not a communist, and like his father critical of the tactics of American communists, Boas refused to permit political discrimination in the face of red-baiting. Boas's insistence on viewing the problem as domestic repression put the Physicians Forum among the few groups in the 1950s that did not see anticommunist rhetoric and tactics as the strategy for survival.

What sustained Boas, permitting him to risk reputation in defense of principle? John P. Peters, head of the Department of Internal Medicine at Yale and a medical reformer, suggested that it was a matter of genetics. From the late 1930s until his death, Franz Boas, a socialist who found much to fault in the Soviet Union, would not permit political discrimination, even as the Committee for Democracy and Intellectual Freedom, which he founded in 1939, was hounded by red-baiting. Like his father, Ernst revealed a tenacious adherence to principle. To his son, Norman, he wrote: "I have no Jewish consciousness or sense of race but I would not forswear myself just to make life easier or pleasanter. I went all thru [sic] that as a young man. The world insisted on labeling me and I would not go thru [sic] some hocus pocus to enable them to patronizingly call me by another name. Your grandfather years ago when it meant something was offered a professorship at the University of Berlin, I believe, if he would have himself baptized. Of course he refused—not because he felt himself a Jew, but because he would not sell himself" (Javitz 1960: 29).

Shy by nature, Boas took the part of medical gadfly at considerable toll. In 1940, he defended his foray into medical politics: "These are critical years in the world we know . . . the struggle in medicine is but a reflection of the struggle in the country at large" (Javitz 1960: 25). With escalating McCarthyism, Boas suffered bouts of depression, as well as a degree of professional isolation, but never doubt: "I am still childish enough to be bothered by the fact that formal recognition and advancement in medicine is closed to me because of my nonconformity; yet I know that I could never . . . buy such preferment by bucking under and playing the game" (Javitz 1960: 36).

BIBLIOGRAPHY

The American Philosophical Society Library in Philadelphia is the repository of the Ernst P. Boas Papers. The fully indexed collection contains twenty-six boxes (cited in text as Boas Papers). The papers illuminate all aspects of Boas's life and career. Among the items of special interest are: "Memorandum on the Desirability of Developing Welfare Island for the Care of the Chronic Sick," 1934; "Chronic Disease," 1944; "Statement before the Committee of Medicine and the Changing Order," January 1944; letter to Allen Butler, February 25, 1951. Some of his letters appear in the Henry E. Sigerist Papers at the Alan Mason Chesney Medical Archives, Johns Hopkins Medical Institutions, Baltimore, Maryland, and in the John P. Peters Papers and the Henry E. Sigerist Papers, Sterling Library, Yale University, New Haven, Connecticut. The archives of the New York County (Manhattan) Medical Society hold the minutes of county society meetings that reveal much of the history of the Physicians Forum. There is no biography of Boas, but Levenson's *Montefiore* covers Boas's tenure at the Hospital, as does Bracker's *Montefiore Hospital for Chronic Diseases*. Brickman, " 'Medical McCarthyism,' " treats Boas's role in combating McCarthyism directed at medical reformers. Brickman's unpublished manuscript, "Minority Politics in the House of Medicine: The Physicians Forum and the Manhattan Medical Leadership, 1938–1965," charts the battles in New York City between the medical establishment and the Physicians Forum, under Boas's leadership.

Writings by Ernst P. Boas

Challenge of Chronic Diseases. New York: Macmillan Co., 1929.
The Unseen Plague: Chronic Disease. New York: J. J. Augustin, 1940.
Treatment of the Patient Past Fifty. Chicago: Year Book Publishers, 1941.
Coronary Artery Disease. Chicago: Year Book Publications, 1949.

Writings about Ernst P. Boas and Related Topics

Bracker, Milton. *Montefiore Hospital for Chronic Diseases. New York. Fiftieth Anniversary 1884–1934.* New York: Privately printed, 1934.
Brickman, Jane Pacht. " 'Medical McCarthyism': The Physicians Forum and the Cold War." *Journal of the History of Medicine and Allied Sciences* 49 (July 1994): 380–418.
Javitz, Romana, ed. *Letters of Ernst P. Boas, M.D., 1891–1955.* New York: Ernst P. Boas Memorial Fund, 1960.
Levenson, Dorothy. *Montefiore: The Hospital as Social Instrument 1884–1984.* New York: Farrar, Straus & Giroux, 1984.

Jane Pacht Brickman

WILLIAM BOYD
(1885–1979)

William Boyd, a Scots-Canadian pathologist, was the most successful pathology teacher and author of his time, and one of the great medical writers and teachers of the twentieth century. Admirers said that he was not simply a writer but a weaver of words. Boyd was born in Portsoy in the northeast of Scotland on June 21, 1885, and trained in medicine in Edinburgh. After graduation, he worked in mental hospitals in the English Midlands and for a short time as a pathologist in Wolverhampton. He was appointed professor of pathology in the University of Manitoba in 1915 but spent a brief, eventful spell in the front line in Flanders as a medical officer before taking up his appointment in Winnipeg. In twenty-two years in Winnipeg, he became an outstanding teacher and a well-known writer of texts on pathology, the scientific basis of the understanding of disease. He became professor of pathology at the University of Toronto in 1937. After retiring from Toronto in 1951 he spent three years as the first professor of pathology in the new medical school of the University of British Columbia. He died on March 10, 1979.

Boyd left behind monuments more enduring than bronze. His books, which ran into many editions, were translated into several languages and influenced innumerable medical students. His neat, confident figure and Scottish accent were well known in the smaller world of pathologists. He was talking, always talking, often emphasizing a point with a twitch of an eyebrow, and often with a cigarette in hand. As a student he had walked the Scottish hills and celebrated his graduation in medicine by sailing "the whole of that perfect June day over the sea to Skye past the enchanted islands." The Cuillins, the mountains of the Island of Skye, stayed in his mind, and thereafter wherever he had the opportunity, and as long as he had the strength, he sought the hills.

His first book recounted his wartime experiences in Flanders. On April 28, 1915, he wrote, "There is only one word in the mouth of everyone today—gas." The picture of a casualty clearing station is burned on to the page: "The hospital is built around a great courtyard, and in the courtyard were two hundred men on stretchers. Some were lying in a state of stupor, the flies buzzing around their faces; some were sitting up gasping for breath, with hands and faces of a deep dusky hue, evidently in the greatest distress; over the countenance of others the pallid hues of death were beginning to creep, whilst a few had fallen back and with gurglings in the throat were passing away into the undiscovered country. They were the first gas cases from Ypres and Hill 60."

He went, in 1915, to the University of Manitoba, in distant cold Winnipeg, as first full-time professor of pathology in the University of Manitoba and chief pathologist to the Winnipeg General Hospital. His career was launched during a wave of particularly virulent epidemics. Hardly had the populace recovered from the influenza pandemic of 1918 when, during the winter of 1919–1920, Winnipeg experienced a major outbreak of encephalitis lethargica. It was Boyd's big chance, and he took it. He published excellent pathological accounts of this and a later epidemic.

It soon became evident that Boyd was a natural and outstanding teacher. The quotations in his Commonplace Book in the early 1920s of passages from great orators show that he was becoming preoccupied with the art of public speaking. He taught in the Scottish manner; his great contribution as a teacher lay not so much in what he taught as in how he taught it, and in particular how he taught the scientific basis of disease as part of human medicine rather than simply morbid anatomy as a dead, circumscribed subject.

In Winnipeg, he developed an excellent pathological museum, rich in correlations between clinical history and pathological specimens. Students flocked to it, to talk about pathology and life among themselves and with the professor and his colleagues. The museum took much space, and many years later his successors dismantled it.

His students and technologists saw and heard a young man with an eager face, the smooth manner of a gentleman, and a splendid lecturer with a pronounced but not broad Scottish accent. The perfection of his lecturing was enhanced rather than marred by an idiosyncrasy in his speech: an inability to trill the letter *r*. He always spoke of "bwonchitis." "Morbid anatomy," he wrote, "is not dead and never has been, except in the hands of those whose dull minds would take the breath of life from the most vital subject."

Boyd had always been a scribbler. His habit of writing out quotations taken from his readings into a Commonplace Book stimulated his literary talent, filling his mind with quotable phrases and influencing his style. He used to write in longhand, mostly early in the morning. From about 1922 writing dominated his life. He first wrote a few papers to prove himself as an academic surgical pathologist and followed these up by a book for surgeons (*Surgical Pathology* first edition, 1925). He wrote steadily over the next few years. *The Pathology of Internal Diseases* (1931) and *Textbook of Pathology* (1932) made his name, followed by *An Introduction to Medical Science* in 1937. His sunset book, *The Spontaneous Regression of Cancer*, was written twenty years after his own parotid cancer had been removed. His cancer was to recur several times, but he survived it, showing a stoical courage.

He was usually well informed, and when he did not know an answer said so. On the cause of tumors: "The essential cause is still unknown; the veil covering the mystery has not yet been rent in twain. . . . Theory after theory cometh up as a flower, only in turn to be cut down like the grass." What was extraordinary was the writing. Only Boyd could transform a mundane object like the gallbladder with the following words: "The graceful, fragile gossamer folds of mucosa are completely altered in appearance, being loaded down by dense yellow opaque masses, much as a delicate birch tree might be weighed down by a load of snow.'' Reflecting on heart disease, he wrote, ''Of all the ailments which blow out life's little candle heart disease is the chief.''

''Influenza travels at an extraordinary speed,'' he wrote, ''but not quicker, as is sometimes imagined, than the speed of man. It crosses a continent as fast as an express train, the ocean at the rate of an Atlantic liner, and the desert as slowly as a camel caravan.'' A consideration of the reasons for the increase in bronchial carcinoma listed possible causes: ''All sorts of irritants including cigarettes. . . . All of these seem highly improbable.'' Epidemiological studies on the relationship between smoking and lung cancer were years in the future. Boyd had little time for immunology: ''The saying that ignorance, however aptly veiled in an attractive terminology, remains ignorance, is particularly applicable to the science of immunology.'' In describing syphilis, he explained that ''tertiary lesions are so widespread that to enumerate them would be like giving the list of the ships in the Iliad or the names of the kings of Judah.'' Some of his prejudices were more picturesque than sustainable: ''Beer and such red wine as port are much more dangerous than whisky; for this reason gout is a rare disease in Scotland.'' On the whole, however, the text was factually reliable.

Patches of vivid human interest capture the attention. On epidemic encephalitis (lethargica) he wrote:

Winnipeg was visited by two epidemics, the first in the winter of 1919–20, the second at the beginning of 1923. In the first epidemic the patient was dull, lethargic, somnolent, and showed oculomotor disturbances. He would lie like a log in bed with drooping lids or closed eyes, the lines of expression all ironed out, sunk in a stupor which no external stimuli could penetrate, the flash and speed of the mind gone, the dim rush light of reason hardly flickering. In the second epidemic the picture had changed completely. Body and mind were now keyed to full activity. The muscles were in a state of constant movement, which was paralleled by a condition of mental excitement. Occupation formed the main topic of conversation: the teacher was continually teaching, the merchant was casting up accounts, the builder planning new houses. The first picture was akinetic, the second hyperkinetic.

Boyd's books stand out among the pathology texts of the time; their prose was clear and readable, and the writing called the mind of the student back, again and again, to the center of pathology, and medicine: the patient. The books sold like hotcakes, ultimately over a million, and made him a wealthy man.

In 1937 Boyd left Winnipeg. For the rest of his life, he spent much time revising and updating his books. ''Old diseases are passing away,'' he wrote, ''but new ones are continually taking their place. . . . The inn that shelters for the night is not the journey's end.'' In many ways, his books held him prisoner; he was fastened to them by a golden chain. They were his children, and he loved them. Of all his family, the *Textbook of Pathology* was his favorite— ''The Textbook,'' he called it.

The books were a constant preoccupation, and his secretaries were kept busy hammering on their typewriters. He borrowed from others sometimes, and not always with generous acknowledgment. A former colleague recalled Boyd's folder:

It played a dominant feature of our lives. In fact we were its willing slaves. The whole department and all our activities were designed to feed it. ''That's a very interesting article'' Boyd would murmur. ''Would you give me your precis of it as I will soon be starting to revise the text book.'' By the time he sat down to the actual revision, a manila folder corresponding to each chapter would be full of references and abstracts, and at five in the morning these would be woven together in narrative form in Boyd's handwriting. His rules for punctuation were simple. ''The comma is only to be put in to make the meaning clear.''

In recognition of his influence and honors, Boyd was elected president of the American Association of Pathologists and Bacteriologists and of the International Association of Medical Museums (1934). He served as chairman of the Committee on Cancer Control and the Canadian Medical Association and director of the Canadian Cancer Society and the National Cancer Institute of Canada (1947). He was elected president of the latter in 1950. In 1962 Boyd was awarded the Gold Headed Cane by the American Association of Pathologists. He received a distinguished award (the FNG Starr Award) of the Canadian Medical Association in 1968. He became an honorary fellow of the American College of Pathologists in 1975.

He was still lecturing in his eighties; his mind stayed bright until late in life, although he was very conscious of the passage of time: ''Water is the fabric for everything that lives. The baby consists mostly of water, whilst the old man or woman shrivels up like a wilted plant.'' He diluted his water well with Scotch whiskey. He spent his old age in his rose garden in Toronto with his beloved wife, Enid. They had no children. Like many another Scot, he found life and fortune far away, but dreamed always of the hills. In the library drawer where his papers are held, his ice axe lies on top.

BIBLIOGRAPHY

The Boyd Papers are lodged in the archives of the Fisher Library, University of Toronto. A videotape of Boyd in his old age is held by the Hannah Institute, Toronto. A complete bibliography of the writings of William Boyd is found in the biography by Ian Carr. I thank the publishers of that biography for permission to quote from it.

Writings by William Boyd

With a Field Ambulance at Ypres. New York: G. H. Doran Co., 1916.
Physiology and Pathology of the Cerebrospinal Fluid. New York: Macmillan, 1920.
Surgical Pathology. 1st ed. Philadelphia: Saunders, 1925.
The Pathology of Internal Diseases. 1st ed., Philadelphia: Lea & Febiger, 1931.
Textbook of Pathology. 1st ed., Philadelphia: Lea & Febiger, 1932.

An Introduction to Medical Science. 1st ed., Philadelphia: Lea & Febiger, 1937.
The Spontaneous Regression of Cancer. Springfield: Thomas, 1966.

Writings about William Boyd and Related Topics

Barrie, H. J. "Sir William Boyd: A Legacy in Print." *Canadian Medical Association Journal* 126 (1982): 421–424.
Carr, Ian. *William Boyd. Silver Tongue and Golden Pen.* Markham, Ontario: Associated Medical Service, Inc. and Fitzhenry & Whiteside, 1993.
McManus, J. F. A. "William Boyd: A Biographical Sketch." *American Journal of Surgical Pathology* 3 (1979): 377–381.

Ian Carr

MIGUEL ENRIQUE BUSTAMANTE
(1898–1986)

Miguel Enrique Bustamante Vasconcelos, one of Mexico's leading public health physicians in the twentieth century, helped design and lead the Ministry of Public Health from the 1920s to the 1980s. From a prominent Oaxaca merchant family that saw its fortunes decline following the Mexican Revolution, Bustamante, born May 2, 1898, was the oldest of fifteen ambitious siblings. Bustamante's early interest in public health and medicine was rooted in family experiences. His mother, Luz Vasconcelos, was a firm supporter of smallpox vaccination and milk pasteurization and the daughter of a physician who died fighting a cholera outbreak in the Isthmus of Tehuantepec. At a time when Oaxaca's infant mortality rate hovered between 400 and 500 per 1,000, all of Luz Vasconcelos's children survived infancy, in large part thanks to her adherence to known public health practices. Unable to become a physician herself, Bustamante's mother encouraged her eldest son's medical studies. After completing his preparatory studies in Oaxaca in 1920, Bustamante went to Mexico City to pursue a medical career at the National University of Mexico. There Bustamante was particularly influenced by his uncle, Angel Brioso Vasconcelos, a prominent public health physician who was the Mexican director of the Rockefeller Foundation's Yellow Fever Commission, which oversaw the eradication of yellow fever from Veracruz and other parts of the country in the early 1920s. Thanks to his uncle's intellectual influence and professional prominence, Bustamante became attracted to the area of public health. As a student, he met the leading public health doctors of the day, who introduced him to the areas of social and preventive medicine, hygiene, and the application of medical knowledge to collective problems.

After completing his medical studies, Bustamante received a Rockefeller Foundation fellowship to study epidemiology and public health at the Johns Hopkins University School of Hygiene and Public Health in Baltimore, Maryland, from 1926 to 1928. Bustamante was among the first handful of Mexican physicians to study in the United States and the first Mexican Rockefeller fellow to study at Johns Hopkins. This was a pioneering move, as the best medical students of this era customarily went to Europe to gain specialty clinical training. He married the former Alice Mary Connolly in 1928, and they had four children.

After receiving his doctorate in hygiene, Bustamante returned to Mexico, where his abilities and ambition led him to a series of instrumental roles in the expanding Department of Public Health. In 1929 he founded the Veracruz city cooperative health unit and moved to Mexico City to become the founder and first head of the Rural Hygiene Service for the Department of Public Health in 1932. In 1934 he wrote a seminal article, "La Coordinación de los Servicios Sanitarios Federales y Locales como Factor de Progreso Higiénico en México" (Coordination of Federal and Local Health Services as a Factor of Sanitary Progress in Mexico) to mark his acceptance to the National Academy of Medicine of Mexico. Published in the *Gaceta Médica de México* (Medical Gazette of Mexico) in 1934, the article called for technical centralization and administrative decentralization of health services, a goal he set as the founder of the Coordinated Sanitary Services in Mexico from 1933 to 1935. Bustamante also called for physicians, visiting nurses, sanitary engineers, and health inspectors to serve as the front line for public health, incorporating geographic, economic, cultural, social, philosophical, racial, and historical factors in their efforts to realize the universal right to health. The article had a tremendous impact in its day and was reprinted in several books more than fifty years after its initial publication; Bustamante's emphasis on the promotion of health as the best societal investment in human capital continues to have relevance. Indeed, the Pan American Health Organization's 1992 *Health Services Research: An Anthology* begins with a reprint of Bustamante's 1934 article.

Following a stint as the director of the Public Health Training School in Xochimilco, Bustamante returned to Mexico City to found the State Welfare Services for the Department of Public Welfare in 1938. In 1939 Bustamante became a research epidemiologist at the new Institute of Health and Tropical Diseases, becoming its director in 1942 and again from 1946 to 1947. In 1947 Dr. Fred Soper, newly elected director of the Pan American Sanitary Bureau, invited Bustamante to serve as the organization's secretary-general in Washington, D.C. As the bureau's chief administrative officer, Bustamante oversaw a tremendous expansion and transformation as the bureau opened three public health research and development institutes in Latin America, reorganized and enlarged its regional offices, and established formal relationships with the Organization of American States and the newly formed World Health Organization. Bustamante was also involved in documenting the Pan American Sanitary Bureau's shift from a small Washington-based office primarily concerned with infectious diseases that threatened commerce to a multinational organization involved in public health administration, education and training, environmental sanitation, health promotion, and communicable disease control. When Bustamante returned to Mexico in 1956, he became director-general of sanitary services and then subsecretary of health for Mexico until 1964. In these positions, as in Washington, Bustamante oversaw a major expansion of public health throughout Mexico, including the extension of health services, large-scale disease-eradication strategies, including a nationwide antimalaria campaign, and the introduction of epidemiological thinking and methods to address the social aspects of health problems.

While Bustamante's appointments reflect a steady progress of accomplishments, this apparently smooth ascent of the professional ladder belies the complexity of his career path. In his early career, for example, Bustamante was a young star as a Rockefeller fellow, but he was unwilling to comply with foundation directives simply because of his association with the prestigious organization. When the Rockefeller Foundation sought to transform its rural hookworm campaign into permanent health units in the late 1920s, Bustamante fought to ensure that Mexicans would have a voice in their design and development. Mexicans had begun to think systematically about rural health services from the time of the 1917 Constitution, which guaranteed every citizen the "right to health." Mobile health brigades, set up during the Mexican Revolution in response to smallpox and malaria outbreaks, had begun by the 1920s to administer vaccines, conduct medical exams, and oversee sanitation efforts, but these efforts were chronically underfunded. In 1926 the federal government issued a new Sanitary Code, which subordinated local health bodies to federal authorities for the first time.

Having demonstrated its dedication to Mexican public health through the joint hookworm campaign, the Rockefeller Foundation actively sought a role in the Departamento de Salubridad Pública's (DSP, Department of Public Health) organization of rural health services. By 1926 Rockefeller Mexico director Henry Carr realized that although his hookworm clinics were well attended, most villagers suffered from multiple health problems. He proposed the transformation of the hookworm campaign into permanent rural health departments to include full-time service of physicians and nurses, employment according to ability instead of political favoritism, attractive salaries, and moral and financial cooperation between the DSP, the state, and the municipality. Carr's plan committed the Mexican government to contribute a growing proportion of its budget to the health units through a system of budgetary incentives. The Rockefeller Foundation (RF) provided only 10 percent of the budget yet specified the services to be offered, the basis for the personnel's local authority, and the parameters of the interaction between health unit staff and patients.

Simultaneously with Carr's efforts, the DSP developed its own extensive plan to replace the country's traveling health brigades with permanent rural hygiene services. The principal architect of this endeavor was Dr. Miguel Bustamante. Although he shared many of Carr's public health ideas, Bustamante's plan was more centralized and supported a broader range of activities for the health units in an effort to address the underlying causes of high death rates, such as unfavorable economic and social conditions and inadequate water provision and sewage disposal. The Rockefeller Foundation (RF) plan concentrated on diseases that could be combated quickly and dramatically, regardless of their epidemiological importance.

Competition over authorship of the cooperative health plan was the first of many differences between Bustamante and the RF. Although Bustamante went on to hold numerous positions connected to local health administration, his desire for Mexican public health sovereignty led to periodic clashes with a succession of RF officers. These policy differences were conceptualized as personality problems by RF officers, who accused Bustamante of being capable yet "strange" and "unscrupulous."

The RF beat out the Mexican government in the race to establish the first cooperative unit, but only because the unit, established in the small port city of Puerto México at the end of 1927, heavily emphasized hookworm diagnosis, treatment, and prevention, activities that had already been carried out during the hookworm campaign. In May 1929 the DSP established its own cooperative health unit in the larger town of Veracruz with Bustamante at its helm. The Veracruz unit had more autonomy and a wider scope than its Puerto México counterpart, training its own personnel, developing popular health education posters, films, and lectures, and collecting, classifying, and analyzing vital statistics. Communicable disease control efforts, largely a continuation of existing measures, included the tracking of typhoid, tuberculosis, venereal disease, vaccination against smallpox and rabies, antilarval efforts against malaria and yellow fever, plague prevention, and the diagnosis and treatment of hookworm. Under Bustamante's leadership, an extensive child hygiene effort was launched, involving prenatal care, visiting nurses, dental care, school physicals, mandatory smallpox vaccination, and the establishment of milk inspection and distribution centers. Market, restaurant, and building inspections were also carried out. Bustamante strove to make Mexico's sanitary units more effective than the Rockefeller Foundation's, often deviating from RF precepts. Although the Veracruz unit was more comprehensive and effective than its RF-sponsored counterparts, Carr repeatedly criticized Bustamante for being too self-important and relying too heavily on central government funding. Writing in the *American Journal of Public Health* in 1931, Bustamante suggested that U.S.-style cooperation with local governments was not a wholly appropriate model for the culturally distinct Mexico, which had limited possibilities for raising revenues locally. When measured by results rather than Bustamante's style, the Veracruz unit's success in improving municipal hygiene was clear, even for RF officials.

Following Bustamante's success in Veracruz, the DSP established the Rural Hygiene Service to administer the growing number of health units, maintain amicable relations between the various levels of government, encourage local initiatives, map the future course of the units, and secure regular state and municipal payments. In 1931 Bustamante was selected to be the service's first director, citing the country's own progress as the basis of achievements in rural health. To Carr's dismay, Bustamante became even less orthodox than in his prior position, advocating the use of teachers in latrine building, water filtration, and health education efforts when medical personnel were unavailable.

The battles between Carr and Bustamante were more than a clash of personalities; they reflected the larger struggles taking place between a government eager to build a modern infrastructure but concerned about its autonomy and a private U.S. philanthropic organization wishing to promote its particular plan. Bustamante optimistically agreed that the RF's "private aid will awaken the nation's sanitary conscience" (Bustamante 1934: 193–195). At the same time, he wished to take pieces of his Hopkins-acquired knowledge and supplement it with sovereign knowledge and experience in the development of local health units. Although Bustamante was a firm believer in modern public health, he sought to bring the maximum benefits possible to Mexican peasants using existing resources rather than await the widespread availability of specialized health workers whose training he also advocated and oversaw.

As the head of the DSP's Coordinated Sanitary Services, Bustamante conducted a nationwide survey of health conditions and sanitary services, which formed the basis for socialist Mexican president Lázaro Cárdenas's health plan issued in August 1935. The president called for the creation of sanitary services throughout the country in order to address poor health conditions, inadequate nutrition, lack of health services, and public ignorance. Cárdenas held that scientific research combined with social goals should guide the country's health activities, and he believed that the RF's expertise should be fully employed in this endeavor. While Bustamante was encouraged to work closely with the RF on the development of a coordinated sanitary services demonstration project in the state of Morelos, he soon moved to direct the Xochimilco Public Health Training Station in an effort to produce trained personnel to fill what were formerly patronage positions.

Throughout his career, Bustamante retained academic appointments and was an active researcher, publishing hundreds of scientific articles on tropical diseases, epidemiology, and health administration. From 1931 to 1947 he was professor of hygiene at the Medical Faculty of the National University of Mexico, also serving as professor of preventive medicine, epidemiology, and health administration at the Rural Medicine School of the Polytechnic Institute and the Superior Normal School in Mexico City. In 1936 and 1937, he was director of the Xochimilco Training School. When he returned to Mexico from Washington, D.C., in 1956, Bustamante served as head of the Department of Medical Sociology and Preventive Medicine at the National University of Mexico. Through these appointments, he taught generations of medical students and public health workers from Mexico and numerous other Latin American countries.

Bustamante's honors include the following: member since 1934 and president of the National Academy of Medicine, Eduardo Liceaga Medal recipient, honorary member of the American Academy of Tropical Medicine, Order of Carlos Finlay,* vice president of the American Public Health Association, president of the Executive Board of UNICEF (1962 and 1963), president of the Mexican Society for Public Health, and president of the Mexican Society for Natural History.

When he looked back at his career, Bustamante considered his work as the first chief of the Veracruz Sanitary to be his greatest achievement. It was to the past that he returned after retiring from the Ministry of Health in the 1960s. While he served as an outside assessor to the ministry until his death in 1986, Bustamante's major occupation became historical inquiry. Like Henry Sigerist,* whose books he read avidly, Bustamante believed that study of the history of medicine is indispensable to good social medicine and public health. Though he never became minister of health, in part due to his fierce independence and the controversies he generated, Bustamante was a major public health figure of his era, influencing public health theory and practice throughout Latin America.

BIBLIOGRAPHY

Bustamante published more than three hundred articles and books. Beginning in the 1930s he wrote a variety of articles about tropical diseases in Mexico, school health, and mental health and countless other public health topics in the leading Mexican scientific journals. In the 1940s he began to publish in the *Bulletin of the Pan American Sanitary Bureau*, where he issued his well-known ''The Pan American Sanitary Bureau. Half a Century of Health Activities'' (1955). Bustamante was instrumental in the publication of the four-volume *Historia de la Salubridad y de la Asistencia en México* (1960), at the time the only history of health and welfare in Mexico. Relatively little has been written about Bustamante other than homages made following his death, such as Soberón Acevedo's ''Miguel E. Bustamante y la Salud Pública'' (1986).

The Rockefeller Archive Center in Tarrytown, New York, has a small amount of biographical information and some correspondence relating to his years as a Rockefeller fellow and his work with the Rockefeller Foundation in Mexico. In Mexico the Archivo Histórico de la Secretaría de Salubridad y Asistencia and the Archivo General de la Nación in Mexico City also have some materials relating to Bustamante's work. The most important archival source is the Fundación Cívico Cultural Bustamante Vasconcelos, located in Oaxaca.

Writings by Miguel E. Bustamante

''Probable Existencia de la Oncocercosis en Chiapas (Probable existence of oncocercosis in Chiapas).'' *Gaceta Médica de México* 56 (1925): 496–498. (Bustamante's first medical publication.)

''Local Public Health Work in Mexico.'' *American Journal of Public Health* 21 (1931): 725–736. (Bustamante's first international publication.)

''La Coordinación de los Servicios Sanitarios Federales y Locales como Factor de Progreso Higiénico en México.'' *Gaceta Médica de México* 65 (1934): 181–228.

''Mortalidad de Menores de un Año por Entidades Federales—México, 1923–1941 (Infant mortality by federal entities—Mexico 1923–1941).'' *Revista del Instituto de Salubridad y Enfermedades Tropicales* (Journal of the Institute of Health and Tropical Diseases) 5 (1944): 101–115.

''Public Health Administration in Latin America.'' *American Journal of Public Health* 40 (1950): 1067–1071.

The Pan American Sanitary Bureau. Half a Century of Health Activities, 1902–1954. Miscellaneous Publications 23. Washington, D.C.: Pan American Sanitary Bureau, December 1955.

(with Alvarez Amézquita, José, Picazos, Antonio L.; and Fernández del Castillo, F.). *Historia de la Salubridad y de la Asistencia en México* (History of health and welfare in Mexico). 4 vols. Mexico, D.F.: Secretaría de Salubridad y Asistencia, 1960.

"Hechos Sobresalientes en la Historia de la Secretaría de Salubridad y Asistencia (Significant events in the history of the Secretariat of Health and Welfare)." *Salud Pública de México* 25 (1983): 465–482.

(with Alvarez Amézquita, José, Picazos, Antonio L.; and Fernández del Castillo, F.). "Servicios Médicos Rurales Cooperativos en la Historia de la Salubridad y de la Asistencia en México." In *La Atención Médica en el Medio Rural Mexicano, 1930–1980* (Medical attention in rural Mexico), pp. 93–107. Edited by Héctor Hernández Llamas. México, D.F.: Instituto Mexicano del Seguro Social, 1984.

Writings about Miguel E. Bustamante and Related Topics

Birn, Anne-Emanuelle. "Local Health and Foreign Wealth: The Rockefeller Foundation's Public Health Programs in Mexico, 1924–1951." Sc.D. dissertation, Johns Hopkins University, 1993.

———. "Public Health or Public Menace? The Rockefeller Foundation and Public Health in Mexico, 1920–1950." *Voluntas* 7(1)(1996): 35–56.

———. "Unidades Sanitarias: La Fundación Rockefeller vs. el Modelo Cárdenas en México (Local health units: The Rockefeller Foundation vs. the Cárdenas model in Mexico)." In *Salud, Cultura y Sociedad en América Latina: Nuevas Perspectivas Históricas* (Health, culture, and society in Latin America: New historical perspectives). Edited by Marcos Cueto. Lima: IEP, 1996.

Chávez Rivera, Ignacio. "Miguel E. Bustamante y la Academia Nacional de Medicina." *Salud Pública de México* 28 (1986): 217–218.

Narro Robles, José R. "Miguel E. Bustamante y la Universidad." *Salud Pública de México* 28 (1986): 215–216.

Soberón Acevedo, Guillermo. "Miguel E. Bustamante y la Salud Pública." *Salud Pública de México* 28 (1986): 212–214.

Anne-Emanuelle Birn

ALLAN MACY BUTLER
(1894–1986)

Allan Macy Butler, academic pediatrician and political activist, was born in Yonkers, New York, one of eight children of parents descended from colonial stock. Butler's father, George Prentice Butler, a banker, raised his family in comfort. Butler's maternal grandfather had moved the family from Long Island to West Virginia, where he ran an oil business that was eventually forced into the Rockefeller domain. His paternal grandfather was a lawyer and chancellor of New York University. Benjamin Butler, Allan Butler's great-grandfather, an author of the New York State Constitution, served as U.S. attorney general and secretary of war.

For five months after graduation from Princeton in 1916, Butler worked as a bond salesman. In January 1917 he left for England, where he took a job with the Cunard Steamship Company until he could join a unit fighting in the world war. Until American entry, he served in an officers' infantry training corps at Oxford. He became a second lieutenant (later captain) in the 6th Field Artillery of the American Expeditionary Force in France. Following the war, he participated in the American Relief Administration in Poland. Discharged in July 1919, Butler returned to Cunard, serving as operations manager in New York, where he expected to oversee the Cunard and New York Central Terminal Corporation under construction in Weehawken, New Jersey. Passage of the high Smoot-Hartley tariff in 1921 and new immigration restrictions derailed plans for the terminal. Without a job, Butler went to Phillipsburg, Pennsylvania, to evaluate the charges of antilabor activity made by the United Mine Workers. For three weeks he mined coal, working alongside a young boy who had just lost his father in a mining accident. This experience, along with his relief work in Poland, drove his decision to become a physician.

Butler entered Columbia University in 1921 to complete prerequisites in chemistry and biology. In the same year he married Mabel H. Churchill, daughter of the American novelist Winston Churchill (among his most popular works were *The Crisis* and *Richard Carvel*). Butler matriculated at Harvard Medical School in September 1922, at twenty-eight the oldest medical student in Harvard history and the first married father, a status that cost him a residency position when he graduated in 1926. He worked a year at the Rockefeller Institute in New York City, leaving to become a tutor in the Department of Biochemical Science at Harvard. In Boston, he began working with Dr. James Gamble at the Infants and Children's Hospital.

In 1930, Butler moved into an academic line in the pediatrics department at Harvard Medical School, while remaining a clinical assistant at the Children's Hospital, working with Dr. Gamble. Promotions followed; he became assistant professor in 1937 and full professor in 1944. In 1942 he joined the Massachusetts General Hospital, where he became chief of the Children's Medical Service, a position he held until his retirement in 1960.

Seemingly successful in every aspect, Butler's career combined components of clinician, administrator, researcher, teacher, reformer, civil libertarian, and cold war critic. His research centered on nutrition and metabolic disease. For twenty years Butler and Gamble collaborated, contributing to understanding the biochemistry of illness and electrolyte metabolism—the critical function of serum electrolytes. He advocated the introduction of multiple electrolyte solutions, especially for infants, to restore the body's normal fluid balance.

Butler was among the first to call attention to the role of high blood pressure in kidney disease and to demonstrate the importance of potassium treatment for starvation and dehydration. He developed methods to determine the level of sodium and vitamin C in body fluids and tissues. In the late 1930s, he established the Adolescent Endocrine Clinic at Children's Hospital. During World War II, Butler supervised a group of conscientious objectors at Massachusetts General, where he led tests of antimalarials and determined the utility of chloroquine, just when quinine supplies became scarce. His studies of the nutritional requirements for survival led to the recognition of the importance of carbohydrates in preventing ketosis.

Butler himself recognized his "Dr. Jekyll and Mr. Hyde roles in medical science and social medicine" (Butler 1969: 475). Like other medical reformers of his generation, he found his intellectual arsenal in such works as the benchmark report of the Committee on the Costs of Medicine (1932), the 1937 statement of the Committee of Physicians for the Improvement of Medical Care, the 1937 publication of *American Medicine, Expert Testimony out of Court*, the 1938 report of the Technical Committee on American Medical Care, sponsored by the Roosevelt administration's Interdepartmental Committee to Coordinate Health and Welfare Activities, and the testimony, culminating in a proposal for a national health program, at the National Health Conference in 1938. Bent on arresting the hegemonistic control over medical policy of the American Medical Association (AMA), Butler collaborated with John P. Peters, Hugh Cabot, Channing Frothingham, Edward Young, and Ernst P. Boas* to present minority medical opinion.

From the 1930s to his death in 1986, Butler remained a stalwart critic of the medical status quo. Profoundly frustrated by AMA opposition to any initiative to involve government in health care, he characterized the AMA as a guild stubbornly protecting outmoded forms and practices (Butler 1946: 264–266). His antagonism was fueled by AMA opposition to experimental prepaid medical delivery plans, including the Ross-Loos Clinic in Los Angeles, the Elk City Cooperative Hospital in Oklahoma, the Permanente Foundation Health Service in Oakland, California, and the Group Health Association in Washington, D.C. (the last resulted in a successful antitrust suit against the AMA). Over the course of his long life, Butler saw the AMA throw its considerable political weight against the Sheppard-Towner Act of 1921, which provided matching funds to the states for prenatal and child health centers; the 1937 Farm Security Administration medical programs; the 1943 Wagner-Murray-Dingell bill, which called for universal and comprehensive national health care; the Emergency Maternal and Infant Care Program of 1944, and the King-Anderson Act (Medicare) in 1965.

Butler railed most passionately against the medical establishment's suppression of minority medical opinion, which robbed the public and medical community of open dialogue. Although the so-called gag rule of the Medical Society of New York State, prohibiting county societies from expressing opinions contrary to official policy, failed in 1938, for Butler the bald attempt to outlaw divergent thought remained emblematic of AMA inhibition of debate. Butler argued that the AMA consistently represented "majority opinion . . . [as] unanimous opinion," ostensibly without violating democratic procedure (Butler 1944: 5–6). Medical journals conspired to present a united front, unwilling to air discord within the ranks. To make minority medical opinion known, Butler and other dissenters joined the Committee of Physicians for the Improvement of Medical Care, the Committee for the Nation's Health, and the Physicians Forum.

In Butler's analysis, advances in medical science made medicine at once more effective and expensive. As more Americans worked for wages or salaries, they became increasingly unable to afford quality medical care. A gap between the actual and the possible sabotaged medicine's effectiveness as it undermined its ethical commitment. Statistics remained nagging reminders: among the industrial nations in the 1940s, the United States ranked eighth in infant mortality, twenty-third in maternal mortality, and sixth in tuberculosis.

Unappeased by the AMA's belated acceptance of voluntary health insurance, Butler collaborated with other medical reformers to promote government sponsorship of health coverage. For Butler, voluntary insurance perpetuated the most insidious feature—fee for service—of medical practice. He warned that by combining fee-for-service with third-party payments, voluntary health insurance invited extravagance, removing checks on patients' malingering and physicians' overtreatment (Butler 1969: 476; Butler 1944: 4) Only with doctors on salaries or contract would, in Butler's view, a national health insurance program be equitable and cost efficient. (Later in his life, he criticized the Canadian health insurance system, which remained fee for service, in effect punishing doctors and hospitals for patients' health and rewarding them for sickness.)

Yet Butler maintained that health insurance alone could not compensate for a delivery system marked by fragmented and uncoordinated services. While medical knowledge had become too vast for physicians practicing alone, 80 percent of illness properly fell within the domain of the general practitioner. Butler envisioned a web of health services, with primary care at community health centers served by a host of health personnel, including doctors, nurses, midwives, social workers, and nurse practitioners. Specialists working in hospitals linked to neighborhood health centers would see patients on referral from primary care physicians. Toward the end of his life, Butler focused his critique on medical education, where specialty training took precedence over preventive and primary care medicine. He continued to urge the reorganization of services to replace the two-tiered system of private and welfare medicine, which was dependent on means testing, fee-for-service reimbursement, and overuse of hospitals (Butler 1969: 476).

Butler was instrumental in establishing one of the first prepaid health groups, the White Cross Health Service, begun in 1939 to give medical care to 20,000 people in the Boston area. (It survived only until 1942, a casualty of the physician shortage caused by World War II.) On his retirement from Harvard and the Massachusetts General in 1960, he became director of clinical services and chief of pediatrics at Metropolitan Hospital in Detroit, providing care for 75,000 members of the Community Health Association, a prepaid comprehensive service.

Butler's activities among the medical insurgents, as well as his involvement in antifascist politics in the 1930s and his critique of cold war policy, enmeshed him in McCarthyism. As the cold war penetrated domestic politics, Butler openly challenged the assault of the House Un-American Activities Committee on civil liberties and a foreign policy that he saw on a collision course with the Soviet Union: "Will our defence [*sic*] of the totalitarian oligarchies of Greece and Turkey strengthen Fascism, Communism or Democracy? . . . Will our aggressive preparedness at home and abroad make Russia more or less aggressive? Will infringement upon civil liberties here at home in order to resist the aggression of Russian totalitarianism protect those rights and traditions?" (Butler Papers).

Beginning in 1951, Butler endured three loyalty trials, resulting finally in exoneration. On February 14, 1951, Butler, who served as a consultant to the Children's Bureau nine days a year, faced an inquiry from the agency loyalty board that began at 10:00 A.M. and ended at 7:45 P.M. The principal charges cited his participation in the Joint Anti-Fascist Refugee Committee, the National Council of American-Soviet Friendship, and the China Aid Council. He also was cited for his work for atomic disarmament under the aegis of the United Nations (a policy the Loyalty Review Board found consonant with the position of the U.S. Communist party and the Soviet Union) with individuals who were members of organizations on the attorney general's list (Boas Papers). Of the last charge, Butler wrote: "One of them was that I was a friend of Harlow Shappley, [*sic*] professor of astronomy at Harvard. And another charge was that 'Dr. Shappley [*sic*] thought highly of Dr. Butler' " ("Dr. Butler" 1977: 7).

After the questioning, the board permitted Butler to speak. His statement stands as an eloquent defense of leftist medical politics. Butler painstakingly traced his political development to World War I, and especially to his work with the American Relief Administration, when he became an ardent advocate of U.S. membership in the League of Nations. From then, he told the board, he believed that citizenship included the obligation of active involvement in public issues. He recalled his opposition to foreign intervention in Russia between 1919 and 1923, believing it to have been ''an unfortunate cause of enmity and suspicion'' that ''may have accentuated the suppressive and totalitarian aspects of that revolution'' (Boas Papers).

Butler spoke of his sympathy for the Spanish Republic and his sorrow that with the fascist success, the defenders of the legally elected government lived in ignominious exile. ''My interest in the medical care of these exiles has reflected no advocacy of Communism but stems from profound loyalty to democracy.'' He reiterated his belief that Americans and Russians must work jointly for peace and rejected the odium of disloyalty. If ''trying to cure a patient of alcoholism [does not] make me an alcoholic,'' he argued, discussion with communists would not subvert him or others. He concluded with an affirmation of American civil liberties: ''These beliefs may be wrong. I am not arguing that they are right. But I do contend that insofar as they are what my experience and considered thought has led me to believe, I have the right and duty to act according to them. Indeed, if I did otherwise through timidity or desire for personal advantage, I would be disloyal to my conscience and country'' (Boas Papers).

Although the agency loyalty board initially dismissed the charges, the Loyalty Review Board revived the case. Butler faced two more hearings that interrupted his work. He was not cowed and never lost his pugnaciousness. In 1952, he lamented to Millicent C. McIntosh: ''The serious thing to me is that only a few individuals who have been attacked . . . have had the courage to say, 'you bet I thought so and I still believe that there is no evidence to show that such advocacy . . . wasn't correct' '' (Butler Papers).

The Jekyll and Hyde dichotomy of Butler's career did not preclude professional recognition. Even as he served as vice chairman and secretary of the Committee for the Improvement of Medical Care, president of the Physicians Forum, and a founder and head of the Boston Committee for a Sane Nuclear Policy (publicizing the hazards of radiation exposure and opposing nuclear testing and the nuclear arms race), he was elected president of the American Pediatric Society and the New England Pediatric Society. Butler won the Ernst P. Boas* Memorial Award for the Advancement of Social Medicine in 1963 and, in 1969, the Howland Award of the American Pediatric Society.

In his last decades, Butler fiercely opposed the war in Vietnam, counseling young men who sought conscientious objector status. In an address entitled ''On Vietnam and the Younger Generation's Opportunity for Social Responsibility,'' Butler, a septuagenarian, defended the ''loyalty of civil disobedience.'' He testified for Benjamin Spock, his friend of thirty years, charged with conspiracy to assist draft resistance. Governments can make mistakes, and unjust laws must be resisted, Butler declared: ''The shibboleth of 'our country right or wrong' was declared at Nuremberg to be no excuse for wrong'' (Butler Papers). Butler died at home on Martha's Vineyard in 1986 at age ninety-two, never wavering from his beliefs.

BIBLIOGRAPHY

The Francis A. Countway Library of Medicine, Boston, holds the Allan Macy Butler Papers. They contain several boxes pertaining to his career in medicine and medical politics. The Ernst P. Boas Papers at the American Philosophical Society Library in Philadelphia contain materials relating to Butler's hearings before loyalty boards during the 1950s. There is no biography of Butler; biographical sketches appeared in various newspapers and obituaries. The Countway Library maintains a list of his publications, with 144 entries. Some of the articles that Butler believed were among his most significant are listed below.

Writings by Allan Macy Butler

(with E. Tuthill). "An Application of the Uranyl Zinc Acetate Method for Determination of Sodium in Biological Material." *Journal of Biological Chemistry* 93 (1931): 171.

(with C. F. McKhann, and J. L. Gamble). "Intracellular Fluid Loss in Diarrhoeal Disease." *Journal of Pediatrics* 3 (1933): 84.

(with M. Cushman). "Distribution of Ascorbic Acid in the Blood and its Significance." *Journal of Clinical Investigation* 19 (1940): 459.

"The Provision of Adequate Medical Care." *State Government* (March 1944): 1–6.

"Minority Views on Improving Medical Care." *New England Journal of Medicine*, February 21, 1946, pp. 260–269.

"Medical Progress: Therapy of Diabetic Coma." *New England Journal of Medicine* 243 (1950): 648.

"Acceptance of the Howland Award." *Pediatric Research* (1969): 475–480.

Writings about Allan Macy Butler and Related Topics

"Dr. Butler: Unrelenting Champion of Improved Medical Care." *Vineyard*, September 20, 1977, pp. 1, 7.

"Allan Macy Butler 1894–1986." *Harvard Medical Alumni Bulletin* (winter 1986–1987): 61–63.

"Dr. Allan Butler, Pioneer in Health." *New York Times*, October 9, 1986, p. 27.

Jane Pacht Brickman

MARY STEICHEN CALDERONE
(1904–)

Mary Steichen Calderone, physician and educator, pioneer in the fields of contraception and sex education, was born in New York City, July 1, 1904, the daughter of Edward Steichen, a struggling artist, and Clara Smith Steichen, a young singer from Missouri. The family moved to France when "Mickie" was very young, where they were able to live on the small income Steichen made from his painting. The Steichens were very poor during Mickie's childhood, but they had a large circle of artistic friends and patrons, and their home was filled with art, music, books, and exciting conversation. Alfred Steiglitz and Carl Sandburg, who married Steichen's sister Paula, were close friends of the family. Mary's younger sister, Kate Rodina, was named for the sculptor Rodin, another friend.

Mickie was an intelligent, strong-willed child. She was very close to her exuberant father, and he adored and was consistently supportive of her. Her relationship with her mother was one of "constant friction and unhappiness" (Calderone 1973: 48), which she remembered with bitterness for years afterward. Late in life she realized that their conflict had reflected that in the Steichens' troubled marriage and Clara's hurt resentment over Mary's strong identification with her father (Gilbert and Moore 1981: 260–261).

The Steichens came to the United States when war broke out in 1914, and the marriage ended soon after. Kate remained with their mother; Mary spent her adolescence with friends and relatives. She lived with the family of Dr. Leonard Steiglitz in New York City while attending the Brearley School and spent summers with her maternal aunt, Charlotte, in Connecticut. She remained close to her father but was separated from him during his war service and as he began his new career in photography. Mary often felt lonely and isolated; she "didn't have a permanent home and family" (Gilbert and Moore 1981: 261) and had to wear hand-me-down clothes. But her father, her aunt, and the Steiglitz family instilled in her a strong belief in her own abilities and capacity for achievement: "Everyone . . . simply took it for granted that whatever I wanted to do, I could do" (Calderone 1973: 48).

Mary began attending classes at Vassar College even before her official graduation from Brearley in 1922. Her talks with Dr. Steiglitz and with her "extraordinary" biology teacher, Ann Dunn, had encouraged her to prepare for a medical career. But she became bored with her scientific classes and turned her attention to dramatics. After receiving her B.A. in 1925, she studied for three years at the American Laboratory Theatre, before finally deciding against an acting career. In 1926, she married a man named Martin (whom she never discussed in later life), and they had two daughters, Nell and Linda, before divorcing in 1933.

Mary Calderone later referred to these years as "a messy period" (Gilbert and Moore 1981: 255), a time of self-doubt and anxiety. As her marriage unraveled, she was forced to work in a department store, selling toasters, to support herself and her daughters, and she began seeing Eunice Armstrong, a psychoanalyst. A more positive venture was a collaboration with her father on two books of photographs for children: *The First Picture Book* (1930) and *The Second Picture Book* (1931). Armstrong pushed her to take the Human Engineering Aptitude Tests offered by the psychologist Johnson O'Connor; the results showed that Mary was a "too many aptitude woman" (Calderone 1973: 48). She credited O'Connor with encouraging her to return to medicine, a field that would fully engage her abilities. A bequest from one of Steichen's wealthy patrons enabled her to take his advice.

Mary sent her daughters to boarding school and spent a difficult year "relearning" chemistry at the College of Physicians and Surgeons in New York. Eight-year-old Nell's death from pneumonia just before she took her final examinations caused her great anguish, but she entered the University of Rochester in the fall of 1934 with renewed determination. In 1939, Mary graduated thirteenth in her class of forty-five and spent a year's internship in pediatrics at Bellevue. But she was anxious to find a specialty that would allow her to spend more time with Linda, from whom she had been separated during much of her training. Dr. Leona Baumgartner and Dr. Margaret Barnard of the New York City Health Department sponsored her for a fellowship to study public health at Columbia University.

Mary was assigned to an internship on the Lower East Side with Dr. Frank A. Calderone, then a district health officer. After a six-month courtship, they were married in November 1941 and bought a home on Long Island. Frank Calderone later served as deputy commissioner of health for New York City. From 1946 to 1951, he was the first chief administrative officer of the World Health Organization, then director of health services for the United Nations Secretariat for five years. He died in 1987.

Although Mary Calderone completed her degree in public health in 1942, she devoted herself for the next ten years to her husband and family. She and Frank had two daughters, Francesca and Maria, and she was determined to give them the attention and care she felt she had not been able to give Linda and Nell. In the late 1940s, she worked part time as a school physician. Her concern for her daughters' religious education drew her to begin attending the Manhasset Friends' Meeting, and she became a committed Quaker.

In 1953, when Francesca and Maria were ten and seven, respectively, Mary Steichen Calderone accepted the half-time position of medical director of the Planned Parenthood Federation of America (PPFA). She later learned that most physicians considered the job "professional suicide" (Calderone 1973: 50). Although the medical dissemination of contraceptive methods and advice was legal in all but two states in the 1950s and had been endorsed by the American Medical Association (1937) and the World Health Organization (1952), the public and the medical profession continued to regard the subject as controversial and the federation as a propaganda organization. Women who visited private physicians had ready access to contraceptive advice; most public facilities offered no such service to poor and working-class women. The latter were usually dependent on the small urban network of PPFA affiliated clinics.

Calderone's job as she saw it was to gain recognition of contraception as a medical and public health field and the federation as the authoritative leader of the field. In addition, she was expected to maintain standards and morale at the affiliates, review the medical content of PPFA publications, and answer the hundreds of letters requesting advice and help that arrived at the federation office each year. She achieved these goals on limited resources through unrelenting determination and the force of her warm and charismatic personality. Within a few years, she was devoting fifty to sixty hours a week to her job, although her position continued to be classified and paid as half-time; she came to resent this inequity deeply. When she left PPFA in 1964, she was replaced by two male physicians, both employed full time.

Part of Calderone's strategy was to raise PPFA's scientific profile by clinical research projects based at the affiliated clinics. "We must get rid of 'the home-made look' [and] do the kind of professional job that the United States and the world is going to expect," she wrote (Calderone 1960, PPFA-SSC). In 1959, she launched the Clinical Investigation Program, a clinical trial of diaphragms and spermicidal products at seven affiliates, with the aid of Christopher Tietze, a medical statistician with the National Committee for Maternal Health. She also facilitated the participation of PPFA clinics in the IUD (intrauterine device) field trials sponsored by the Population Council and cooperated with the Food and Drug Administration in the evaluation of oral contraceptives.

Calderone sought stronger and clearer endorsements of family planning as essential to public health and sound medical practice from the American Public Health Association (APHA) and the American Medical Association (AMA). To build her case, she presented contraception as preventive medicine against the "diseases" of abortion and teenage pregnancy. In 1955, she organized the Arden House Conference, Abortion as a Preventable Disease, bringing together clinicians, sociologists, clergy, and other authorities for the first scholarly examination of this taboo subject. Among the new facts established at the conference were that some 90 percent of abortions in the United States were performed not by unskilled quacks but by physicians, at the referral of medical colleagues, and that most of the patients were married women.

Calderone edited the conference proceedings, published in 1958 as *Abortion in the United States*, and continued to press the argument in speeches and papers, including two major 1959 presentations: "Illegal Abortion as a Public Health Problem," at the American Public Health Association (Calderone/AJPH 1960:

948–954), and at the Virginia Public Health Conference, "Health Is a State . . . (An Inquiry into Certain Dark Corners)," in which she described illegal abortion and out-of-wedlock pregnancy as problems of "social health" for which contraception was one effective therapy (Calderone 1959, MSC-SLRC).

Calderone combined her talks and writing with private contacts with APHA and AMA members. Her untiring efforts over several years contributed to a strong resolution by the APHA, calling for "full freedom . . . for the selection and use of such methods for the regulation of family size" ("The Population Problem" 1959) as individual families found acceptable, and to the revision of the AMA's thirty-five-year-old position, strongly identifying contraception with "responsible medical practice" ("AMA Policy Statement" 1964). Contraception's new respectability in this period is often credited to the growing concern with population control, but Calderone played a key role; associates detected "your fine hand" in the endorsements (Phelps 1964, MSC-SLRC).

In her "dark corners" paper, Calderone cited another hazard to public health: the ignorance, fear, and guilt many Americans felt about their own sexuality. She saw ignorance and fear over sex as contributing not only to increases in teen pregnancy and venereal disease, but to the unhappiness of the married women who wrote her about the problems of sexual incompatibility and frigidity they could share with no one else; and the confusion she saw among teenagers, including her own daughters. In 1960, she wrote a very frank and personal book about healthy sexuality, *Release from Sexual Tensions*, which brought her to the attention of clergy concerned with the same problems. The following year, she was invited to attend the North American Conference on Church and Family, sponsored by the National Council of Churches. She and a small group of colleagues from this conference began planning a new organization to study, educate about, and "establish man's sexuality as a health entity." This organization, incorporated in 1964, was SIECUS, the Sex Information and Education Council of the United States. Mary Calderone became its first executive director.

At SIECUS, Calderone felt she had come into her own. She crisscrossed the country, traveling some 50,000 miles a year, sometimes giving ten talks in two days. Her emphasis was on developing mature, responsible, healthy attitudes toward sex, based on education—an education that, she argued, should begin in childhood but was possible at any age. SIECUS, dependent on gifts and grants, was often in financial straits, and she was working twelve-hour days, but she rejoiced in the full support of her associates and warmly positive responses from her audiences. She believed that she had a special covenant with young people, and cherished comments such as the one reported from a young man who heard her speak in 1969: "I'll never again be able to make out with the girls the way I used to" (Timberlake 1969, MSC-SLRC).

Calderone's ideas about sexual health contained a strong measure of conservatism; even some of her supporters called her a "puritan." She believed that the locus of responsible sexuality was the monogamous marriage, and her thinking about homosexuality was conflicted. But the positions she did take as the voice of SIECUS, in support of early sex education and of masturbation as a useful outlet, aroused a storm of protest from conservative groups such as the John Birch Society and the Christian Coalition. These attacks, calling Calderone "an aging libertine" and accusing SIECUS of distributing pornography to schoolchildren, became particularly virulent during 1968–1970. (SIECUS supplied information only to teachers, principals, and PTAs to aid them in preparing curricular materials.) Calderone was deeply distressed by the campaign but heartened by the consistent support of clergy and other allies.

She maintained her forthright stance into her eighties, even as she eased her heavy public schedule, accepting the presidency of SIECUS in 1975. She "retired" from this post in 1982, only to undertake a lecture tour of the Soviet Union and study computer programming. Calderone has received several honorary degrees and awards, including the 1968 Woman of Conscience award from the National Council of Women of the United States; the 1973 award from the American Association of Sex Educators and Counselors; and the Elizabeth Blackwell Award in 1977. But she is most proud of the gratitude and confidence shown her by men, women, and teenagers everywhere she has gone. "Thank you," one woman wrote. "You make us proud to be women and to be human" (Gilbert and Moore 1981: 263).

BIBLIOGRAPHY

Mary Steichen Calderone's papers have been deposited at the Schlesinger Library of the History of Women at Radcliffe College (cited as MSC-SLRC). The bulk of the documents relate to her professional career with the Planned Parenthood Federation and SIECUS, but Calderone has also donated personal materials and memoirs. Additional documents of interest are in the Planned Parenthood Federation of America Papers at Smith College, Northampton, Massachusetts (cited as PPFA-SSC). Other biographical sources are the several accounts she gave in interviews during the SIECUS years; see Calderone (1973) and Gilbert and Moore (1981). Calderone's personality comes through vividly in these recollections, but they are inconsistent, and sources should be checked against each other. Calderone wrote extensively on contraception, sex education, and related issues. Besides the works cited here, see her talks to college students (Calderone 1964) and her books on sex education for families (Calderone 1981). The most useful secondary source on the contraception revolution is Reed (1978).

Materials cited in this essay include: Mary Steichen Calderone, "Health Is a State . . . (An Inquiry into Certain Dark Corners)," 1959 Virginia Public Health Conference, Box 13, Folder 224; Mrs. Stowe C. Phelps, letter to Mary Calderone, December 14, 1964, Box 10, Folder 176; Virginia Timberlake, letter to Mary Calderone, January 3, 1969, Box 14, Folder 230: all MSC-SLRC. Planned Parenthood Federation of America Papers, Sophia Smith Collection, Smith College, cited as PPFA-SSC. Material from this collection cited in the essay is from Mary Steichen Calderone, "Medical Director's Comments on Medical Program," November 7, 1960, in Medical Committee Reports.

Writings by Mary Steichen Calderone

Abortion in the United States. Edited by Mary S. Calderone. New York: Hoeber-Harper, 1958.

(with Phyllis Goldman and Robert Goldman). *Release from Sexual Tensions.* New York: Random House, 1960.

"Illegal Abortion as a Public Health Problem." *American Journal of Public Health* 49 (July 1960): 948–954.

"A Doctor Talks to Vassar College Freshmen about Love and Sex." *Western Journal of Surgery, Obstetrics and Gynecology* 72 (March–April 1964): 112–117.

"Physician and Public Health Educator." In Ruth B. Kundsin, ed., "Successful Women in the Sciences: An Analysis of Determinants." *Annals of the New York Academy of Sciences*, March 15, 1973, pp. 47–51.

(with Eric Johnson). *The Family Book about Sexuality.* New York: Harper & Row, 1981.

Writings about Mary Steichen Calderone and Related Topics

Gilbert, Lynn, and Gaylen Moore. *Particular Passions: Women Who Have Shaped our Times.* New York: C. N. Porter, 1981.

Reed, James Wesley. *From Private Vice to Public Virtue: The Birth Control Movement and American Society since 1830.* New York: Basic Books, 1978.

"AMA Policy Statement." *Journal of the American Medical Association*, December 21, 1964, pp. 31–32.

"The Population Problem." *American Journal of Public Health* 49 (December 1959): 1703–1704.

Marcia Meldrum

MAUDE E. CALLEN
(1900–1990)

Maude E. Callen, an African American public health nurse midwife, delivered over 1,000 babies and provided pre-and postnatal care for their mothers in rural Berkeley County, South Carolina. From 1923 until her retirement in 1971, Callen was often the sole accessible provider of maternal and infant care for the mostly black population of the Low Country, isolated from coastal population centers by marshlands, tidal rivers, and swamps. Callen also served residents of Pineville and St. Stephens, South Carolina, as a teacher and nutritionist. Although herculean efforts to ease the health care problems of a poor and disfranchised population earned "Miss Maude" accolades and an honorary doctoral degree from Clemson University, Callen's story is especially significant for what it tells us of black and white medical women's joint efforts to create a network of maternal and infant health care providers in one of the most isolated corners of the Jim Crow South.

Born in Quincy, Florida, Callen arrived in Berkeley County in 1923 as a missionary nurse for the Protestant Episcopal church under the auspices of the United Thank Offering. Years later she recalled, "There wasn't a paved road in this area. There were no telephones or electric lights. There was no hospital" (Thomas 1983). As late as 1967, there were only four physicians in the county (one doctor for every 7,500 residents), and only three of them delivered babies. In the 1920s, however, few white physicians in the rural South would see black patients in any case, forcing African Americans requiring hospitalization to attempt a thirty-mile wagon trip to Charleston that required crossing several unbridged tidal creeks.

Callen was a graduate of Florida A&M College and the Georgia Infirmary in Savannah. She studied care procedures for patients with tuberculosis in St. Louis at the Homer G. Phillips Hospital and trained as a nurse midwife at the Tuskegee Institute in Alabama. Shortly after her arrival in Berkeley County, Callen began teaching children to read and write in a one-room schoolhouse on the grounds of the mission that became her home. She also designed classes to teach nutrition to mothers on meager budgets. Callen held clinics during which she vaccinated children against smallpox and diphtheria. During one epidemic, she gave over 1,500 inoculations to schoolchildren in a single day. But she was best known for her work with Low Country midwives. Callen began giving lectures for local midwives in 1926 and accompanied many on their deliveries. She recalled that most had no formal training. Midwives who encountered problems during a delivery could rarely expect the assistance of a doctor. As a result of the midwives' lack of training and the poverty and isolation of their patients, maternal and infant mortality rates in the region were among the highest in the

United States. In 1929, the Berkeley County infant death rate was 121.5 per 1,000 live births (compared with a South Carolina rate of 91 and a rate of 68 for the national registration area). The mortality rate for African American babies in Berkeley County was 141.4 per 1,000 live births (South Carolina Council 1931: 7–9).

Callen organized two-week resident institutes for midwives in Berkeley and neighboring counties. Her work in an empty school house was cosponsored by the church mission and the state, which had begun to register and train midwives in 1920. Callen urged the "granny" midwives of the region to focus on cleanliness and "scientific" methods instead of depending on traditional practices, such as prohibiting new mothers from bathing for nine days. New mothers were traditionally kept inside the house, told not to brush their hair for a month after their deliveries, and given potions made from dirt daubers' nests to ease pain. Knives were also placed under new mothers' pillows to "cut" pain. Instead of a frontal assault on the "grannies," Callen and her supervisors with the state board of health sought to raise the women's status in their own communities through registration, licensing, and the wearing of uniforms.

Callen's programs were adaptations of those designed by Ruth Dodd, R.N., who was sent to South Carolina by the U.S. Children's Bureau and became the first director of the State Bureau of Child Hygiene in 1920. Dodd wrote a set of regulations governing the practice of midwifery and an outline of ten lectures, which became the first course of instruction for South Carolina's lay midwives. With funding from the Sheppard-Towner Act between 1922 and 1929, a midwife supervisor and a nutritionist were hired by the state bureau, and over 4,000 midwives voluntarily registered. Attendance at state-sponsored prenatal clinics, a series of lectures on maternal and infant care conducted during the Presbyterian Conference for Colored Women in 1927, and a month-long course in midwifery and nutrition at Voorhees School (now Voorhees College) indicated that lay midwives were eager to learn. Most traveled across several counties in rough wagons, and some walked more than 100 miles in order to receive formal training.

During the Great Depression, Sheppard-Towner funds were discontinued and the state's general assembly made no appropriations for the Bureau of Child Hygiene. After the position of midwife supervisor was discontinued, the training and supervision of lay midwives was turned over to county public health nurses. Without a federally funded state agency that focused on the health care needs of women and children, infant mortality rates and tuberculosis rates rose for the first time since 1915. Maternal mortality increased to its highest level in eighty years (Hilla Sheriff Papers, Box 4, Folder 129).

Maude Callen continued her work in Berkeley County with only church and community support until 1935, when Social Security Act funds enabled the state board of health to establish the Division of Maternal and Child Health. The new federal funds allowed the Berkeley County health department to hire Callen as a public health nurse the following year, institutionalizing the training and supervision of area midwives until her retirement in 1971. She also established the county's first prenatal and venereal disease clinics. Callen was authorized to make difficult deliveries and acted as a resource for lay midwives. During the late 1930s, she was among the first county public health nurses to receive special training in the care of premature infants from the state Division of Maternal and Child Health. Graduates of this program remained on call twenty-four hours a day to assist physicians and midwives in the delivery and care of premature infants in their counties. Callen served as a professional mentor to Eugenia Broughton, the county's second nurse midwife, who conducted a generalized nursing program with an emphasis on maternal care. Callen's and Broughton's lay charges delivered approximately 85 percent of the babies in Berkeley County well into the 1950s.

Callen worked closely with Dr. Hilla Sheriff,* who joined the Division of Maternal and Child Health in 1940 and became its director during World War II. Unlike many physicians and public health officials, who blamed midwives for high infant and maternal death rates and sought their eradication, Sheriff recognized that to eliminate lay midwives from a segregated South would be to deny most African American women access to any form of legal medical assistance during and after their deliveries. According to Sheriff, problems were most often not caused by the midwives but stemmed from the poor general health of women who had little access to prenatal care. In addition to tuberculosis and nutritional deficiencies, malaria and venereal diseases were rampant throughout much of the state. It was not unusual for midwives to be called only after hard labor had begun. Sheriff was moved by black women's demonstrated concern for their communities and committed her agency's resources to standardizing the sporadic programs that had provided midwife training since the 1920s.

Maude Callen and seven other graduate nurse midwives played crucial roles in Sheriff's two-week Midwife Training Institutes, held at the Penn Community Center on St. Helena Island near Beaufort. Sheriff relied heavily on Callen, Broughton, and Eula Harris, an African American nurse midwife who practiced near Augusta, Georgia, to design a program that would effectively disseminate medical knowledge to black lay midwives, many of whom did not read or write. Callen persuaded Sheriff to secure Penn Center, originally a school for newly freed slaves, as a site for the institutes because of its symbolic value in the Low Country communities served disproportionally by midwives. Training took place in the historic school buildings beneath moss-draped live oaks on a barrier island claimed by black farm families after the Civil War. Participants frequently described the experience as "inspirational."

South Carolina midwives were required by law to attend one of the summer institutes every four years. By the early 1950s, midwives spoke fondly of the "reunions" that maintained their legitimacy and raised their status among peers and patients. A day began with breakfast at 7:30 A.M., followed by chapel. Classes were held from 9:00 A.M. until noon and again from 2:00 P.M. until 5:00 P.M. Laura Blackburn, a nurse midwife who directed the program for the

Division of Maternal and Child Health, Callen, and several county public health nurses were the teaching staff and remained on call throughout the institutes, but most activities were designed by peer group leaders. Since many midwives were illiterate, Callen persuaded Sheriff to send a reading and writing teacher to the institutes. As a result, midwives who had refused to obtain state licenses because they lacked the literacy skills to register births with county health departments were brought into the fold. As Callen predicted, the midwife license became a source of pride. Black women felt a sense of ownership toward the institutes; in their own space, they acquired the long-sought-after skills of literacy and medical knowledge and received instruction from role models with whom they identified. Callen encouraged the singing of spirituals, and Eugenia Broughton even wrote a ''Birth Certificate Song'' to be sung to a familiar tune:

> Whenever you deliver perhaps a baby boy
> Remember he is human, not just a little toy
> His birth should be recorded within ten days or less
> And in years to come you will be blessed.
> We know that it's important, a solid standard rule
> He'll need birth registration to enter any school
> To prove he is the right age to marry or to vote
> So be sure his birth date you report.
> He'll need it for enlistment or maybe go abroad
> Producing his birth record will prove he's not a fraud
> It'll make him mighty happy if he can really say
> ''I'm a native of the U.S.A.''
> He'll then be eligible to earn an honest wage
> Receive a monthly pension if he can prove his age
> When sixty-five or over, he then will in due time
> Live in comfort, peace and sweet sublime.
>
> CHORUS
> Be sure his name, the date, the place are right
> If not, in time he'll be in quite a plight
> Check and recheck, then have the mother sign
> And you will have great peace of mind
> (Hilla Sheriff Papers, Box 4, Folder 121)

The Division of Maternal and Child Health's program to train and license lay midwives was an effective partnership between two groups of medical women: white public health officials who provided supplies, funding, and training and African American nurse midwives and peer leaders, most significant, Maude Callen, who contributed their expertise, experience, and cultural awareness. An interim step in a society historically unwilling to recognize the equality and basic human rights of almost half its population, South Carolina's Midwife Training Institutes continued to operate throughout the period during which southern medical facilities opened their doors to black patients (as late as 1967, 306 midwives delivered 3,000 babies in South Carolina).

In 1951, Callen's work in Berkeley County was featured by photographer W. Eugene Smith in a pictorial essay in *Life* magazine. Readers touched by the photos sent Callen $27,000. She used the money to build the county's first permanent clinic. After "Miss Maude's" retirement, the facility was abandoned temporarily until Callen persuaded the local director of the Agency on Aging to allow her to reopen it as a nutrition site. She spent the last decade of her long life preparing and serving meals each weekday to about fifty of her fellow senior citizens. Maude Callen died at the age of eighty-nine, shortly before her induction into the South Carolina Hall of Fame.

BIBLIOGRAPHY

Callen's career in Berkeley County and contributions to the state midwife training institutes are documented in the papers of Dr. Hilla Sheriff, housed at the South Caroliniana Library of the University of South Carolina in Columbia. Materials in topical files on Midwives, Pediatrics, and the State Board of Health are especially helpful in an analysis of the relationships between state officials, nurse midwives, and lay midwives. The Sheriff Papers contain many photographs of state programs to educate mothers and midwives (including the Institutes) that feature Callen. Mildred Hood (Berkeley County historian), Sinclair Richard Callen (Maude Callen's adopted son), and Bob Hirsch (South Carolina Hall of Fame) can supply information. Callen discussed the Midwife Training Institutes in "Carrying Health to the Country," a 1988 profile of Dr. Hilla Sheriff by South Carolina Educational Television.

Writings about Maude E. Callen and Related Topics

Adkinson, Austin. "SC's Graduate Nurse Midwives Travel into Remotest Nooks and Corners; Job Not for Faint-Hearted Clock-Watchers." *State* (Columbia, S.C.), December 30, 1951.

Borst, Charlotte G. "The Training and Practice of Midwives: A Wisconsin Study." *Bulletin of the History of Medicine* 62 (1988): 606–627.

"Clemson Honors Miss Maude." *State* (Columbia, S.C.), December 21, 1983.

Litoff, Judy Barrett. *The American Midwife Debate: A Sourcebook on its Modern Origins.* Westport, Conn.: Greenwood Press, 1986.

Sadler, Betty. " 'I Just Loved That Job of Delivering a Baby.' " *State* (Columbia, S.C.), November 24, 1968.

———. "Midwives Still 'Catch' S.C. Babies." *State* (Columbia, S.C.), November 21, 1968.

Thomas, Jamie. "Maude E. Callen." (Charleston, S.C.) *Post and Courier*, May 22, 1983.

Smith, Susan L. "White Nurses, Black Midwives, and Public Health in Mississippi, 1920–1950." *Nursing History Review* 2 (1994): 29–49.

South Carolina Council. Committee on Health. *A Study of Health Education, Maternal Death Rate, Infant Mortality, Nutrition and Degenerative Diseases.* Cheraw, S.C., 1931.

Waring, Joseph I. "American Academy of Pediatrics Study of Child Health Services in South Carolina." *Journal of the South Carolina Medical Association* 45 (September–October 1949).

Patricia Evridge Hill

KATE CAMPBELL
(1899–1986)

Kate Campbell, Australian pediatrician and pioneer in neonatology, is best known for her discovery of the role of oxygen as a cause of blindness in infants due to retrolental fibroplasia. Campbell was born in Melbourne, Australia, in 1899 and graduated in medicine in 1922.

Australia's first medical schools were founded toward the end of the nineteenth century: Melbourne in 1862, Sydney in 1883, and Adelaide in 1886. There was considerable opposition to the admission of women to medical courses, except for the University of Adelaide, where in 1880 women were admitted on equal terms by adding to its constitution: "words imparting the masculine gender shall include the feminine." The first woman to practice medicine in Australia was Constance Stone, who had traveled to Philadelphia in 1884 and later also graduated in England, where she worked with Elizabeth Garrett Anderson. Stone commenced practice in Melbourne in 1889. The first women graduates in medicine in Australia were Claire Stone (Constance's sister) and Margaret White in Melbourne and Grace Robinson in Adelaide in 1891. In 1896, ten women graduates met at Constance Stone's home and made plans to establish a hospital that was to be exclusively administered by women for female patients along the lines of Anderson's New Hospital for Women in London. Initially called the Victoria Hospital for Women, it became Queen Victoria despite her majesty's well-known opposition to the suffragettes and women's rights in general—"this foolish folly," as she described it. The hospital opened its doors in 1899 with the motto *Profeminis A Feminis''* (For Women by Women). The initial battle for women's place in medicine in Australia had thus been won before Campbell entered the war. One of the chief obstacles for women was difficulty in obtaining training positions in hospitals, often on the grounds that hospitals lacked appropriate bedrooms or toilet facilities for women doctors. These barriers were still in place when Campbell arrived on the scene. She participated in the second wave in the assault on the bastions of male privilege and was one of several whose successful careers and achievements eventually led to the current position in Australia where approximately 50 percent of medical school students are female, although women are still underrepresented in all the specialist and academic areas.

Campbell's parents, both of Scottish origin, had met and married in New Zealand before settling in Australia, where they raised Kate and her three brothers. Although Campbell's father worked as a clerk and money was always short, her parents retained the Scottish belief in the importance of good education and academic achievement, but neither of the two elder children showed ability or interest in schoolwork. The parents' ambitions were more than fulfilled by their two younger children. While at Hawthorn State School, Campbell won a scholarship to the more prestigious Methodist Ladies College. She was dux of the college (top student of the year) and won a bursary (scholarship) to study at the university as a resident in Janet Clarke Hall, a nondenominational woman's college. Initially, she contemplated science, but her mother discouraged her because a friend's daughter had found difficulty finding a job on graduation. Her mother suggested medicine, which appealed to Campbell's instinctive altruism. Campbell enrolled in the Faculty of Medicine in 1916, a time when many young Australian doctors and students had volunteered for military service in World War I.

Women doctors were refused enlistment in the Australian armed forces. Some women managed to circumvent this prohibition and saw service with volunteer groups such as the Red Cross. The lack of manpower caused some teaching hospitals to forgo their embargo on employing female resident medical officers, but at the end of the war, the lack of toilets and bedrooms miraculously returned. Although the male medical students regarded their female counterparts as somewhat eccentric, and society in general still regarded medicine as an unsuitable occupation for women, they were well treated except for some curious attitudes of the administration. Administrators saw no contradiction in forbidding women from attending casualty rooms (emergency rooms), because of the unsavory situations they might encounter, but at the same time scheduling naive young women to attend the male venereal disease (VD) clinic as their first experience in outpatient care.

Campbell had an excellent undergraduate record and shared first place in physiology with Frank MacFarlane Burnet, winner of the 1960 Nobel Prize in Medicine. Apart from the occasional crudity on the part of some lecturers and the traumatic experiences encountered at the VD clinic, Campbell enjoyed her student days immensely, graduating in 1922 in eighth place. With another brilliant young woman graduate, Jean McNamara, she was appointed as a junior resident (intern) at the Melbourne Hospital attached to Sir William Upjohn's medical unit. Many observers thought that Campbell and McNamara were the best residents in their year, but nevertheless they were not given appointment to continue work at the Melbourne Hospital. With recommendations from Upjohn, they were appointed to the resident staff of the Children's Hospital.

While examining "a little child of two, the dearest little thing," Campbell came to the conviction that she wanted to specialize in pediatrics. Although she appeared slight, shy, and rather delicate, Campbell had a keen sense of humor, and her energy and dedication to her duties were prodigious. After a particularly strenuous day in the labor ward at the Women's Hospital during her training in obstetrics, Campbell's male counterpart collapsed. She recalled that when she suggested that he lie down while she fetched him a brandy, "His masculine pride stung to the quick he sat bolt upright and shouted 'You'll not get me brandy. You look like three halfp'worth of God help us, and you're as tough as an old boot.' " This inner energy served her well throughout her life.

Although she gained a foothold on the lowest rung of the career ladder at the Children's Hospital with her appointment as a clinical assistant, she soon recognized that her gender prevented further promotion when she saw less competent male colleagues promoted. In 1924, she resigned from the hospital to join the staff of the Women's Hospital, a move that was encouraged and supported by the professor of obstetrics and gynecology, Marshall Allan. She was appointed to the staff of the Queen Victoria Hospital as pediatrician in 1926 and went into general practice in the Melbourne suburb of Essendon. Some male patients made it obvious that they were uncomfortable with a woman doctor, but this was more than compensated for by the relief expressed by women who saw her as someone who sympathized with them and understood their fears and did not adopt a superior attitude. Initially she did all her rounds on foot; when her practice was more established, she was able to borrow the money for a car.

At Queen Victoria Hospital, Campbell took over the training program for the infant welfare nursing sisters who staffed the Victorian Baby Health Association, established in 1917 by Vera Scantlebury to provide suburban centers to give advice to mothers and to monitor the baby's progress in the postnatal period. Campbell became the medical officer of the Baby Health Association. Campbell and Scantlebury met while they were medical students and became fast friends. Both women strongly encouraged a relaxed and natural approach to infant care, opposing other popular schools of the day, which advocated extremely rigid regimes and banned cuddling during the day, apart from a period termed "the mothering hour." "We believed in human warmth and contact," Campbell said, "not in disciplining the baby from the day of its birth. We fed and cuddled babies when they wanted feeding and cuddling" (Grimshaw and Strahan 1982: 166). Their jointly authored book, *A Guide to the Care of the Young Child* (1945), was an enlarged revision of Scantlebury's earlier *Guide to Infant Feeding* (1929). The book was an immediate success. After Scantlebury's death in 1945, it went through seven editions, the last in collaboration with Dr. A. Elizabeth Wilmot in 1972.

Together with her unpaid position as pediatrician at the Queen Victoria, Campbell built up a busy practice. Marshall Allan, the first professor of obstetrics and gynecology in Australia, recognized the lack of know-how in the management of the newborn and in 1929 established a university lectureship to promote this area. He had planned to ask a senior pediatrician to fill this post, but after hearing Campbell speak at a meeting, he appointed her, believing that she would grow with the job and be less traditional in her approach. Soon her advice was being sought by all the obstetricians at the hospital, and babies were no longer regarded as simply a necessary by-product of the process of childbirth. Her attendance at all autopsies and meetings to voice the question, "Why did the baby die?" became a feature of the hospital. She commented at a valedictory dinner at her club, the Lyceum, that she learned later that she had earned the title of "The Pediatric Policeman." She commented, "I realized early that the first time one made a suggestion nothing would happen. It was just a softening up process. It was necessary to introduce the subject at intervals as occasions offered.'' She related that after one such occasion, a male colleague said, ''Do you know what happens to nagging women?'' When she replied that she did not, he answered, ''They get things done!''

What had started as a formal commitment of only three lectures per year rapidly grew into seminars and demonstrations to all of the student groups and consultations on any problem that obstetricians encountered with the babies. Thus became established her famous evening rounds. Problems in the newborn had to be seen promptly, and because of Campbell's other commitments, only the evening remained. Apart from the standard clinical duties, Campbell would take time to discuss issues with the night staff, both medical and nursing, in a delightfully friendly and informal fashion; she was always willing to listen to their suggestions and respond to queries. Often she would return home exhausted, but she built up a rapport and reputation for her legendary approachability and wisdom that earned her the universal title of ''Auntie Kate.''

In 1937, the demand for her opinion in pediatric problems was so great that she abandoned general practice and became a consultant (a specialist). That same year, with the support of Marshall Allan, she established the first Department of Neonatology at the Women's Hospital; it was one of the earliest such departments in the world. Campbell now had three major clinical commitments: pediatrics at the Queen Victoria, neonatology at the Women's Hospital, and her private practice. She carefully collected and correlated data from all three, while introducing and monitoring new drugs, such as the sulfonamides, and new medical technology for infants and children. With the outbreak of World War II in 1939, her workload increased. Queen Victoria, with its all-female staff, had always been less well funded than Melbourne's other hospitals. Because the hospital was so understaffed, the residents were exhausted from obstetrics work. According to Campbell, ''The honoraries [unpaid visiting staff] at the hospital insisted that the residents get their full night's sleep and took it in turns to do night duty. That sort of thing would never happen anywhere else. The hospital really meant something to those women.'' Campbell never forgot her debt to the ''Queen Vic'' and the opportunities that this all-female institution had given her.

While pursuing the busy life of a consultant and teacher in the late 1940s, Campbell noted that there seemed to be an increasing incidence of blindness among neonates and found that in the majority, the cause was ascribed to retrolental fibroplasia, an entity she had not encountered in the past. The condition was first described in Boston and was noted to be most common among neonates of three to four pounds or less (Terry 1942). The condition had a curious geographical distribution; careful epidemiological studies confirmed the geographical variations between cities in the United States and its rarity in England (Kinsey and Zacharias 1949). Researchers noted only three significant variations in the treatment of the infants: ''first, administration of a multiple vitamin preparation in which the fat-soluble vitamins are made miscible with water; secondly, administration of iron in greatly increased quantities, and thirdly, more frequent administration of oxygen.'' Researchers focused their attention on the oral preparations administered and ignored the use of oxygen as a possible factor, but Campbell noticed that the incidence of the disorder was most common at the Women's Hospital, was lower at Queen Victoria, and was least frequent in her own private practice. An arrogant clinician might have concluded that this result was a function of his or her own innate superiority and proper handling of cases in comparison to that of residents and other staff at a public institution, that is, the superiority of private versus state medicine. However, Campbell astutely realized that her findings provided a way to identify the cause of this new affliction. She examined the differences in treatment in the three groups and concluded that the only factor that differed significantly was the use of oxygen. The Women's Hospital, better funded and equipped, had oxygen piped in at the bedside, and its use for neonates was lavish, universal, and at high concentrations. At Queen Victoria, oxygen cylinders were the only source, and oxygen was therefore used much less frequently. In her private practice in small hospitals, oxygen was supplied even more sparingly; the cost limited it to situations where it was clearly essential. The lowering of oxygen concentration and amount administered resulted in a dramatic decrease in the incidence of retrolental fibroplasia and blindness in neonates.

Campbell was not a laboratory worker, and she was distressed by the slowness of the acceptance of her work, which was in part independently supported by others (Crosse 1951; Evans 1951; Jefferson 1952). Campbell reasoned on physiological grounds that oxygen is toxic to the blood vessels of premature infants and therefore should be administered only when there were clear-cut indications. One study that particularly upset her was done at Bellevue Hospital, New York, in 1954. Neonates were randomly allocated to oxygen treatment for a controlled clinical trial that resulted in an increase of retrolental fibroplasia and blindness in the group given oxygen. Thirty-six premature infants were given high concentrations of oxygen for two weeks; eight developed irreversible blindness in both eyes, and two others had possible damage to one eye. None of the infants in the control group that was given oxygen at low concentrations became blind. This work has been cited as an example of an ill-conceived and unethical investigation (Papworth 1969: 221). It illustrates Campbell's comment: ''It is interesting how the basic and fundamental things one knows by intuition, get recognition and respectability only when they come out of a laboratory.'' Although this statement can be debated, it illustrates her commitment to a clinical approach to medicine and her deep belief in the rights and sanctity of each patient and the doctor's duty to follow the famous Hippocratic aphorism, *primum non nocere* (first do no harm).

Conscious of the continuing struggle that women have to compete at the higher levels of the profession, Campbell identified the ''3 Ms'' as the main obstacles to be overcome: muscle, maternity, and money. In 1964, she was awarded the Britannica Award jointly with Sir Norman Gregg, who had discovered the link between rubella and congenital defects. In 1954 she was awarded the title Commander of the British Empire and in 1971 that of Dame of the British Empire, a title that is the equivalent of a knighthood. These awards for outstanding service to the community involve the recommendation of the Australian government to the queen. Melbourne University awarded her an honorary L.L.D. in 1966.

Although justly proud of her many contributions to neonatology, she considered her most important achievements the help, hope, and succor she gave to her young patients and their parents. Campbell always acknowledged the help she received from her mother and from her lifelong friend and companion, Win (Winifred) Crick (1904–). Crick had trained in general nursing at the Alfred Hospital and also earned certificates in midwifery and infant care at the Royal Women's Hospital. In 1940 Crick became matron in charge of infant care training at the Royal Women's Hospital, a position she held until 1945.

Campbell said, "I owe Sir William Upjohn my entry into pediatrics, Vera Scantlebury my entry to infant welfare and Marshall Allan my entry to the neonatal area. I'll always be in debt to those three people." Renowned for her stories and sense of humor, this pioneer of neonatology served as a role model for generations of students and doctors who affectionately remembered her as "Auntie Kate." She concluded one interview by saying, "I have learned three things in my life: firstly, you can't have everything; secondly, nothing for nothing—you (or somebody else) has to pay for everything; thirdly, there's a back and a front, a good and a bad side to everything. I am always grateful that it has been my good fortune to spend my life in the satisfying, rewarding and fascinating field of pediatrics. Such fulfillment is the lot of few people" (Grimshaw and Strahan 1982: 169).

BIBLIOGRAPHY

Much of the information for this essay has been derived with the assistance of Win Crick, whose cooperation and patience I gratefully acknowledge. An obituary by Margaret A. Mackie was published in the *Medical Journal of Australia* 146 (1987):161–162. A complete list of Campbell's writings was included in "Dame Kate Campbell: An Appreciation." *Australian Paediatric Journal* 10 (1974): 48–55.

Writings by Kate Campbell

"Intensive Oxygen Therapy as a Possible Cause of Retrolental Fibroplasia: A Clinical Approach." *Medical Journal of Australia* 2 (1951): 48–50.
(with Vera Scantlebury-Brown). *Guide to the Care of the Young Child.* 2d ed. Melbourne: W. M. Houston, Government Printer, 1947.

Writings about Kate Campbell and Related Topics

Crosse, V. Mary. "The Problem of Retrolental Fibroplasia in the City of Birmingham." *Transactions of the Ophthalmological Societies of the United Kingdom* 71 (1951): 609–612.

Evans, P. Jamieson. "Retrolental Fibroplasia." *Transactions of the Ophthalmological Societies of the United Kingdom* 71 (1951): 613–615.

Grimshaw, Patricia, and Lynne Strahan, eds. *The Half-Open Door: Sixteen Modern Australian Women Look at Professional Life and Achievement.* Sydney, New South Wales, Australia: Hale and Iremonger, 1982.

Jefferson, Eirlys. "Retrolental Fibroplasia." *Archives of Disease in Childhood* 109 (1952): 329–336.

Kinsey, V. Everett, and Leona Zacharias. "Retrolental Fibroplasia. Incidence in Different Localities in Recent Years and a Correlation of the Incidence with Treatment Given the Infants." *Journal of the American Medical Association* 139 (1949): 572–578.

Neve, M. Hutton. *The Mad Folly. The History of Australia's Pioneer Women Doctors.* Sydney: Library of Australian History, 1980.

Papworth, M. H. *Human Guinea Pigs.* Harmondsworth: Penguin, 1969.

Terry, T. L. "Extreme Prematurity and Fibroblastic Overgrowth of Persistent Vascular Sheath behind Each Crystalline Lens." *American Journal of Ophthalmology* 25 (1942): 203–214.

Barry G. Firkin

ROBERT DAVIES DEFRIES
(1889–1975)

Dr. Robert Davies Defries, known as Canada's Mr. Public Health, played a central role in the development of public health in Canada during the first half of the twentieth century. He possessed a rare combination of scientific knowledge, keen judgment, and organizational, administrative, and teaching skills, along with the ability to provide leadership and inspiration to those around him. At the same time, Defries remained unassuming and kindly, with a deep religious commitment, a quiet sense of humor, and a complete dislike of ostentation. He had an encyclopedic knowledge of applied bacteriology, epidemiology, immunology, and public health administration, all of which were efficiently tapped during his long service with the University of Toronto's Connaught Medical Research Laboratories and the intimately connected School of Hygiene, especially while director of both institutions between 1940 and 1955.

From seeds planted in 1913, "Dr. Bob," as he was affectionately called, became the primary architect of, and was personally inseparable from, these internationally renowned institutions, particularly Connaught, and its unique public health mission: medical research, noncommercial production and distribution of essential biological products, and public service. Under Defries's leadership, Connaught played a key role in the international control of numerous infectious diseases, especially through its pioneering development of methods for the large-scale production of such essential products as insulin, diphtheria toxoid, heparin, penicillin, combined antigens, and both types of polio vaccines. Moreover, Connaught's unique university structure and close links to the federal and provincial governments, reinforced by Defries's professional and personal relationships, ensured that the public health benefits of Connaught's many products were kept within the reach of everyone.

Defries was born in Toronto, Ontario, on July 23, 1889. His family's Canadian roots extend back to 1829, when his great-grandfather Robert William Defries arrived from England and established a small brewery in Toronto's east end. His great-uncle, Robert Davier, owned a large brewing business, operating five of the city's thirteen breweries in 1885. His father, Thomas William, worked at the Davier brewery until his untimely death at age thirty-eight. His mother, Agnes (Lumsden), a deeply religious woman, was determined that her two sons stay out of the brewery business and go to university. Both Robert and his brother, William attended the University of Toronto and graduated in medicine. Robert graduated in 1911 with his M.B., followed by an M.D. in 1913, and a diploma in public health (D.P.H.) in 1914. Indeed, Defries was the first candidate and first graduate of the D.P.H. program, a situation that developed fortuitously and with some resistance, but with enormous implications for the subsequent evolution of public health in Canada.

Public health education in Toronto began in 1875 with undergraduate instruction in sanitary science at the Toronto School of Medicine, a forerunner of the University of Toronto's faculty of medicine that amalgamated in 1903. In 1910 a new professor of hygiene was appointed, Dr. John A. Amyot (1867–1940), who was also director of the Provincial Board of Health Laboratory. Efforts to introduce graduate education in public health by offering a D.P.H. at the University of Toronto had been initiated as early as 1901, but a diploma was not offered until 1904 and not granted until 1911. Only physicians were eligible, but it involved passing only one examination with no formal course work.

A more structured D.P.H. program with specific courses was initiated in 1912 with the appointment of Dr. John W. S. McCullough (1868–1941) as Ontario's provincial health officer, who was interested in improving local health services across the province. However, he needed more qualified health officers and turned to Amyot for help. Initially, the University of Toronto was reluctant to establish a formal D.P.H. graduate course. This situation changed when the young Defries, after a year of postgraduate study in biochemistry, approached Amyot to apply for a postgraduate course at Toronto. With a qualified and enthusiastic candidate in hand, Amyot finally convinced the faculty of medicine to establish a new D.P.H. course, and Defries was the sole student for the first academic session of 1912–1913.

The curriculum Defries studied was based on the British model that emphasized sanitation, quarantine, ventilation, and the clinical study of fevers, supplemented by studies in geology, microbiology, meteorology, and an apprentice course in bacteriology in the Provincial Board of Health laboratory. In 1913, Defries was appointed as a demonstrator for the D.P.H. course and was joined by Dr. John G. FitzGerald (1882–1940).

From this point, Defries and FitzGerald worked closely together to establish what would become Connaught Laboratories in 1913–1914, while at the same time overseeing the growth of the Department of Hygiene and Preventive Medicine and its transformation into the School of Hygiene in 1927. FitzGerald and Defries were a unique and complementary team: the former an inspired, and even a reckless, public health visionary, the latter an eminently practical medical missionary and a prudent administrator.

The unique vision of an institution devoted to medical research and the noncommercial production of essential health products within a university environment originated with FitzGerald. It emerged out of a long period of education and travel driven by a strong desire to develop and apply the latest methods of preventive medicine at the lowest possible cost and for the largest public benefit. FitzGerald's first opportunity emerged in the summer of 1913 when he prepared the Pasteur rabies treatment in the Ontario Board of Health laboratory. Hitherto, this product had been imported from New York at a much greater cost. Fitzgerald then presented his vision for a university-based laboratory for biologicals production and research, but encountered resistance from the university governors, who were concerned that such an enterprise seemed to involve commerce more than academics. However, FitzGerald was keenly aware of the tragic toll of diphtheria in Canada. Diphtheria antitoxin imported from U.S. commercial suppliers was accessible only to the rich.

Undaunted by the university's hesitancy, FitzGerald used his own money to build a stable and buy horses and laboratory equipment for the production of diphtheria antitoxin. Within a few months, he won his first contract to produce the life-saving antitoxin for the Ontario Board of Health for free provincial distribution; he produced it at one-fifth to one-tenth the cost charged by American producers. Finally, recognizing the obvious public service benefits, on May 1, 1914, the University of Toronto assumed full financial responsibility for Fitz-Gerald's work, gave him laboratory space, and appointed him director of this new Antitoxin Laboratory in the Department of Hygiene. Despite some early opposition from commercial manufacturers and druggists, by 1920 all provinces were freely distributing Connaught's public health products.

The outbreak of World War I at first threatened the survival of this fledgling laboratory, but the war soon generated the national interest necessary to ensure its rapid growth. Defries played a key role in this process through the expedited production of tetanus antitoxin that was urgently needed by the Canadian Expeditionary Forces. The Canadian Red Cross tried to purchase the antitoxin in the United States, but supplies were limited, and each dose cost $1.35. The savior of FitzGerald's vision was Colonel Albert E. Gooderham (1861–1935), a wealthy Toronto distiller, who served on the Canadian Red Cross Executive Committee and was a University of Toronto governor. Prompted by the federal government, Gooderham approached FitzGerald to prepare the tetanus antitoxin, but the capacity of the new Antitoxin Laboratory was thought insufficient to meet the growing demand for it as well as other essential health products. Nevertheless, beginning in February 1915, tetanus antitoxin production was stepped up under Defries's personal direction and was made available to the army at $0.34 a dose. In total some 250,000 doses were manufactured during the war, meeting all the Canadian military needs.

Gooderham's most important legacy came in 1915 with his gift of a fifty-seven-acre farm property that would include a modern laboratory building. These new facilities were officially opened on October 25, 1917, and, by request of Gooderham, were christened the Connaught Antitoxin Laboratories and University Farm, after the Duke of Connaught, Canada's governor-general during the war. The Ontario government matched Gooderham's gift with a grant of $75,000 to support medical research. To ensure a national character for Connaught, FitzGerald set up the Advisory Committee on Scientific Work with representatives from each province. In 1920, soon after the establishment of a Department of National Health, a more formal Dominion Council of Health was established; it included the federal and provincial deputy ministers of health and five other members, including FitzGerald, and then Defries (1940–1962), affording a regular national health forum in which the work of Connaught was integrated into provincial and federal health programs.

Connaught's practical value to public health became especially prominent with the discovery of insulin at the University of Toronto in 1921–1922. This story is well known (Bliss 1982), but less appreciated is Connaught's pioneering role, largely under Defries's direction, in developing methods to produce insulin on a large scale and at the lowest possible cost to those with diabetes. Defries played a critical role in securing a patent for the University of Toronto to ensure high international production standards and the direction of insulin proceeds to the expansion of medical research across Canada. Defries worked closely and unselfishly with the discoverers of insulin, as well as Eli Lilly and Company of Indianapolis, to ensure expanded production. This cooperative approach was also applied to the production of diphtheria toxoid, heparin, protamine zinc insulin, penicillin, typhus vaccine, combined antigens, and the Salk polio vaccine.

Insulin was the most significant product to Connaught's financial health and physical growth until the development of polio vaccines. Moreover, "the discovery of Insulin was a stimulus of first importance" to the establishment of the School of Hygiene and its endowment by the Rockefeller Foundation (Defries 1957: 289). In addition to being associate director of the school until 1940, Defries was also head of the Department of Epidemiology and Biometrics and later the Department of Public Health Administration. The new School of Hygiene building provided a national center for public health teaching, expanded facilities for Connaught, and an administrative focus for both institutions. This building also served as the heart of the Canadian Public Health Association (CPHA), founded in 1910, and its journal, especially when Defries became its editor in 1928, a position he held until 1964. Defries was the backbone of the CPHA and is widely credited with reenergizing its journal.

World War II placed heavy demands on Connaught and resulted in a major period of expansion in staff and capacity. In addition to supplying the military with tetanus and gas gangrene toxoids and a new typhus fever vaccine developed by Connaught, the war placed the greatest demands on Defries's administrative skills to produce dried human blood serum to treat shock among soldiers. This work required additional space, and in 1943 Defries expedited Connaught's acquisition of a large building on campus that became the Spadina Division. The new division was also urgently required to develop methods to produce penicillin on a large scale for the federal government in time for D-Day in June 1944.

During the postwar years Defries led Connaught through a period of accelerated expansion, driven largely through cancer and virus research, financed most significantly by federal public health research grants and the National Foundation for Infantile Paralysis (NFIP) or U.S. March of Dimes. While Connaught conducted research in many fields, its comprehensive polio research program, which began in 1947 under the direction of Dr. Andrew J. Rhodes (1911–

1995), paid the greatest scientific, public health, and political dividends. Methods that proved essential to the large-scale production of Salk's inactivated polio vaccine were developed at Connaught.

The first step was Connaught's development of the world's first synthetic medium, known as "Medium 199," for cancer research by J. F. Morgan, H. J. Morton, and R. C. Parker in 1949. In 1951, through a close friendship between Morgan and Dr. A. E. Franklin of Rhodes's group, Franklin discovered that 199 proved ideal for cleanly culturing the poliovirus in monkey kidney cells. This made Salk's vaccine safe for the first human clinical trials in 1952. The NFIP then financed a major pilot project at Connaught to cultivate poliovirus in larger quantities. In 1953, this effort led to the "Toronto method," developed by Dr. Leone N. Farrell (1904–1986), which involved culturing the poliovirus in a suspension of monkey kidney cells in 199 using large bottles incubated on special rocking machines. Salk's vaccine could now be produced in large quantities. In July 1953, as Defries took direct control of the polio work, the NFIP asked Connaught to carry out what Salk called the herculean task of supplying all the bulk poliovirus fluids that were inactivated in the United States for the 1954 field trial. Despite some reservations within the university over the speed of the trial and the safety of the vaccine, Defries efficiently carried out this unusual project.

Soon after the NFIP field trial began in April, Defries turned his attention to preparing vaccine for Canadians and planning for its introduction in the light of its still-unknown value. Gambling that the vaccine was safe and at least somewhat effective, in October 1954, the Dominion Council of Health agreed to Defries's plan for the national use of the vaccine on an experimental basis, regardless of the U.S. trial results. The cost of the vaccine was to be shared equally between the federal and provincial governments, ensuring free vaccinations for some 500,000 children across Canada.

The start of this Canadian program coincided with the much anticipated April 12, 1955, announcement of the NFIP field trial results in Ann Arbor, Michigan, which revealed that the vaccine was safe and 60 to 90 percent effective against paralytic polio. However, high public expectations and unprecedented media coverage generated the popular perception that the vaccine was completely successful and that the long war against polio was over. This attitude was particularly strong in the American press, and it worried Defries. Dr. G. D. W. Cameron (1899–1983), deputy minister of national health, who, with Defries, sat well toward the back of the room at the Ann Arbor event, was more concerned that "throughout the performance there was no recognition of what the Connaught had done." He later remembered "being furious but Bob, of course, was philosophical" (Rutty 1995: 345).

Canada's foresight in planning early for the vaccine's orderly introduction, orchestrated largely through Defries's leadership, was prominently vindicated in the wake of the infamous "Cutter incident." By early May 1955, some eighty cases of paralytic polio in the United States were directly associated with vaccine prepared by Cutter Laboratories of Berkeley, California, touching off a national crisis that resulted in the cancellation of the entire American vaccination program. In Ottawa, Paul Martin, the minister of national health and welfare, faced one of his most difficult political decisions: What should Canada do? The prime minister was reluctant to let the Canadian trial continue, but based on Defries's counsel and experience, Martin maintained his confidence. Canada maintained a strict testing procedure; Connaught and the federal Laboratory of Hygiene tested each vaccine lot, unlike the United States, after the vaccine was licensed. The Canadian success story generated significant American media attention and political debate, sharply highlighting the differing levels of government interest in controlling the vaccine. The prominence of the Canadian Salk vaccine program also played a major role in ensuring its future international use in the control of polio.

The Salk vaccine introduction was Defries's swan song. He retired as director of Connaught and the School of Hygiene on September 30, 1955. On November 17, Defries was the 1955 recipient of the prestigious Albert Lasker Award from the American Public Health Association. He was the first Canadian so honored. While the award was given in recognition of Defries's polio vaccine leadership and his distinguished career in Canadian and U.S. public health, the award was expedited by an American-led "effort to make up for the omission at Ann Arbor" (Rutty 1995: 358–359).

After his retirement, Defries remained as director emeritus and consultant for Connaught, actively supporting the efforts of his successor, J. Kenneth W. Ferguson (1907–) to expand production of the Salk vaccine and develop the first trivalent Sabin oral polio vaccine. Defries also worked closely with his successor at the school, A. J. Rhodes, who faced perhaps the greater challenge of maintaining the public health mission of the school in the shadow of a rapidly expanding Faculty of Medicine. In recognition of Defries's enormous legacy, in 1965 the Canadian Public Health Association established the R. D. Defries Award to honor outstanding individual contributions to public health. Defries received many other honors, including the Companion of the Order of Canada in 1970. Defries's personal life was inseparable from his work. He never married, and his spare moments were devoted to his passion for flowers and photography, and to helping others, particularly employees. Defries was the first official historian of Connaught, and he spent much of his retirement preparing a history of the laboratories (Defries 1968).

Robert D. Defries, Canada's Mr. Public Health, died quietly at his home on October 25, 1975, leaving an indelible impact on Canadian public health through his writings and the institution he largely created, Connaught Laboratories. Connaught was sold by the University of Toronto in 1972 and has since been transformed into the North American component of the world's largest fully integrated biologicals company, Pasteur Mérieux-Connaught of Lyons, France. Defries's medical missionary spirit still resides in Connaught's public health research and its continuing efforts to protect the public from the tragedy of infectious disease.

BIBLIOGRAPHY

Information pertaining to Defries is held in the Archives of Connaught Laboratories Ltd., 1755 Steeles Avenue West, North York, Ontario. The collection contains numerous medical journal and newspaper articles, correspondence and reprints of Defries's articles, and a personal papers file. More information can be found in various accessions in Connaught's Archives (especially 83–005). Also important are Defries's Connaught and School of Hygiene *Annual Reports of the Director* (formally published after 1948). The Archives of the University of Toronto and the National Archives of Canada in Ottawa (RG29) also contain some of Defries's correspondence. Dr. J. Kenneth W. Ferguson, Defries's successor as director of Connaught (1955–1972), was another important source of information on Defries's life. I thank Dr. Ferguson for his kind assistance. Very little secondary material has been written on the life and work of Defries. The most significant sources are by Bator (1990, 1995) and Rutty (1995). Craig Defries has recently written a substantial essay on the early life and work of his great uncle, which remains unpublished.

Writings by Robert Davies Defries

The Federal and Provincial Health Services in Canada. Edited by Robert D. Defries. Toronto, Canadian Public Health Association, 1940, 1956, 1962.
"The Connaught Medical Research Laboratories, 1914–1948." *Canadian Journal of Public Health* 39 (August 1948): 330–344.
"The Connaught Medical Research Laboratories during the Second World War, 1939–1945." *Canadian Journal of Public Health* 40 (August 1949): 348–360.
"Postgraduate Teaching in Public Health in the University of Toronto, 1913–1955." *Canadian Journal of Public Health* 48 (July 1957): 285–294.
The First Forty Years, 1914–1955: Connaught Medical Research Laboratories, University of Toronto. Toronto: University of Toronto Press, 1968.

Writings about Robert Davies Defries and Related Topics

Bator, Paul A., with Andrew J. Rhodes. *Within Reach of Everyone: A History of the University of Toronto School of Hygiene and the Connaught Laboratories*. Vol. 1, *1927–1955*. Ottawa: Canadian Public Health Association, 1990.
Bator, Paul A. *Within Reach of Everyone*. Vol. 2: *A History of the University of Toronto School of Hygiene and Connaught Laboratories Limited, 1955–1975, with an Update to the 1990s*. Ottawa: Canadian Public Health Association, 1995.
Bliss, Michael. *The Discovery of Insulin*. Toronto: McClelland and Stewart, 1982.
Editorial. "Dr. R. D. Defries Retires." *Canadian Medical Association Journal*, August 15, 1955, pp. 300–301.
Hare, Ronald. *The Birth of Penicillin and the Disarming of Microbes*. London: George Allen and Unwin Ltd., 1970.
Kapp, Richard W. "Charles H. Best, the Canadian Red Cross Society, and Canada's

First National Blood Donation Program.'' *Canadian Bulletin of Medical History* 12 (1995): 27–46.

Rutty, Christopher J. '' 'Do Something! . . . Do Anything!' Poliomyelitis in Canada, 1927–1962.'' Ph.D. dissertation, University of Toronto, 1995.

Wilson, R. J., and A. M. Fisher. ''Obituary: Robert Davies Defries.'' *Canadian Journal of Public Health* 66 (November–December 1975): 510–512.

Christopher J. Rutty

PAUL HENRY DE KRUIF
(1890–1971)

Paul Henry de Kruif, medical writer and microbiologist, was born in Zeeland, Michigan, the son of Dutch immigrants, Hendrik and Hendrika J. de Kruif (the family name rhymes with "life"). His father was a farm implement dealer in Zeeland. He received a B.A. from the University of Michigan in 1912 and a Ph.D. in bacteriology in 1916. His thesis, prepared under the guidance of Frederick G. Novy, was entitled "Primary Toxicity of Normal Serum."

De Kruif served as a private in the U.S. Army with General John J. Pershing's expedition in 1916 to retaliate against the raids of Pancho Villa from Mexico into U.S. territory in the Southwest. He then joined the Sanitary Corps of the U.S. Army and went to France when the United States entered World War I. In his work for the army, he had contacts at the Pasteur Institute, and during the course of the war he met many eminent European bacteriologists. De Kruif's war work involved the immunological study of *Clostridium perfringens (Bacillus welchii)*, the microbe responsible for gas gangrene, a major problem in the bloody trench fighting in the Great War. The goal of this work was to develop an antitoxin to prevent the devastating effects of this infection, which often resulted in limb amputations.

After the war, de Kruif returned to Novy's department in Ann Arbor, where he was assistant professor of bacteriology. His work with Novy on studies on the mechanisms of anaphylaxis was published as a series of seven papers in the *Journal of Infectious Disease* in 1917. They identified a substance they called anaphylatoxin, now known as components C_{5a} and C_{3a} of the complement system. They had found an alternative pathway of complement activation. Even though his work in Michigan was going well, in the fall of 1920 de Kruif moved to the Rockefeller Institute in New York to join the laboratory of Simon Flexner as an assistant in bacteriology. This move was partly motivated by the breakup of de Kruif's marriage to Mary de Kruif and partly by his attraction to the elegant and famous laboratories of the Rockefeller Institute. In Flexner's group he joined a newly conceived research program on laboratory epidemiology of respiratory infections in rabbits.

De Kruif's research at the Rockefeller Institute focused on the variations in pathogenicity among strains of *Streptococcus* of rabbit septicemia. He analyzed the changes in virulence in this organism and observed that the colony morphologies on agar plates (smooth and rough) correlated with the pathogenicity in animals. He also showed that a "pure" culture of virulent organisms could give rise to avirulent variants. This phenomenon, in which a homogeneous culture gave rise to two types of colonies, was called "microbic dissociation" (i.e., the single type dissociated into two types). De Kruif's interpretation was that these variants were mutations, analogous to those observed in plants by Hugo DeVries. Others, however, interpreted dissociation in terms of bacterial life cycles (the cyclogeny theory). De Kruif's experiments were the first to explain this phenomenon in the framework of genetic mutations in bacteria, and he was among the first to recognize that attention must be given to individual organisms within the bacterial culture rather than to the culture as a whole. This work was published in a series of four papers in the *Journal of Experimental Medicine* and one with John H. Northrop in the *Journal of General Physiology.*

While in New York, de Kruif made the acquaintance of several literary figures including H. L. Mencken, Clarence Day, and Norman Hapgood. These friends encouraged him to try his hand at writing on medical and scientific topics for a popular audience. His first opportunity came in the form of an invitation from Harold Stearns who was editing a book for Harcourt, Brace and Co. aimed at poking fun at America's cultural pretensions. Other contributors included Mencken, Lewis Mumford, Ring Lardner, and Van Wyck Brooks. De Kruif was asked to write a chapter on American medicine. This he did, but he asked that it be published anonymously, because he feared the reaction of his colleagues at the Rockefeller Institute. In this short essay, de Kruif took medicine to task for its claims of scientific authority while ignoring the basic notions of modern science. Two themes that de Kruif used in much of his later writing first appeared in this essay: the tension between science and medicine, and the military metaphor for medicine and science. This article is sprinkled with references to "soldiers of health," "the armamentarium of modern science," and "battalions of hygienists." While chiding his medical colleagues for their self-proclaimed image as "men of science," he described "science" as "concerned with the quantitative relationship of the factors governing natural phenomena. No favourites are to be played among these factors." To illustrate his claim that medicine is not a science in the modern sense, de Kruif decried the lack of controls in medical research. This criticism, in almost the same form, would later appear in *Arrowsmith*: the medical researcher failed to "divide his cases of pneumonia into two groups of equal size, to administer his serum to group A and to leave group B untreated. He almost invariably has a *parti-pris* that the serum will work and he reflects with horror that if he withholds his remedy from group B, some members of this group will die, who might otherwise be saved. So he injects his serum into all of his patients (A and B)."

This essay brought de Kruif to the attention of Glenn Frank, then the editor of *Century Magazine*, who asked de Kruif to write a set of essays on medicine, which were later published together under the title *Our Medicine Men*. Simon Flexner, de Kruif's chief at the Rockefeller Institute, interpreted these articles as a veiled attack on the institute, as well as an embarrassment to him. In the fall of 1922 de Kruif resigned his position at the Rockefeller Institute and left laboratory science to become a full-time writer.

Morris Fishbein, the associate editor of the *Journal of the American Medical Association*, introduced de Kruif to Sinclair Lewis in late 1922 while de Kruif was in Chicago researching material for his *Century Magazine* pieces. De Kruif and Lewis took a quick liking to each other and agreed to collaborate on a novel about American medicine. De Kruif would provide the scientific material and character sketches based on physicians and scientists he knew, and Lewis would supply the plot and dialogue. They spent two months sailing in the Caribbean from port to port discussing the book, working on scenes, with de Kruif teaching Lewis about microbiology, and Lewis trying to construct characters and plots for the book that would become *Arrowsmith*. By all accounts, this offshore locus allowed for much drinking, even during the time of U.S. prohibition. Their contract with Harcourt, Brace and Co. apparently stipulated that Lewis and de Kruif would share authorship and that de Kruif would receive one-fourth of the royalties from the book. This literary collaboration became something of an event in itself, described at length in de Kruif's autobiography, in Mark Schorer's biography of Lewis, and in various introductions to editions of *Arrowsmith* (e.g., "How *Arrowsmith* Was Written" by Barbara Grace Spayd). In 1925 when the book was published, however, Lewis objected to recognizing de Kruif's role with the suggested phrase "in collaboration with Paul H. de Kruif" and insisted instead on sole authorship with a paragraph acknowledging de Kruif's "help." In spite of this lost recognition, de Kruif did receive the agreed-upon royalties from this book.

De Kruif built on the narrative style he was developing with Lewis, and in 1926 he published a collection of heroic accounts of famous microbiologists: *Microbe Hunters*. This book, critically acclaimed and a huge commercial success, has been in print for almost seventy-five years, has been translated into at least eighteen languages, and has been cited for its major influence on popular perceptions of microbiology. Although his writings were apparently carefully researched, de Kruif's embellishments and exaggerations render them frankly hagiographic. One of his subjects, Ronald Ross, still alive when the book appeared, was so incensed at de Kruif's portrayal of him and his work that he sued de Kruif and managed to prevent publication of the offending chapter in the version sold in the United Kingdom. De Kruif was convinced of the power of science to solve health problems, and of the message of public health that militant attacks on germs would conquer infectious diseases. He wrote with the fervor of a talented and enthusiastic true believer.

The phenomenal success of *Microbe Hunters* won de Kruif a platform from which to carry on his crusades for health. He became a staff writer on medical subjects for *Country Gentleman* and the *Ladies' Home Journal*, published by the Curtis Publishing Co., while he poured forth a stream of books on important health issues of the day. Nutrition and agriculture were featured next in *Hunger Fighters* (1928), followed by ten more titles dealing with such diverse topics as the health effects of poverty, hormones, syphilis, prepaid health care plans, and mental illness. In most of his writings, de Kruif's style and approach closely followed that used to great effect in *Microbe Hunters*: narrative essays on heroic feats involving men of science, locked in mortal combat against ignorance and disease. This style was easily adapted to magazine articles, and de Kruif had a long career as a writer of many short pieces on medicine for the *Reader's Digest*.

De Kruif was widely respected for his ability to communicate the excitement of science along with the essential scientific and medical facts. His solid background in medical research, his broad enthusiasms, and his careful study of his subject matter uniquely informed his articles. His military and playing-field metaphors could be counted on to elicit positive responses from the American readers of his time.

As a national spokesman for the exciting advances in modern medicine, de Kruif was enlisted by Franklin Roosevelt to help in the war on poliomyelitis. In 1934 de Kruif was appointed secretary to the Commission for Infantile Paralysis, which included such captains of American industry as Edsel Ford, Jeremiah Milbank, and James Couzens. On this committee, he was an effective voice in promoting funding for basic research on polio prevention. De Kruif convinced the commission to direct most of its funds to medical research under the guidance of himself and a board of medical advisers. De Kruif used his magazine articles to advocate the cause of the battle against polio and to support the work of the commission. A few years later, this commission was reconstituted as the National Infantile Paralysis Foundation, a model for public medical action and philanthropy.

De Kruif's final book, *The Sweeping Wind*, was his autobiographical memoir written in 1962 on the occasion of the death of his second wife, Rhea Barbain de Kruif. Although not deeply introspective, this autobiography shows de Kruif as aware of his personal flaws, drinking and infidelity, while holding fast to his social and scientific enthusiasms. His flair for a good story, his unshakable faith in scientific progress for human welfare, and his robust enjoyment of life are all hallmarks of his journalistic style. As an advocate for medical research and the advances in medicine that follow, Paul de Kruif reached several generations of Americans and significantly shaped perceptions of science, medicine, and health.

BIBLIOGRAPHY

The most extensive sources for information about Paul de Kruif are his autobiography, *The Sweeping Wind* (1962), Mark Schorer's account of de Kruif's relations with Sinclair Lewis, in *Sinclair Lewis* (1961), and Ben Hibbs's short book on de Kruif as seen by his editor, *Two Men on a Job* (1938). Brief biographical articles, none with references to sources, include those by Kunitz (1942), Bradley (1943), Maizel (1946, 1947), and Bendiner (1979). His scientific papers extend from his Ph.D. dissertation in 1916 until his departure from the Rockefeller Institute in 1922. His papers are held in the Netherlands Museum, Holland, Michigan, by the Holland Historical Trust, Holland, Michigan.

Writings by Paul Henry de Kruif

"Dissociation of Microbic Species. I. Coexistence of Individuals of Different Degrees of Virulence in Cultures of the Bacillus of Rabbit Septicemia." *J. Exptl. Med.* 33 (1921): 773–789.

"Medicine." In H. E. Stearns, ed., *Civilization in the United States: An Inquiry by Thirty Americans*, pp. 443–456. New York: Harcourt, Brace and Co., 1922.

Our Medicine Men. New York: Harcourt, Brace and Co., 1922.

Microbe Hunters. New York: Harcourt, Brace and Co., 1926.

Hunger Fighters. New York: Harcourt, Brace and Co., 1928.

Seven Iron Men. New York: Harcourt, Brace and Co., 1928.

Men against Death. New York: Harcourt, Brace and Co., 1932.

The Sweeping Wind. New York: Harcourt, Brace and Co., 1962.

Writings about Paul Henry de Kruif and Related Issues

Bendiner, E. De Kruif. "From Practitioner to Chronicler of Science." *Hospital Practice* 31 (1979): 35, 39–41, 45–46, 51–52, 57.

Bradley, J. "Paul De Kruif: Guerrilla Fighter against Death." *Knickerbocker Weekly* (New York), August 23, 1943, pp. 20–25.

Chernin, E. "Paul de Kruif's Microbe Hunters and an Outraged Ronald Ross." *Reviews of Infectious Diseases* 10 (1988): 661–667.

Hibbs, B. *Two Men on a Job.* Philadelphia: Curtis, 1938.

Kunitz, S. J. "Paul De Kruif." In *Twentieth Century Authors*, pp. 363–364. New York: H. W. Wilson, 1942.

Lewis, S. *Arrowsmith.* New York: Harcourt, Brace and Co., 1925.

Maizel, A. Q. "Fighter for the Right to Live. I." *Reader's Digest* 49 (1946): 91–96.

———. "Fighter for the Right to Live. II." *Reader's Digest* 50 (1947): 43–49.

Schorer, M. *Sinclair Lewis: An American Life.* New York: McGraw-Hill, 1961.

Spayd, B. G. "How Arrowsmith Was Written." Preface to *Arrowsmith* by Sinclair Lewis. New York: Harcourt, Brace and Co., 1945.

Summers, W. C. "On the Origins of the Science in *Arrowsmith*: Paul de Kruif, Felix d'Herelle and Phage." *Journal of the History of Medicine and Allied Sciences* 46 (1991): 315–332.

William C. Summers

ROBERT LATOU DICKINSON
(1861–1950)

Robert Latou Dickinson presents an interesting example of a person whose major accomplishments came after his retirement from the private practice of medicine. Dickinson was born in Jersey City, on February 21, 1861, to Horace and Jeannette (Latou) Dickinson. His father was a hat manufacturer. The family home was in Brooklyn, New York, where he grew up and spent most of his life. After attending the Brooklyn Polytechnic Institute, he went on to study medicine in Switzerland and Germany for four years, after which he returned to the United States, and received a doctor of medicine degree in 1882 from the Long Island College Hospital (later Long Island College of Medicine). He interned at Williamsburg Hospital and Long Island College Hospital. Although he started his practice of medicine as a staff member in the chest department dispensary of Long Island College Hospital in 1883, he became affiliated with the obstetrics and gynecology department in 1884 and from 1886 to 1918 was a member of its obstetrics-gynecology faculty. He was also on the staff of King's County Hospital and the Methodist Episcopal Hospital, both in Brooklyn, as well as Brooklyn Hospital, during much of this period.

An innovative specialist in obstetrics and gynecology, Dickinson introduced several new surgical procedures, including the use of electric cauterization in the treatment of cervicitis, and he was among the first to use aseptic ligatures for tying the umbilical cord. He also gained widespread prominence during this part of his career for his innovative teaching methods for medical students—particularly for his use of rubber models, as well as his own sculpted models to teach female anatomy and fetal growth from fertilization to birth. During World War I, he went to Washington, where he was appointed in 1917 as assistant chief of the medical section of the National Council of Defense with the rank of lieutenant colonel. During 1918–1919, he served as medical adviser to the general staff, followed by missions to China in 1919 and to the Near East (1926) for the U.S. Public Health Service.

In his sixtieth year, Dickinson retired from practice to devote himself to causes, particularly birth control and sex education, and to the publication of his studies, the data for which he had gathered during his practice. In the process, he moved from a closeted researcher of human sexuality to its dominant medical figure. In 1923, he founded the Committee on Maternal Health (after 1930 known as the National Committee on Maternal Health), which began compiling data on contraception. He tried to persuade Margaret Sanger to allow physicians to have more control in her New York clinic, but she did not take his advice; nevertheless, he remained one of her major supporters.

Dickinson broke new ground in the medical profession in 1920 with his presidential address to the American Gynecological Society in which he urged his fellow physicians to do more work in the fields of contraception, infertility, artificial impregnation, and voluntary sterilization. In 1939 he became senior vice president of the Planned Parenthood Federation of America and the senior consultant of the Margaret Sanger Research Bureau. He was also active in the euthanasia movement, serving as president of the society from 1946 until his death.

Probably his most significant contributions were to the study of female sexuality, and although he had written scholarly articles on some of his data during the course of his active medical career, most of his data were published late in his life. As a young physician, Dickinson had been dissatisfied with the inadequacy of the illustrations in medical books, and after some self-training in illustration, he did the drawings for and coedited a popular textbook on obstetrics (Cameron, Davis, Norris, and Dickinson 1895).

Dickinson also applied his artistic ability to his patients' problems. During the years of his most active gynecological practice, 1890–1920, he would not see patients until they had filled out a four-page questionnaire that accounted for general and family history. As he examined the patient, he also made at least five drawings: one each of the uterus, cervix, and vulva, and two of the pelvic difficulty for which the woman had sought his assistance. The maximum number of drawings for any one patient was sixty-one. Later, as photography improved, he supplemented the drawings with photographs. His standard practice was to read the patient's answers to the questionnaire before he examined her and then use the answers as a basis to probe deeper. He quickly found that his patients often confided in him information about sexual problems, which he recorded and treated, if possible.

By the time of his retirement, Dickinson had compiled data on more than 5,000 cases, which he turned over to the Committee on Maternal Health, which had agreed to help him publish. Lura Beam, a writer with a background in education and applied psychology, made a preliminary review of the data, and two ground-breaking books were published: one consisting of data based on four thousand married women (Dickinson and Beam 1931) and the other of twelve hundred single women (Dickinson and Beam 1934).

One of the advantages of Dickinson's data was that he often saw his patients at different points in their lives and could plot changes in their attitudes on sexual issues. For example, he illustrated with twenty cases how "passion and frigidity" could appear and disappear. At age thirty-four, one of his patients became disgusted with coitus, but her husband did not. Later the husband lost interest, but after six years without an orgasm, the woman again became orgasmic, and the husband and wife found it difficult to remain apart.

Data from Dickinson's studies included information on frequency of intercourse, which was usually two to three times a week in his married sample. Some 11 percent, however, had intercourse once a year or less. He had information on length of intromission before ejaculation and on the attitudes of brides. Dickinson also collected data on more treatment-oriented issues, such as "frigidity," dyspareunia (pain during intercourse), minor menstrual disturbances, sexually transmitted diseases, and fertility, as well as on such psychological issues as anxiety and fear. One in twelve of his patients in the married sample had a venereal disease, usually gonorrhea, emphasizing just how widespread the disease was among his upper-middle-class patients.

In comparing single women with married women, Dickinson found that relatively more wives than single women reported masturbating. Twenty-eight of the sample of single women had been involved in same-sex relations, but he found no evidence of "maleness of feelings" (i.e., lesbians were believed to have masculine qualities) in his subjects, some of whom he examined in the period before 1900. He also reported that seventeen of those who had lesbian experiences later married and had ordinary fertility.

Among his other major publications in human sexuality were a guide to contraception (1931), a birth atlas (1940), and an illustrated study of sex anatomy (1949). Along with W. F. Robie and LeMon Clark, Dickinson was responsible for the introduction of the electrical vibrator, or massager, into American gynecological practice. This device produced intense erotic stimulation, and even orgasm, in some women who previously had been anorgasmic. Dickinson and his collaborators theorized that once a woman had achieved orgasm, even with a vibrator applied to her genitals, she was more likely to proceed to orgasm during coitus or through digital masturbation.

Dickinson married Sara Truslow on May 7, 1890. The couple had three daughters, two of whom, Dorothy (Mrs. George B. Barbour) and Jean (Mrs. T. S. Potter), survived him. He died November 20, 1950, in Amherst, Massachusetts.

BIBLIOGRAPHY

Writings by Robert Latou Dickinson

(with J. C. Cameron, E. P. Davis, and R. C. Norris). *American Text Book of Obstetrics.* Philadelphia: Saunders, 1895.
Control of Conception. Baltimore: Williams and Wilkins, 1931.
(with L. Beam). *A Thousand Marriages.* Baltimore: Williams and Wilkins, 1931.
(with L. Beam). *The Single Woman.* Baltimore: Williams and Wilkins, 1934.
Birth Atlas. New York: Maternity Center Associates, 1940.
Human Sex Anatomy. Baltimore: Williams and Wilkins, 1949.

Writings about Robert Latou Dickinson and Related Topics

Bullough, V. L. *Science in the Bedroom: A History of Sex Research.* New York: Basic Books, 1994.

Current Biography. New York: C. W. Wilson, 1950.
Dictionary of American Biography, Supplement 4. New York: Scribner, 1945–1950.
National Cyclopedia of American Biography. New York: J. T. White, 1898–1981.
New York Times, November 30, 1950.
Who Was Who in America. Vol. 3. Chicago: Marquis, 1960.

Vern L. Bullough

LAVINIA LLOYD DOCK
(1858–1956)

Lavinia Lloyd Dock, nurse, reformer, and author, entered nursing in 1884. She exerted a profound influence on health care until her death seventy-two years later. Described in one obituary as a "catalytic agent," Dock helped to shape public health nursing, nursing education, and several American and international nursing organizations (*Nursing Outlook* 1956: 298). Her books, articles, and columns also influenced several generations of nurses. Dock's concern for health and well-being led her to broaden her interests and work for such causes as international peace and women's suffrage.

Dock was born on February 26, 1858, in Harrisburg, Pennsylvania's capital. Her family was civic minded and somewhat prominent in this riverside city. One grandmother was a Quaker, a member of a religious group well known for its interest in humanitarian causes. Both grandfathers were active in local affairs. One helped found Harrisburg State Hospital, and the other served as a municipal judge. Dock's parents, Gilliard and Lavinia Lloyd Bombaugh Dock, raised their six children in middle-class comfort and in a fairly liberal environment. Young Lavinia, the second child, received, what for the time, was an extensive education in a Harrisburg girls' academy. After her mother's death in 1876, she helped raise her younger siblings.

According to Dock, her interest in nursing stemmed from an article she read in the *Century* in 1882. This article, "A New Profession for Women," discussed the need for trained nurses in New York City's slums and praised the new nurses' training program at Bellevue Hospital. Dock was intrigued. It took her two years to convince her father that nursing was a suitable occupation for a respectable young woman. In 1884 she finally entered Bellevue, and she graduated two years later.

Dock engaged in a variety of pursuits in the first few years after completing her education. In 1886 she worked as a visiting nurse for the United Workers of Norwich, Connecticut. During 1888 and 1889 she undertook disaster nursing, first at a Jacksonville, Florida, hospital during a yellow fever epidemic, then in Johnstown, Pennsylvania, in the aftermath of the famous flood.

Later in 1889 Dock joined her former teacher, mentor, and lifelong friend Isabel Hampton at Johns Hopkins University Hospital, serving as Hampton's assistant superintendent. In this capacity she supervised the nurses' training school. Here Dock also found another friend in her student Adelaide Nutting. Frustrated with the exploitation of nurses, these three women collaborated on key approaches to the professionalization of nursing, including the establishment of the collegiate program at Columbia University, the *American Journal of Nursing (AJN)*, and several professional organizations. While she clearly envisioned the *AJN* as a vehicle through which the profession could "hear our members speak," Dock also relished using the pages of her column, the "Foreign Department," as a vehicle for her own strong opinions (Dock 1901–1922: 637).

While at Hopkins, Dock wrote her first book, the drug manual *Materia Medica for Nurses* (1890). Her reasons for writing the book were twofold. Turn-of-the-century nurses lacked an adequate manual, and patients often became nauseated by the drugs prescribed for them. *Materia Medica* addressed both problems: it provided nurses with both reliable information and recipes that made drugs more palatable. The book proved to be a success. First published in 1890, it sold over 150,000 copies—6,000 a year at its peak. (James 1985: 26; Marshall 1984: 6–7). It became the standard text for at least one generation of American nurses (James 1985: viii).

In 1893 Dock relocated to Chicago to become superintendent of the Illinois Training School. During her two years in the Windy City, she helped organize the American Society of Superintendents of Training Schools (ASSTS), a forerunner of the National League for Nursing. From 1896 to 1901 she served as the organization's secretary. Dock saw the society as a vehicle for separating medicine from nursing, an organization through which nurses could set standards and control their own affairs (James 1985: ix–xii). Dock decried the subordination of nurses to doctors. In a 1906 *AJN* column she even referred to physicians who meddled in nursing affairs as "political bosses" (Dock 1901–1922: 980; James 1985: 55). Dock always insisted that nurses' first obligations were to patients, not doctors. She urged nurses to stop being a "silent sister-hood" and "a flock of sheep" (Dock 1901–1922: 980; James 1985: 55). For Dock, voluntary association was the perfect antidote to the "pointless obedience" practiced by many nurses (James 1985: 44, 55–56).

Dock urged the ASSTS to promote nursing's autonomy in two ways. First, she wanted a registration system in which nurses sat for an examination and were then licensed by the state. Standards for educational programs and the licensing exam would be developed by a state examining board composed of nurses (Dock 1901–1922: 466–467). Dock argued that a registration system also protected the public by allowing consumers to distinguish between a fully trained, licensed nurse and an amateur (Dock 1901–1922: 872). Dock also insisted on the need for nurses to manage their own educational programs. In a 1901 letter to the *American Journal of Nursing*, she argued, "Physicians, be they men or women, cannot teach nursing, any more than nurses can teach medicine. Medicine and nursing are not the same" (Dock 1901–1922: 64). Through both the ASSTS and her extensive writings, she called for a number of improvements. She supported a three-year graded curriculum, an eight-hour day for nursing students, and more classroom instruction (Dock 1901–1922: 320, 468; James 1985: 51–52). Concerned about the ability of small and specialty schools to provide a quality education, Dock advised hospital affiliation and student rotation through a prescribed course of studies (Dock 1901–1922: 709). She vehemently opposed the practice of sending out students as private duty nurses, a policy she referred to as "sweating" (James 1985: 24). Finally, Dock advocated postgraduate college education for nurses, particularly those interested in teaching, administration, or public health (James 1985: 11; Dock 1901–1922: 120).

During her two years in Chicago, Dock discovered that she was not suited temperamentally to administrative work and left the city in 1895. After spending a year in Harrisburg to arrange her deceased father's affairs, Dock returned to New York. Here she embarked on one of the defining experiences of her life. She joined Lillian Wald's Henry Street Settlement and labored as a public health nurse among working-class, immigrant families. Dock lived at the settlement for twenty years until her militancy over women's suffrage led to disagreements with the more moderate Wald (James 1985: x; Marshall 1984: 7). The camaraderie and independence of the settlement house, the intellectual stimulation, and the female-dominated environment appealed greatly to her. She counted these years as among the happiest of her life, once describing the Henry Street environment as "full, free, and untrammeled in its cooperative independence . . . the pleasantest type of family life—a family, to be sure composed only of women" (James 1985: 29).

Dock also enjoyed the autonomy and challenges of public health nursing. Henry Street nurses, under Wald's supervision, made the rounds of the New York City tenements, visiting families, treating illnesses, and dispensing advice. As Dock described it, each woman had relative independence, since patients themselves usually called the nurse rather than relying on a physician's referral. Dock also liked the opportunities available for utilizing a wide variety of skills. Besides treating patients, visiting nurses dealt with family concerns, much as social workers would do later in the century. They also taught hygiene, cooking, and home nursing classes (James 1985: 30–32). In 1902 Wald placed nurses in the New York City school system to treat simple cases and make home visits, an experiment Dock believed to be "eminently satisfactory" (Dock 1901–1922: 108–110). Dock saw public health nursing as an effective way to provide comprehensive health care for Americans of modest means. To this end she advocated a number of measures that have since been enacted: municipally supported visiting nurse agencies, licensed school nurses, and a formal postgraduate public health nursing curriculum (Dock 1901–1922: 109–110, 131, 391–392).

As a public health nurse, Dock saw so many cases of tuberculosis that she believed the disease was "practically endemic" among New York City's poor (Dock 1901: 631). With other Henry Street nurses, she developed effective techniques for managing tuberculosis cases: hospital admittance for the infected patient, disinfection of clothing and household furnishings, and fumigation of the home (Dock 1901–1922: 529). In 1903, she visited a sanitarium located in Pennsylvania's Mount Alto Park and was so impressed that she urged other states to establish similar facilities in their state forests (Dock 1901–1922: 188–191). Dock also promoted a number of measures to prevent the spread of tuberculosis. Believing unsanitary tenement conditions fostered the disease's spread, she recommended better housing construction, more diligent examination of factories, and the employment of nurses as housing inspectors (Dock 1901: 540–541, 631–634). Furthermore, she advocated that nurses trained in tuberculosis prevention and treatment teach public school courses on the disease (ASSTS 1909: 934–935).

Dock believed that venereal disease was as serious a threat to American health as tuberculosis, and, in 1905, she joined the American Society of Sanitary and Moral Prophylaxis (James 1985: xiv). As a society member and author, Dock argued the need for sex education, public discussion and dissemination of information, and free treatment for infected individuals (Dock 1901–1922: 189; James 1985: 33, 83). Concerned about congenital syphilis and the infection of unsuspecting spouses, she called for a public health program that investigated cases and notified persons who might unknowingly have contracted a disease (Dock 1901–1922: 658). Not content simply to treat the problem as a health care issue, Dock also decried the sexual double standard (James 1985: 60–61). In her book *Hygiene and Morality* (1910), Dock treated venereal disease as a moral problem and called for the elimination, rather than the regulation, of prostitution (James 1985: 68–76, 95–107, 130–131, 144–159).

At Henry Street, Dock, in her own words, "saw injustice and oppression" for the first time (James 1985: 24). These experiences led to her involvement in a wide variety of social causes. Dock supported shorter working hours, the enactment of minimum wage legislation and widows' pensions, and the abolition of child labor. She argued that such measures eradicated the poverty that contributed to tuberculosis and prostitution (Dock 1901–1922: 581). To promote these reforms Dock helped trade unionist Lenora Reilly organize garment workers and actually picketed during the New York City shirtwaist strike of 1909. While at Henry Street, Dock became a socialist and supported the Woman's Peace party (Dock 1901–1922: 665; Marshall 1984: 8–9). One of her most pervasive frustrations was her failure to interest more nurses in trade unionism, progressive reforms, and women's rights (Dock 1901–1922: 230, 925; James 1985: 899–900, 971–973).

Through her social reform work, Dock became an enthusiastic proponent of women's suffrage. In 1911 she wrote, "Efficacious care for popular health is impossible without women partaking in legislation" (Dock 1901–1922: 129). She deplored the ineffectiveness of voteless female reformers whom she believed "play one man [politicians] against another to gain our ends" (Dock 1901–1922: 574). She also linked the well-being of her own profession to suffrage, arguing that since nurses worked "out in the world" they "must stand on a level with men" (Dock 1901–1922: 47). During the 1910s, Dock was increasingly involved in the women's movement. She joined the National Woman's party in 1912 and participated in suffrage parades in New York City, Albany, and Washington, D.C. On June 27, 1917, Dock was one of six American women jailed in the infamous Occoquan Workhouse of Virginia for picketing the White House (Marshall 1984: 8–10). In 1923 Dock became one of the first American feminists to support the equal rights amendment (James 1985: xvi, 834).

During her years in New York City, Dock involved herself with a number of other nursing projects. She served as an unpaid lecturer for ten years in the nursing education program at Teachers College, Columbia University. She also helped found the Nurses Associated Alumnae (NAA), later the American Nurses Association (ANA), in 1896. Dock saw the NAA as a way for rank-and-file nurses to protect themselves and improve their position. Unlike other nursing leaders who wanted an exclusive organization composed of graduates from the best training schools, Dock preferred a broad-based, inclusive association (Dock 1901–1922: 470–471; Nurses Associated Alumnae 1900: 89–90). She wanted the NAA to take up issues of concern to the average nurse who struggled to make a living doing irregular, often poorly paid private duty work. In 1905, for example, Dock urged members to consider establishing reasonably priced boardinghouses that would provide comfortable lodging for residents and pay dividends to nurse-stockholders (Dock 1901–1922: 251–252). A year later, she advocated the creation of city-wide, private duty directories controlled by nurses, through which members could secure work and protect wages (Dock 1906: 13). Dock argued that although nurses were professionals, they were also workers and as such were entitled to band together for self-protection (James 1985: 971). She had little patience for physicians who badmouthed the NAA by calling it a union. She referred to these opponents as "reactionaries" (Dock 1901–1922: 458).

In 1899 Dock represented the United States at the founding meeting of the International Council of Nurses (ICN). Her service to the ICN was indispensable. She wrote the organization's constitution and bylaws and served as its unpaid secretary for the next twenty-two years (James 1985: xii; Marshall 1984: 8; Roberts 1956: 178). Through the ICN she formed lifelong friendships with prominent nurses from around the world, such as Great Britain's Ethel Bedford-Fenwick (Roberts 1956: 177). The ICN soon became one of Dock's favorite projects. She saw it as a radical, feminist organization with "progressive" views but also as a means through which nurses from all nations could find mutual support and solidarity (Dock 1901–1922: 684–685, 813–814. In 1901 she argued that an international federation was the best way "to make our united influence felt" (Dock 1901–1922: 444). Through the ICN, Dock called on members from Europe and the United States to promote nursing education, improve nurses' economic position, and work for health-related social reforms (Dock 1901–1922: 52, 114, 317–318, 996). Above all she urged nurses to follow "the principle laid down by Florence Nightingale" (the control of nursing by nurses) and use the ICN to exert their independence from medicine (James 1985: 23).

Dock's involvement in the *American Journal of Nursing* and other publications reflected her interest in internationalism. A stockholder and contributing editor of the *AJN*, Dock saw the "nursing press as the chief engine of nursing progress" (Dock 1901–1922: 293). From 1901 until 1922 she used the

"Foreign Department" to report on nursing and public health developments in Europe, Asia, Latin America, and Australia and New Zealand (James 1985: xi–xii; Marshall 1984: 8). As a staunch pacifist, Dock refused to report on World War I. In 1914 she announced her intention to "boycott" the war, fearing that covering it might be interpreted as "a tacit giving of moral support" (Dock 1901–1922: 47, 847).

In 1907, with Adelaide Nutting, Dock wrote the two-volume *History of Nursing*. Dock added two more volumes in 1912. In order to write the *History*, Dock traveled to Europe on many occasions to gather and translate important archival materials (James 1985: xii–xiii; Marshall 1984: 8). As one of her last professional projects, Dock collaborated on *The History of the Red Cross Nursing Service* (1922), which contained information on both European and American agencies (Marshall 1984: 6; Roberts 1956: 178).

In later life Dock became increasingly deaf. She retired in 1922 to the family farm in Fayetteville, Pennsylvania. Even in retirement Dock continued to write about nursing, revising the *History* and occasionally writing for the *AJN*. In 1947 the ICN honored her with a citation for distinguished service. The characteristically modest Dock attended the ceremony in Atlantic City but could not understand what the fuss was all about (*AJN* 1947: 442; Roberts 1956: 176). Nine years later she died of bronchopneumonia in Chambersburg Hospital. Even in death Dock proved generous to nursing. In her will she bequeathed half the royalties from the first two volumes of *A History of Nursing* to the ANA (*AJN* 1956: 1447).

BIBLIOGRAPHY

Some of the most useful writings on Lavinia Dock are those she penned herself. In addition to the monthly "Foreign Department" column, she contributed numerous articles to the *AJN*, as well as occasional letters to the editor. The *AJN* contains other pertinent material such as proceedings of the ASSTS and NAA meetings at which she was present. Other useful writings by Dock include *Short Papers on Nursing Subjects* (1900) and her venereal disease treatise, *Hygiene and Morality* (1910). These works, along with others, have been compiled by Janet Wilson James in *A Lavinia Dock Reader*. Valuable biographical articles include Alice Marshall's "Little Dock: Architect of Modern Nursing" (1984), Susan M. Posluny's "Feminist Friendship: Isabel Hampton Robb, Lavinia Lloyd Dock and Mary Adelaide Nutting" (1989), and Mary M. Roberts's obituary in the *AJN*, "Lavinia Lloyd Dock—Nurse, Feminist, Internationalist" (1956). The Library of Congress houses Dock's papers, including material dealing with the ICN, the Red Cross, Henry Street, and Dock's international correspondence. Other useful collections at the Library of Congress include the Mira Lloyd Dock Papers, the National American Woman Suffrage Association Records, and the National Woman's Party Records. The Dock Family Papers at the Pennsylvania State Archives and the Adelaide Nutting correspondence at Teachers College, Columbia University, have relevant materials as well.

Writings by Lavinia Lloyd Dock

Textbook of Materia Medica for Nurses. New York: G. P. Putnam's Sons, 1890.
"Foreign Department." *AJN* 1–20 (1901–1922).
"Extracts from the Report of the Tenement House Commission, New York, 1901." *AJN* 1 (May 1901): 538–541, (June 1901): 631–634.
"Central Directories and Sliding Scales." *AJN* 7 (October 1906): 10–13.
(with Adelaide Nutting). *A History of Nursing.* New York: G. P. Putnam's Sons, 1907.
"Report of the Seventeenth Annual Meeting of the American Society of Superintendents of Training Schools for Nurses." *AJN* 10 (1910): 758–792.
Hygiene and Morality. New York: G. P. Putnam's Sons, 1910.
A History of Nursing. Vols. 3–4. New York: G. P. Putnam's Sons, 1912.
The History of the Red Cross Nursing Service. New York: Macmillan, 1922.

Writings about Lavinia Lloyd Dock and Related Topics

James, Janet Wilson. *A Lavinia Dock Reader.* New York: Garland Publishing, 1985.
"Lavinia Lloyd Dock." *Nursing Outlook* 4 (May 1956): 298–299.
Marshall, Alice K. "Little Dock: Architect of Modern Nursing." *Pennsylvania Heritage* 10 (spring 1984): 5–11.
NAA. "Proceedings of the Twelfth Annual Convention of the Nurses' Associated Alumnae of the United States. Minneapolis, Minnesota. June 10–11, 1909." *AJN* 9 (1909): 877–991.
"News about Nursing." *AJN* 56 (November 1956): 1447–1470.
Posluny, Susan M. "Feminist Friendship: Isabel Hampton Robb, Lavinia Lloyd Dock, and Mary Adelaide Nutting." *Image: Journal of Nursing Scholarship* 21 (summer 1989): 64–67.
Roberts, Mary M. "Lavinia Lloyd Dock—Nurse, Feminist, Internationalist." *AJN* 56 (February 1956): 176–179.

Susan Rimby Leighow

ERIK HOMBURGER ERIKSON
(1902–1994)

Erik Homburger Erikson, born June 15, 1902, in Frankfurt-am-Main, Germany, psychoanalyst, writer, lecturer, scholar, and clinician, popularized and modernized analytic principles. Upon the occasion of Erikson's eighty-second birthday, the medical director of Austen Riggs Center in Stockbridge, Massachusetts, Daniel Schwartz, said, "Erikson began as a young artist. He became an analyst who helped all of us to see more clearly. In studies of dreams, of children's play, in the explication of the regularities in our sense of psychological space as influenced by our bodies and our cultures, he has helped us define crucial configurations" (Schlein 1987: xxvi).

Erikson's parents were Danish. They separated before his birth, however, and the details of his biological father's identity and the circumstances of his birth are mired in contradictions. Some sources say that Erikson was the result of an extramarital affair. Others cite his mother's first husband as his father. They differ, though, on the issue of whether he abandoned Erik's mother or simply died around the time of Erik's birth. In any event, Erikson never saw either of his alleged birth fathers.

When Erik was three years old, his mother married a German pediatrician, Theodore Homburger, and throughout Erik's childhood he used the name Erik Homburger. He grew up in comfortable surroundings in southern Germany. Theodore Homburger was Jewish. His mother's heritage has also been disputed, with some claiming it to be Lutheran and others claiming that she too was Jewish. Regardless of the truth, Erikson was rejected by both groups. His German schoolmates expressed anti-Semitic attitudes toward him; the local Jewish community did not accept him because of his Nordic features. Erikson completed high school in Karlsruhe and was expected to pursue a medical career. Instead, he meandered about the Continent after school, studied art in Munich, earning money by sketching children, and spent time in Florence. His sense of being rejected by those around him, and his decision to decline the projected medical career in favor of wandering about Europe, may have contributed to his ability later to depict and define that adolescent period.

At age twenty-five, in 1927, when Erikson was living by painting children's portraits, his lifelong friend Peter Blos asked him to come to Vienna. Blos was the director of a small, progressive school, actually run by two women, Dorothy Tiffany Burlingham and Eva Rosenfeld, who were closely associated with Freud's daughter Anna. Originally Blos simply asked Erikson to paint the portraits of Burlingham's four children, but then, as he was going on holiday, he asked Erikson to tutor for him at the school.

The school itself remains of interest and was unique. It had begun when Blos was hired to tutor Burlingham's four children. However, afraid that the tutoring served as an isolating experience, Burlingham expanded the teaching to encompass all of the children whose parents were in analysis or who were themselves in analysis. As such, the school was multinational and experimental. At the school, Erikson functioned as a tutor and supervisor for Burlingham's four children in Blos's absence while she was working with Sigmund Freud. After observing Erikson's work with the schoolchildren, both Burlingham and Anna Freud asked Erikson to consider becoming a child analyst, a field hitherto unknown to him.

As the first step toward this profession, Erikson had a training analysis with Anna Freud. She worked with him at the reduced fee of seven dollars per month and he received a fifty-minute session nearly every day. This analysis took over three years and was completed in 1933. During the sessions, Anna did some handiwork. After the birth of Erikson's first son, Kai, she knitted the infant a small blue sweater. The analysis process liberated Erikson from his fears and greatly expanded his self-awareness. It also allowed him entrance into Freud's inner circle.

Erikson married a Canadian woman, Joan Serson, an artist and a dancer, in 1930. They had two sons, Kai and Jon, and, in 1938, a daughter named Sue. In 1933 Erikson moved with his family to Copenhagen and in 1934 to the United States. On the boat from Europe to America, George F. Kennan, an American diplomat, taught him eight hundred words in English so that he arrived in the United States with the necessary linguistic skills to commence work. He settled in Boston and became the city's first child analyst. Upon becoming an American citizen, he changed his name to Erik Homburger Erikson.

As the first child analyst in Boston and a member of Freud's inner circle, he was accepted at Harvard Medical School and did research with the Harvard Psychological Clinic. While there, he made several key associations with anthropologists Margaret Mead, Gregory Bateson, and Ruth Benedict and psychologists Henry Murray and Kurt Lewin. In 1936, he became a full-time teacher and researcher at the Yale University Institute of Human Relations. Subsequently, in 1938, he visited a Sioux Indian Reservation in South Dakota with Scudder Mekeel, an anthropologist, and studied Sioux child-rearing practices. In 1939 he moved to the University of California, Berkeley, and spent the next ten years on the West Coast undertaking a number of significant projects. He became engaged in longitudinal study of childhood development, as well as working as a child and training analyst in San Francisco.

During the war he did analyses of Adolf Hitler's speeches and investigated the psychological facets of submarine life. He also took a trip with Alfred Kroeber to northern California to study Yurok Indians, whose childhood training emphasized a strenuous lifestyle. His observations of children at play, war veterans, and the two Indian cultures all contributed to his later theories.

In the early 1950s Erikson came to Austen Riggs Center, Stockbridge, Massachusetts, and worked with affluent children who had severe and persistent mental illness. Those patients often had been hospitalized for as much as a decade. At the same time he worked with Dr. Benjamin Spock biweekly in Pittsburgh treating poorer troubled children. In the 1960s, he again worked at Harvard, this time as professor of human development. He formally retired in 1970 and lived in both Marin County, California and Cape Cod, Massachusetts. In 1987, he moved to Cambridge, Massachusetts, to be part of the Erik Erikson Center, a division of Cambridge Hospital, a Harvard Medical School teaching hospital. He died on May 12, 1994, in Harwich, Massachusetts.

Erikson defined himself and his work as post-Freudian, as opposed to the terms *anti-Freudian* and *neo-Freudian*. In his theory of the ages of man, he celebrated nine stages: (1) Trust vs. Mistrust; (2) Autonomy vs. Shame and Doubt; (3) Initiative vs. Guilt; (4) Industry vs. Inferiority; (5) Group Identity vs. Alienation; (6) Individual Identity vs. Identity Confusion; (7) Intimacy vs. Isolation; (8) Generativity vs. Stagnation; and (9) Integrity vs. Despair. These nine stages provided many new insights into human psychological development. The culmination of each step required the integration of three issues: a somatic or constitutional contribution, often referred to as organic or biologic issues; the social matrix and context in which, through which, and by which the events occur within the person's social environment; and an identity or ego process, how the person views, adapts, and resolves the conflict.

As a result of these three convergent and interacting issues, there emerges at each stage a resolution that is important in and of itself and also as a building block toward the next stage. The solution of each step requires the ultimate balancing of the three qualities, so the best possible resolution becomes a series of critical answers. For example, as the infant struggles in the world for survival and comfort, his best solution to issues of trusting and not trusting results not only in a sense of trust but also a hopeful view of himself, his world, and his future. Therefore, (1) Trust vs. Mistrust leads to Hope (first year). (2) Autonomy vs. Shame and Doubt results in Will. Free will emerges in the feelings of self-control without the loss of self-esteem (second and third year). (3) Initiative vs. Guilt produces Purpose. Here, one constructs and moves toward a goal without the sense of defeated fantasies, guilt, or perceived looming retaliation and retribution (third to sixth year—the age of play). (4) Industry vs. Inferiority results in a sense and feeling of Competency—the joy and individual celebration of the person's skills, abilities, and intellect (six to twelve or thirteen years—puberty and school age). (5) Group Identity vs. Alienation produces a sense of Participation and Involvement in society and the world. The result here yields to feelings of loyalty and fidelity (early adolescence). (6) Individual Identity vs. Identity Confusion produces a sense of total integrated self with goals, identity, and directions (e.g. career; later adolescence to early twenties). (7) Intimacy vs.

Isolation leads to the flowering of Love. The person starts to move beyond self and into close, sharing, and committed relationships (young adulthood—middle to late twenties). (8) Generativity vs. Stagnation leads to a resolution that extends into another generation and the ability to care. (9) Ego Integrity vs. Despair is a stage in which one looks back with consolidation and pride and sets the stage for a sense of wisdom and fulfillment.

These stages dramatically advanced and expanded concepts of human growth and the developmental process. They offered a lifelong process of change, opportunity, maturity, and development. The stages themselves became a rich source of individual fulfillment, destiny, and hope. The coupling of hope and wisdom also demonstrates the full cycle and circle of life.

Erikson's major contributions use the nine stages as the basis of the other ideas and the paradigm on which he influenced mental health views. The stages helped to frame his biographies of Mahatma Gandhi and Martin Luther. In each Erikson emphasized the developmental challenge as the center of the story.

The influence of the nine stages on personality development remains Erikson's hallmark and landmark. He extended, popularized, and modernized the basic works of Freud. He moved the libido from sex, to power, to energy. He depicted the maturation sequence as lifelong and not limited to the first five years. His views of the interaction of biology, society, family, personality, and culture as the prime integrates of the personality remain the key and cornerstone of current concepts of the individual. He drew upon anthropology and sociology and wove them into the tapestry of psychodynamics.

BIBLIOGRAPHY

The work of Erikson is readily available. All of his previously unpublished works have been collected in a single volume by Stephen Schlein, *A Way of Looking at Things: Selected Papers from 1930 to 1980 Erik H. Erikson* (1987). This volume contains forty-seven papers and includes a complete bibliography of Erikson's work. Schlein has divided the book into eight subject sections: Psychoanalysis and Enlightenment; Configurations in Play and Dreams; War Memoranda; Cross-Cultural Observations: The Communal Environment; Thoughts on the Life Cycle; Reflections on Identity, Youth, and Young Adulthood; Portrait Sketches; and Configurations on Human Potential. Robert Coles's biography of Erikson, *Erik H. Erikson: The Growth of His Work* (1970) is the most accessible secondary work, although it lionizes Erikson. Richard Isadore Evans's *The Making of Psychology: Discussions with Creative Contributors* (1976) features a strong interview with Erikson, as well as an effective review of his stages of man and his biohistorical writings. Paul Roazen's *Erik H. Erikson: The Power and Limits of a Vision* (1976) provides a balanced view and biography of Erikson and cites the therapeutic usefulness of Erikson's approach in contrast to that of Freud. The author questions, however, many of Erikson's assumptions, particularly about women. Richard Stevens's *Erik Erikson: An Introduction* (1983) provides a basic, balanced conceptual framework of Erikson's work. He emphasizes the interplay of the somatic or constitutional contributions, the social matrix and context, and the identity or ego process in Erikson's theories. Finally, John W. Nichols, in "Ego Psychology: Erik Erikson" (1993) offers a brief but thorough review of Erikson's life and the contributions of his book *Childhood and Society.*

Writings by Erik Homburger Erikson

Childhood and Society. New York: Norton, 1950, 1963, 1985.
Young Man Luther: A Study in Psychoanalysis and History. New York: Norton, 1958.
Identity and the Life Cycle. New York: Norton, 1959, 1980.
Gandhi's Truth: On the Origins of Militant Nonviolence. New York: Norton, 1969.
Life History and the Historical Moment. New York: Norton, 1975.
Adulthood: Essays. New York: Norton, 1978.
(with Joan M. Erikson and Helen Q. Kivnick). *Vital Involvement in Old Age.* New York: Norton, 1986.
A Way of Looking at Things: Selected Papers from 1930 to 1980 Erik H. Erikson. Edited by Stephen Schlein. New York: Norton, 1987.

Writings about Erik Homburger Erikson and Related Topics

Coles, Robert. *Erik H. Erikson: The Growth of His Work.* Boston: Little, Brown, 1970.
Evans, Richard Isadore. *The Making of Psychology: Discussions with Creative Contributors.* New York: Alfred A. Knopf, 1976.
————. *Dialogue with Erik Erikson.* Westport, CT: Praeger, 1981.
Nichols, John W. "Ego Psychology: Erik Erikson." In *Survey of Social Science Psychology Series,* 2: 867–873. Edited by Frank N. Magill. Pasadena, CA: Salem Press, 1993.
Roazen, Paul. *Erik H. Erikson: The Power and Limits of a Vision.* New York: Free Press, 1976.
Schlein, Stephen. *A Way of Looking at Things: Selected Papers from 1930 to 1980 of Erik H. Erikson.* New York: Norton, 1987.
Smelser, Neil J., and Erik H. Erikson, eds. *Themes of Work and Love in Adulthood.* Cambridge, MA: Harvard University Press, 1980.
Stevens, Richard. *Erik Erikson: An Introduction.* New York: St. Martin's Press, 1983.

Stephen Soreff

ALICE CATHERINE EVANS
(1881–1975)

Alice Catherine Evans, microbiologist, played a crucial role in the recognition of the disease brucellosis as a public health problem and in the acceptance of the need to pasteurize milk. Evans was born on January 29, 1881, on a farm in Neath, Pennsylvania, the younger of two children of William Howell and Anne (Evans) Evans. Both of her parents were of Welsh descent, and her father was a surveyor and teacher, as well as a farmer. Evans received her secondary education at a private school, the Susquehanna Collegiate Institute, in Towanda, the county seat, where she played on an early women's basketball team at a time when the sport was still considered to be unladylike by many. After graduating from Susquehanna in 1901, Evans became an elementary school teacher. She later recalled that lack of financial means prevented her from attending college, and teaching was one of the few professions open to women at the time.

Evans's life was changed when she learned about a two-year course at the College of Agriculture of Cornell University given free of tuition to rural teachers. The purpose of this program was to train teachers in nature study so that they might foster in rural schoolchildren a love of nature and an appreciation for their country life. Using the money she had saved in four years of teaching to pay her subsistence expenses, Evans enrolled in this course in 1905. Students in the two-year course joined the regular agriculture students in classes for basic studies, and Evans found herself taking classes with a number of distinguished members of Cornell's faculty. Her interest in science, especially biology, was so stimulated by the nature study course that upon its completion, Evans decided to continue on at Cornell for a B.S. degree in agriculture. Her study was made possible with the aid of a scholarship and a College of Agriculture policy that waived tuition in order to train more leaders for the nation's agricultural industry.

Most of the major subjects available in the College of Agriculture were branches of applied science, such as horticulture and dairy science. These subjects did not interest Evans, so she chose to specialize in bacteriology, a science still in its infancy at this time, even in Europe and certainly in the United States. At the end of her senior year, William A. Stocking, Jr., professor of dairy bacteriology, encouraged Evans to apply for a scholarship to undertake graduate work at the College of Agriculture of the University of Wisconsin. This university scholarship, for a student specializing in agricultural chemistry or bacteriology, had never been held by a woman before Alice Evans became the recipient in 1909. At the end of the 1909–1910 academic year, Evans received her M.S. degree from Wisconsin. She was encouraged by Professor Elmer V.

McCollum, who taught the course in the chemistry of nutrition and was later to achieve fame as the discoverer of vitamin A, to continue her graduate studies for a Ph.D. degree. Evans declined the opportunity because her five years of higher education had been both a financial and a physical strain, and at the time a Ph.D. did not seem to be a prerequisite for success in a scientific career.

Another opportunity opened at this point for Evans to pursue scientific research. The Dairy Division of the Bureau of Animal Industry (BAI), U.S. Department of Agriculture (USDA), was expanding its research staff. Because of space limitations at the USDA laboratories in Washington, D.C., temporary arrangements were being made for research on a cooperative basis to be carried out at several agricultural experiment stations associated with state universities. The USDA provided the salaries of the investigators, and the state provided laboratory facilities and oversight of the research. Although the scientists hired under this program were federal civil service employees, they were selected by the professors at the experiment stations who were in charge of the projects. Professor Edwin G. Hastings, of the University of Wisconsin Department of Bacteriology, offered Evans the federal position as bacteriologist on the team that was searching for methods to improve the flavor of cheddar cheese. She accepted the offer, beginning work in Madison on July 1, 1910. Over the next three years, her name appeared as a coauthor on four scientific papers based on dairy science research.

In July 1913, Evans left Madison when she was called to Washington, D.C., to work in the newly completed laboratories of the Dairy Division. On her way east, she stopped at the University of Chicago to meet with faculty in the Department of Bacteriology. One of the faculty members was surprised to learn that she had a position with the Dairy Division; he had visited the Washington laboratories a short time before and was told that it did not want any women scientists. When Evans arrived in Washington, she found that there were a number of women scientists employed by the USDA, but only one had preceded her in the BAI, and she had remained only a year or two. Evans concluded that she had been hired essentially by accident. When cooperative arrangements were made with state experiment stations that allowed the faculty members in charge of research projects to select their own staff, it had apparently not occurred to some BAI members that a woman might be chosen for such a position. Having been employed for three years as a civil service employee, however, Evans could not be readily dismissed. She later stated, "According to hearsay, when the bad news broke at a meeting of BAI officials that a woman scientist was coming to join their staff, they were filled with consternation. In the words of a stenographer who was present, they almost fell off their chairs" (Evans 1965: 14).

Despite the inauspicious circumstances of her arrival, Evans found that the Dairy Division was a good place to work. Her immediate supervisors and coworkers did not seem to share the antagonism of higher officials in the bureau to women scientists. While serving as a junior collaborator on investigations already in progress, Evans was also assigned a problem of her own: a study of the bacteria that multiply within the cow's udder and are excreted in the milk.

Evans soon found her attention drawn to one particular species of bacteria, the causative organism of contagious abortion (Bang's disease) in cows, then designated *Bacillus abortus*. Previous reports on the isolation of this organism from apparently healthy animals had warned that there was a possibility that these bacteria might be hazardous to human health, and Evans decided to investigate this subject. She consulted with Adolph Eichorn, chief of the bureau's Division of Pathology, about whether he knew of any example of an apparently healthy animal excreting in its milk bacteria that were harmful to humans. Eichorn informed her that milk from apparently healthy goats could carry the organism that caused human undulant fever or Malta fever, *Micrococcus melitensis*.

Comparing the characteristics of *M. melitensis* and *B. abortus*, Evans found that they both behaved remarkably alike in the culture tests used at the time for the identification of bacteria. She also arranged for comparative tests of cultures of both organisms on pregnant guinea pigs and found that both caused three of four animals to abort. Her findings were reported at the 1917 meeting of the Society of American Bacteriologists and published the following year in the *Journal of Infectious Diseases*. Evans raised the question of whether this close relationship between the causal organisms of human undulant fever and bovine contagious abortion might mean that the bovine organism, if present in raw milk, could also cause disease in humans.

Her results were greeted with skepticism. It was argued that if the two organisms were really that similar, this fact would have been noted by earlier investigators. Presumably the fact that Evans was a woman, relatively unknown, and without a Ph.D. degree counted against her credibility. In addition, the apparent absence of undulant fever in this country argued against the idea that the two microorganisms were practically identical and thus both capable of causing the disease. It was later shown, however, that undulant fever is far more common in this country than had been realized. Milder forms of the disease resemble influenza, and severe cases were often mistaken for typhoid fever, malaria, or other diseases.

The dairy industry particularly objected to Evans's claims that raw milk might be the source of disease, and it resisted recommendations that all milk be pasteurized. The most vocal scientist opposing Evans's views was Theobald Smith,* the eminent bacteriologist who had been one of the first to isolate *B. abortus* from milk and had warned of its possible pathogenicity in humans. The opposition of a scientist as prominent as Smith served to support those who doubted Evans's work. She refused to back down on her convictions, however, and over the course of the 1920s her results were confirmed in several laboratories around the world. Another bacterial genus, *Brucella*, was introduced to include the bacteria then designated as *M. melitensis* and *B. abortus*, and the name *brucellosis* came into use to describe the disease caused by infection with this organism (replacing terms such as *undulant fever* and *Malta fever*). The work of Alice Evans played a pivotal role in the recognition of brucellosis as a significant public health problem and in the acceptance of the need to pasteurize milk.

In 1918, Evans became interested in contributing to the war effort, and she applied to the Hygienic Laboratory (forerunner of the National Institutes of Health and a part of the U.S. Public Health Service). She was accepted for an opening as a bacteriologist and joined a team working to improve the serum treatment for epidemic meningitis. The Hygienic Laboratory was then under the direction of George McCoy, who went out of his way to hire women scientists and encourage and support their work. Evans was one of the first of a group of exceptionally capable female scientists to be hired by McCoy, though she had been preceded by another bacteriologist, Ida Bengston, in 1916. In spite of the generally supportive environment created by McCoy, however, women scientists at the Hygienic Laboratory still tended to earn less and to be promoted less readily than their male counterparts.

At the Hygienic Laboratory, Evans continued her studies on brucellosis (as it was later called), and she contracted the disease herself in 1922. For the next twenty years, her health was impaired by the disease, with periods of incapacitation alternating with periods of partial or complete recovery. Since chronic brucellosis was not recognized at the time, Evans at first had to put up with diagnoses suggesting that she was suffering from imaginary or pretended ills. One can only speculate as to whether her gender was a factor in this situation as well. When she was undergoing surgery for another reason in 1928, however, doctors found lesions from which *Brucella* was cultivated, thus supporting the view that Evans was suffering from brucellosis. Her own later research helped to provide a better understanding of the chronic form of the disease.

Although her work on brucellosis was her most important research accomplishment, Evans also made contributions to the study of other infectious diseases, such as meningitis and streptococcal infections. She retired in 1945 from the National Institute (later Institutes) of Health, which had been created from the Hygienic Laboratory in 1930. Never one to back down on her beliefs, Evans protested in 1966, at the age of eighty-five, that the disclaimer of communist affiliation on the Medicare application violated her right of free speech. In January 1967, the Department of Justice conceded that this provision was unconstitutional, and it was never enforced.

Evans's accomplishments were recognized through various honors. In 1928, she was elected the first woman president of the Society of American Bacteriologists. She also received honorary doctoral degrees from the Women's Medical College (later the Medical College of Pennsylvania), Wilson College, and the University of Wisconsin. She died at the age of ninety-four on September 5, 1975, in her retirement home in Alexandria, Virginia, after suffering a stroke.

BIBLIOGRAPHY

The National Library of Medicine holds one box of manuscript and printed materials relating to Evans, including several letters, newspaper clippings, the script of a 1947 radio play about Evans's work on brucellosis, published articles by and about her, and the typescript of Evans's unpublished "Memoirs" (1965). There is also some Evans correspondence in the Cornell University Libraries and the Department of Bacteriology of the University of Wisconsin-Madison. The best published articles about Evans are by Elizabeth O'Hern: "Alice Evans, Pioneer Microbiologist" (1973) and "Alice Evans and the Brucellosis Story" (1977). A bibliography of Evans's publications appears in her "Memoirs," and a somewhat less complete version was published in *Annali Sclavo* (1977).

Writings by Alice Catherine Evans

"Further Studies on *Bacterium abortus* and Related Bacteria. II. A Comparison of *Bacterium abortus* with *Bacterium bronchisepticus* and with the Organism Which Causes Malta Fever." *Journal of Infectious Diseases* 22 (1918): 580–593.
"Publications by Alice C. Evans." *Annali Sclavo* 19 (1977): 7–11.

Writings about Alice Catherine Evans and Related Topics

Bums, Virginia. *Gentle Hunter: A Biography of Alice Evans, Bacteriologist.* Laingsburg, MI: Enterprise Press, 1993.
Harden, Victoria. *Inventing the NIH: Federal Biomedical Research Policy, 1887–1937.* Baltimore: Johns Hopkins University Press, 1986.
O'Hern, Elizabeth. "Alice Evans, Pioneer Microbiologist." *ASM News* 39 (1973): 573–578.
———. "Alice Evans and the Brucellosis Story." *Annali Sclavo* 19 (1977): 12–19.
———. "Evans, Alice Catherine." In Barbara Sicherman, Carol Hurd Green, Ilene Kantrov, and Harriette Walker, eds., *Notable American Women, the Modern Period: A Biographical Dictionary*, pp. 219–221. Cambridge, MA: Belknap Press of Harvard University Press, 1980.
Rossiter, Margaret. *Women Scientists in America: Struggles and Strategies to 1940.* Baltimore: Johns Hopkins University Press, 1982.

John L. Parascandola

CARL EMIL FENGER
(1814–1884)

The new medical ideas and insights developed above all in Paris during the first decades of the nineteenth century were gradually spread to the outskirts of Europe. From the late 1830s, Carl Emil Fenger, together with a few other doctors, introduced experimental physiology and medical statistics in Denmark. These ideas were characterized by quantitative methods, experiments, observations, and a reductionist approach, while rejecting personal experience and undocumented theories as the basis for medicine. Fenger maintained the superiority of these ideas with great emphasis and consequence, and this led to resistance among his colleagues representing vitalistic and humoralistic views. The study of his work can thus elucidate both old ideas and the new "scientific" medicine that has constituted the basis of medical thought and health care during the past 150 years. Fenger also took part in the democratization of Danish society. In 1848, Denmark was one of the first countries in Europe to get a constitution granting the right to vote to most men, and a parliament was established. The following year, Carl Emil Fenger was elected as a member of the first parliament. Thus Fenger participated actively in at least two fundamental processes of change in Danish society: (1) the introduction of new ideas in medical research, disease therapy, and the politics of health care and (2) the introduction of democracy for the majority of males.

Carl Emil Fenger graduated as a surgeon in 1835; between 1836 and 1839 he made a "study-journey" through Europe—a journey that at the time was common among academics who could afford it. He was appointed a professor in 1845 and chief of the Medical Department of Frederiks Hospital in 1852. He participated on a voluntary basis in organizing the medical and public health work during the cholera epidemic in 1853. In 1859 he left all his medical tasks and became a full-time politician as minister of finance. Later, between 1875 and 1883, he was finance and hospital mayor of Copenhagen. Thus, his career was characterized by several shifts from surgery to internal medicine, from medicine to politics, and from national to local politics, and he had several parallel sidelines such as membership in the Sundhedscollegiet, the highest authority on medical issues, directorship of the Royal Veterinary and Agricultural High School, membership on the board of the Institute for the Blind and the Public Health Board of the City of Copenhagen, and a number of other posts. Until he became a full-time politician, he had a large private practice besides his other activities. The importance of Fenger in a Danish context can be said to be his ability to pick up and reformulate ideas created by others and to convince many of his contemporaries of their relevance. He had an enormous working capacity and could present ideas in an instructive way. The majority of Fenger's publications were on medical statistics and demography, but he also published some articles on methodology and medicine and a few on specific medical topics. In his political life, as a physician and a scientist, and in his private life, Fenger demanded the truth and empirical proofs.

Complete devotion to what could be empirically proven and to accuracy in detail characterized all Fenger's activities, even when dealing with his own children. In remembering her father, Fenger's youngest daughter said: "we were always afraid of telling a story which was not completely true, since it rendered us a sharp reprimand" (Bock 1914: 99). He was sometimes accused of being more concerned with details than with the whole, not least in the budget discussions. Fenger possessed the classical Protestant virtues: diligence, thrift, and honesty. His father was a minister in a Copenhagen parish. Although religion does not seem to have played a prominent role in his life, Protestant morals obviously did.

For the Copenhagen middle class, the decades around the middle of the nineteenth century were characterized by a strong feeling of progress and change in many areas. The rationalism of the Enlightenment prevailed, and romanticism was fading out. Intellectually and culturally, this period has been labeled Denmark's golden age, with new currents in music, art, and literature. Outside Denmark, the period's most famous Danes were Hans Christian Andersen and the philosopher Søren Kierkegaard. The intellectual climate was lively. The city of Copenhagen was small, about 125,000 inhabitants in 1845; academic and cultural circles were closely connected. Urbanization was increasing, and industrialization was just beginning. Between 1845 and 1880, the population of Copenhagen increased by more than 60 percent; the city was characterized by overcrowding and slums, which became very visible during the cholera epidemic in 1853. New disease problems occurred due to poor housing and occupational hazards. The growth of a proletariat increased the need for publicly organized care for the ill. Health care for the poor had since the late eighteenth century been provided by the state and local authorities; charity played only a minor role.

Copenhagen had two big hospitals: Frederiks Hospital from 1757, with three hundred beds, where medical and surgical students got their clinical education, and the General Hospital, owned by the city. In 1863 the latter was replaced by the Municipal Hospital, with 844 beds. The aim of the hospitals and publicly employed doctors was to ensure a large and healthy population, to reduce the number of people entitled to poor relief, and to provide clinical education to the medical and surgical students and young doctors (Vallgårda, 1989: 95–105).

Fenger's contribution to the introduction of new ideas about research and methodology into medicine was achieved by both writing and teaching medical students. His pedagogical capacity was repeatedly praised. The young doctors in his department were encouraged to undertake research, and most of them did so. Fenger's pedagogical abilities can also be seen in his writings, where his style was both polemic and very instructive.

On his study-journey through Europe, Fenger visited Vienna, where therapeutic nihilism was the dominant medical philosophy of the time. In Zurich, he studied with Johan Lukas Schönlein, who had developed many different methods for the clinical examination of patients. In Paris, François Magendie, with his experimental physiology and study of the effect of drugs, and the medical statistician Jules Gavarret exerted a strong influence on his thinking. While in Paris, Fenger also studied political economy. He brought new ideas back to Denmark about scientific methods, medical statistics, pathological anatomy, and experimental physiology. Obviously he had a strong feeling of living in a period of transition, where all old ideas should be replaced, and one of his central tasks was to spread new ideas to Danish doctors.

In Denmark, humoralism, combined with romantic vitalism, still dominated medical thought. Humoralists considered knowledge of the patient's individual traits, constitution, and surroundings important for diagnosis, therapy, and prognosis. They believed that therapeutic measures designed to restore the balance of the body fluids were central to medical practice. The degree of interference, however, varied widely. A vital force was seen as the main feature distinguishing organic from inorganic materials; this vital force was also considered crucial in the healing of diseases.

Fenger opposed humoralism in terms of both theory and therapeutics, and he strongly criticized the "scientific" methods of his contemporaries. In his first article on the new medical theories and above all on medical statistics, or the "numerical method," as it was then called, published shortly after he had returned from Paris, Fenger described how a new disease could be identified, and he typically enough started by assuming that a doctor made findings when carrying out autopsies. The next step, according to Fenger, would be a number of quantitative observations such as the duration of the disease, mean temperature, and pulse, thus using statistical methodology. He stressed the importance of counting as opposed to labels, such as "seldom," "frequent," "several," or "common," when describing diseases. Fenger continued with epidemiological research into the distribution of the disease in various ages, sexes, temperaments (he had not totally abandoned the humoralistic way of thinking), crafts, and social classes (Fenger 1839: 305). Hospitals, according to Fenger, constituted the best settings for this research. If the number of patients was not sufficient, he suggested cooperation between several hospitals where observations could be made according to his carefully elaborated instructions. Today this method is known as multicenter studies.

His ideas were met with resistance. One of his friends and antagonists in a debate on medical science and practice, Andreas Buntzen, chief surgeon at Frederiks Hospital, argued that the numerical method, which depended on autopsies, could be carried out only in hospitals. Because of this change of focus from the individual person to anatomical observations, medicine had changed so that "disease replaced the sick person." Buntzen warned that when doctors stopped seeing patients as individuals, "the art of medicine ceases to exist" (Buntzen 1859: 46).

According to Fenger, the unique and individual were, on the contrary, not the object of science. He called for medical science to "put forward rules and nothing else" and to consider individualities as "the worst enemy of science" (Fenger 1840: 55). Fenger was heading toward positivism, where general laws should be derived from observations. He wanted to see medicine established as a science at the same level as physics and chemistry and rejected the "idealism" championed by Buntzen (Fenger 1859: 9). Fenger asked for the empirical, observable evidence and criticized the old theories, such as the existence of a vital force, as merely speculative constructions. His opponents accused him of being atheoretical and too absorbed by detail. The same accusation was applied to his political work.

Fenger criticized his colleagues not only for sticking to old dogmas but also for accepting novelties without the necessary skepticism. Following his reductionist way of understanding the world, Fenger would rather strive to find one cause of a disease than attempt to explain it by a complexity of factors, as did the humoralistic tradition. According to the humoralists, the constitution of the individual, determined by internal and external factors, was decisive for the development of diseases. Fenger, on the contrary, maintained that efforts to improve disease resistance in the population through improved living conditions had not resulted in a single discovery that could destroy disease or prevent its transmission between individuals (Fenger 1866–1868: 144).

Fenger denied the normative approach to disease, which considers health as a norm and disease as a deviation from this norm (Fenger 1843: 1). His definition of disease was functional; that is, disease prevented the individual from functioning in an appropriate manner (Fenger 1843: 2). His main humoralist opponent, Buntzen, called it a philosophy devoid of all idealism, but to Fenger normality was a statistical average rather than an ideal standard as the individual was one in a row rather than something unique.

The middle of the nineteenth century saw new trends in ideas about medical treatment and increased scientific discussion of therapeutic practices throughout the civilized world. Regional and international variations in therapeutic practices, however, caused concern and uncertainty about which were the best. Fenger argued that the history of medicine also supported the same lack of trust in therapies. He believed that the history of medicine provided evidence of a number of revolutions that produced new ideas that did not build on previous experience (Fenger 1859: 13). One could say that Fenger represented a new revolution of the same kind. The only part of medicine where he saw continuity and ability to learn from previous periods was care or nursing, which relieves pain and sometimes contributes to cure (Fenger 1859: 22). Fenger promoted the introduction of educated nurses to the Municipal Hospital in Copenhagen in the 1870s.

Fenger accused his colleagues of being irresponsible because they used therapies, the effects of which had not been proven. He warned against using dubious remedies to "break the disease," because they might instead injure the patient (Fenger 1859: 30). He did, however, understand the reasons for his colleagues' behavior. It was much more satisfactory to act and to believe one's actions actually did cure patients than do nothing.

Fenger noted that there was a rather short list of scientifically valid treatments for certain diseases, such as quinine for malaria and iron for anemia. For diseases where knowledge of cause and effect of the treatment was not at hand, he recommended an expectative treatment; not the same as doing nothing, this meant concentrating on activities intended to relieve pain, remove symptoms, and strengthen the patient. Thus he did not accept the accusation of being a nihilist.

Although the body-soul relationship was important in the humoralistic understanding of disease, mind or soul did not play a role in Fenger's universe of disease and medical science. In accordance with his exclusively biological concept of disease, he denied that the faith a doctor could inspire among his patients would have an effect on the cure. To a limited extent, Fenger used humoralistic therapies, such as laxatives, means to increase transpiration and urination, and emetics for some diseases such as pneumonia. Fenger also presented a long discussion of the appropriateness of bloodletting and ended by saying that he would continue to use it on many occasions. Interestingly enough, in this case he referred only to his own experience rather than statistical studies.

It was Fenger's hope that quantitative methodologies would raise medical research to a scientific level. To achieve this goal, data of good quality had to be carefully collected—clinical data from hospitals and vital statistics on the population level. Fenger was involved in improving data collection and analysis of data for both medical and administrative purposes. In 1845 he initiated and became chairman of a committee on statistics set up by the Royal Medical Society. From 1846 and onward, the committee published papers in *Bibliotek for Læger* (Archives for physicians), now held to be the oldest medical journal in the world, on a variety of medico-topographical and statistical topics, many written by Fenger himself. The committee sent questionnaires to all Danish doctors in order to collect information on age of menarche, causes of death, epidemic diseases, and obstetric cases in medical practice and to all midwives about obstetric cases in their practices. The information was to be used for writing a medical topography (i.e., descriptive epidemiology) of Denmark containing data on physiology, pathology, and preventive and therapeutic measures in the population (Fenger 1847: 37).

In one of his publications, Fenger presented different ways of calculating the Danish population's mortality and life expectancy, ending with the average length of life being the most appropriate. To a modern reader, his presentations seem sometimes exhaustive, but to readers not acquainted with statistical reasoning, this level of detail was probably helpful. Each step of his investigation was described, along with tables. Not only did he analyze data, he also showed imaginativeness in trying to validate data. For example, when analyzing the data from the censuses, he found that there was incongruence between the number of inhabitants in each five-year group in one census compared with the same cohort five years earlier. There were too many people. He argued that the most likely explanation was that people gave incorrect information on their age. To validate this assumption, he looked at a Nyboder, a smaller community in Copenhagen. He compared the age people had stated when they were admitted to Frederiks Hospital and the age data available from a special register of the inhabitants. This validation showed that the information on age that people reported was often wrong and that the deviations increased as people grew older (Fenger, 1848: 3–71).

As finance and hospital mayor of Copenhagen, he initiated improved statistical work in the city and employed a young political economist to undertake the collection and analysis of data. A separate office was, however, not established until Fenger had resigned. His antagonists did not want to give him more power than he had already.

Fenger was elected to the first Danish parliament and immediately became a leading figure in financial politics. His professional interest in political economy as a science rather than his political vision apparently led him to enter politics. To a present-day observer, medicine and political economy seem far apart. That was not the case for Fenger and his contemporaries. When on his medical study-tour, Fenger also studied political economy in Paris, as did his fellow traveler C. J. Kayser, also a medical doctor, who in 1848 became the first professor of political economy at the University of Copenhagen. Strict boundaries between disciplines did not yet exist. For Fenger, the link between the two disciplines was most likely his interest in statistics. His political work was characterized by thoroughness and logical clarity (i.e., scientific virtues), rather than visions and new ideas (Bille 1884: 26). He seems to have been painstaking and almost parsimonious in his administration of the government's, and later of Copenhagen's, finances, virtues probably more called for in scientific work than in politics.

One of his most important suggestions was to change the departments of the Copenhagen Municipal Hospital from being specialized according to treatment, surgery, and internal medicine, to being specialized according to which parts of the body the diseases affected, such as the eyes, the urinary tract, thorax, diseases of the brain and nerves, and women's diseases. Two reasons for this change were put forward by Fenger: (1) by spreading the surgical cases, the risk of hospital infections was reduced, and (2) specialization would lead to scientific progress. Most doctors resisted this new form of specialization and saw the plan as a threat to the survival of surgery as a specialty. Only one of the suggested departments was established, but even this department was eventually closed. Fenger's power in the city was not great enough to counteract the resistance from the doctors. He was more successful in introducing educated nurses to the Municipal Hospital in order to improve the care and surveillance of patients.

The process started in 1876; not until 1905, however, were nurses employed in all the hospital's departments.

As hospital and finance mayor of Copenhagen, Fenger took part in several changes in the public health area. After the cholera year, he and his colleagues established an association to work for better housing conditions for the poor. As hospital mayor he continued his work against infectious diseases by promoting the building of a quarantine hospital, which opened in 1875, and an isolation hospital in 1879. In order to prevent disease, he also furthered the building of slaughterhouses and the introduction of control of meat and milk in Copenhagen.

Fenger's achievements are more characterized by the introduction and promotion of new ideas than by their creation. He did so with much emphasis and diligence and in every way was preoccupied with documentation and accuracy in detail. He was successful when he furthered ideas where the soil was already prepared, especially new ways of medical thinking and acting, less so when he came up with new ideas such as changing the principles of specialization. His work was much admired, but he also succeeded in making enemies, both by steadily maintaining his opinions, becoming less and less inclined to listen to other people's opinions, and by criticizing those who did not live up to his standards. He died in 1884, two years after the death of his wife, a sick and broken man.

BIBLIOGRAPHY

Fenger's correspondence can be found in Rigsarkivet (the National Archive) in Copenhagen.

Writings by Carl Emil Fenger

"Betænkning fra det i Mødet den 21de Juni i Sagen angaaende Forandringer i forskjellige Communehospitalet vedrørende Forhold." In *Kjøbenhavns Borgerrepræsentanters Forhandlinger 1869–70*, pp. 209ff. Copenhagen 1870. (Report from the committee set up to deal with various changes in the municipal hospital. Proceedings from the Copenhagen city council, 1869–1870. Fenger wrote the report as the chair of the committee, but his authorship is not explicitly stated in the report.)

"Om den numeriske Methode (On the numerical method.)." *Ugeskrift for Læger* (Physicians weekly) 1 (1839): 305–315, 321–325.

"Modbemærkninger imod Dr. Djørups Critik af den numeriske Methode (Reply to Dr. Djørup's critique of the numerical method)." *Ugeskrift for Læger* (Physicians weekly) 2 (1840): 49–64.

Plan til en Forelæsningscyklus over den almindelige Pathologie (Plan for a cycle of lectures on general pathology). Copenhagen: Jens Sostrup Schultz, 1843.

"Første Halvårsberetning fra det kongelige medicinske Selskabs statistiske Komite (First

half-yearly report from the Statistical Committee of the Royal Medical Society).''
Bibliotek for Læger (Archives for physicians) 3 Rk, 1 Bd (1847): 32–82.

"Om Dødelighedsforholdene i Danmark (On mortality in Denmark).'' In *Det kongelige medicinske Selskabs Skrifter* (Publications from the Royal Medical Society,) pp. 3–71. Copenhagen: Ny Række, 1. Første Bind, 1848.

"Bidrag til Oplysning af vor Tids therapeutiske Bevægelse (Contribution to the information about the therapeutic movement of our time).'' *Hospitalstidende* (Hospital journal) 1 (1859): 9–10, 13–14, 17–18, 21–22, 25–26, 29–30, 33–34.

"Om det Virksomme ved Gjæringen, Foraadnelsen og visse Arter af Sygdomssmitte (On the activity of fermentation, putrefaction, and some types of contagion).'' *Hygieiniske Meddelelser* (Hygienic communications) 5 (1866–1868): 127–230.

Writings about Carl Emil Fenger and Related Topics

Bille, C. St. A. "Carl Emil Fenger.'' *Illustreret Tidende* (Illustrated journal) 26 (1) (1884): 1–2.

Bock, Alma. *Min Far og hans Hjem* (My father and his home). Copenhagen: C. C. Petersens Bogtrykkeri., 1914.

Buntzen, Andreas. "Therapie og pathologisk Anatomie. Betragtninger over den nyeste Tids Retning i Lægekunsten (Therapy and pathological anatomy. Considerations on the newest trends in medicine).'' *Hospitalstidende* (Hospital journal) 1 (1859): 41–50.

Lesky, Erna. "Von den Ursprungen des therapeutischen Nihilismus (On the origin of therapeutic nihilism).'' *Sudhoff Archiv für Geschichte der Medizin und der Naturwissenschaften* (Sudhoff's archive for the history of medicine and the natural sciences) 44 (1960): 1–20.

Neergaard, Niels. *Under Junigrundloven I* (Under the June constitution). Copenhagen: Philipsens forlag, 1892.

Petersen Ester. *Fra opvarter til sygeplejerske* (From servant to nurse). Copenhagen: Dansk Sygeplejeråd, 1988.

Vallgårda, Signild. "Hospitals and the poor in Denmark, 1750–1880.'' *Scandinavian Journal of History* 13 (1989): 95–105.

Signild Vallgårda

CARLOS JUAN FINLAY
(1833–1915)

Carlos Juan Finlay, physician, clinical investigator, and discoverer of the role of the *Aedes egypti* mosquito in the transmission of yellow fever, was born in Camagüey, Cuba, on December 3, 1833. His father, Edward Finlay (1795–1872), was a Scottish physician, and his mother, Elizabeth de Barrés (b. 1811), was a French woman from the island of Trinidad. After being tutored at home by a maternal aunt, he was sent to France (1845) for his secondary education. An attack of chorea left him with a slight but permanent speech impediment. Political unrest in France forced him to spend a year in Mainz, where he learned German and swam in the Rhine. He graduated from the highly reputable Lycée de Rouen in 1851.

As a student at Jefferson Medical College of Philadelphia, Finlay was greatly impressed by a lecture delivered by John Kearsly Mitchell, who believed that a botanical agent was the cause of tropical fevers. Mitchell pointed out the inconsistencies in the theories of the environmentalists, who believed that diseases were transmitted by miasmas, and the contagionists, who believed that one patient could give a disease to another. Drawing the conclusion that yellow fever was portable but not contagious, Mitchell indirectly suggested the existence of a vector. The professor's son, Silas Weir Mitchell,* was Finlay's prosector and lifetime friend.

Receiving his M.D. degree in 1855, Finlay declined an invitation to establish himself in the United States and gladly returned to Cuba. After passing the required examination to revalidate his American diploma, he went to Paris for postgraduate studies in internal medicine under the direction of Armand Trousseau (1801–1867) in Paris. Returning home in 1863, he established a practice in the community of El Cerro and published the first observation of hyperthyroidism in Cuba. He was interested in public health and wrote a learned survey of the world literature on cholera.

Finlay's encyclopedic memoir on the etiology of yellow fever, published in 1865, revealed the mind of a keen epidemiologist. He also began a careful and original study of the alkalinity of the air in relation to seasons, climate, and health. In 1865 he met and married Adelaîde Shine (1833–1916), a native of Trinidad. By 1876 the Finlays had three children: Carlos Eduardo (b.1868), Jorge Enrique (b.1870), and José María Francisco (b.1876). In 1872 he was elected to the Science section of the Real Academia de Ciencias Médicas, Físicas y Naturales. His choice of universal gravity as the subject of his inaugural dissertation revealed his knowledge of physics and mathematics. His knowledge of French, German, and English kept him abreast of the current literature. He was an exemplary academician and an active participant in discussions of a large variety of subjects. In 1875, when the Royal Academy of Havana celebrated its fifteenth anniversary, Finlay presented the commemorative lecture, a philosophical essay entitled "La Verdad Científica (Scientific Truth)," which dealt with experimental hypotheses, experimental methods, invention, and relative and absolute scientific truth.

Yellow fever, endemic in the Caribbean islands, made frequent visits to southern ports in North America; the dreaded scourge also made unpredictable incursions as far inland as St. Louis, Cincinnati, and Pittsburgh. In a few summer weeks, the disease could decimate and demoralize entire populations. These epidemics made evident the appalling lack of knowledge about the cause of the fever, means of transmission, and preventive measures. In 1879, an official U.S. Yellow Fever Commission was sent to Cuba, where the disease was endemic. The chairman of the commission, Stanford E. Chaillé (1830–1911) of New Orleans, brought a medical student, Rudolph Matas (1860–1957), as a scribe; George Sternberg (1836–1915), a noted bacteriologist, was secretary, and Juan Guiteras (1852–1925), of Pennsylvania, was the pathologist. The Spanish government designated Finlay as local liaison officer. Matas later wrote "The image of Carlos Finlay remained in my mind as the model of exemplary wisdom, of the laborious worker wealthy in strength of knowledge, in rectitude of principles, in conscientiousness and intellectual integrity." The official report of the commission's three-month investigation mentioned Finlay's views on the alkalinity of the air.

Finlay had long held an anticontagionist point of view concerning yellow fever, but following his work with the American commission, he developed an additional concept that required preliminary investigation and experimental verification. An International Sanitary Conference was called in Washington, and Finlay was appointed a member of the Spanish delegation. During the discussion, Finlay pointed out that the sanitary measures generally adopted to prevent the spread of yellow fever were inconsistent with a number of observed facts. According to Finlay, an independent agent was needed to transmit the disease from a sick person to a healthy one; to prevent the transmission of the disease, this agent would have to be destroyed or diverted from its path. There is no record of further discussion of Finlay's hypothesis and its clear suggestion of a vector.

Finlay suspected that a mosquito served as the vector of yellow fever, and, by logical analysis, chose to investigate the *Culex mosquito* (later *Stegomyia fasciata* and now *Aedes egypti*), one of the numerous possible species. This small, nocturnal pest has a short flight span and lays its eggs in the stagnant waters of cisterns and flower vases. He learned that it was the female that sucks blood; the male prefers fruits. With careful experimental methodology, he hatched the eggs of the suspected culprit, kept the mosquitoes in individual fastened test tubes, and allowed them to fill themselves with the blood of a patient with yellow fever. The next step was to have the infected insects bite a normal, nonimmune subject to verify transmission of the disease. The ideal subjects were recent immigrants.

Finlay obtained permission from the military authorities to test twenty volunteers, soldiers who had recently arrived from Spain. In groups of four, the volunteers were brought to his office to be interviewed, examined, and inoculated by the bites of infected mosquitoes. The soldiers were quartered in La Cabaña, across the bay from Havana. On June 10, 1881, Finlay inoculated his first volunteer, Francisco Beronat, who nine days later developed fever, jaundice, and albuminuria. Gaining confidence from Beronat's illness and recovery, Finlay inoculated others, but the results were not consistent.

On August 14, 1881, Finlay gave a report on his research to the Royal Academy with details of the specific mosquito, its habitat, and the geographical distribution. Experimental inoculations continued, with Jesuit priests and nonimmune Spanish immigrants. Finlay kept detailed records of 104 such trials. Only 3 of the inoculated Jesuits later developed yellow fever. Finlay concluded that a single bite from an infected mosquito resulted in an abortive form of the disease, which usually conferred immunity. He published about forty papers, mostly in British or American journals, and hailed the inoculations as a plausible means of vaccination. But Finlay was to face long years of skepticism. In an article devoted to Finlay's inoculations, Sternberg, who was considered an authority on yellow fever, stated that "no one has felt sufficiently impressed to repeat the experiment of Dr. Finlay." In 1894 at the Eighth World Congress of Hygiene and Demography, in Budapest, Finlay presented his recommendations for the prevention of yellow fever epidemics: prompt isolation of patients, fumigation of houses to keep mosquitoes away, and thorough destruction of sites where eggs could be laid.

Finlay was in Tampa, Florida, in April 1898 when the United States declared war on Spain. He went to Washington and, despite his age, volunteered as a contract surgeon. He was sent to Cuba on a hospital ship. The American troops suffered more from yellow fever, malaria, and imported typhoid fever than from warfare. In Havana, Finlay often talked to members of the U.S. Army, Navy, and Public Health Service.

In 1897 Giuseppe Sanarelli of Uruguay claimed to have discovered the causal agent of yellow fever, which he called *Bacillus icteroides*. With Cuba under military occupation following the Spanish-American War, Surgeon General of the U.S. Army George Sternberg was granted authority to appoint a board for special studies of infectious diseases prevailing in Cuba. The board was composed of Major Walter Reed (1846–1902) as chairman and contract surgeons James Carroll (1846–1907), Jesse Lazear (1866–1900), and Arístides Agramonte (1869–1931). Within five weeks, the board proved that Sanarelli's agent was simply *Bacillus cholerae suis*, a frequent contaminant in cadavers. The board was about to embark on a study of the intestinal flora of yellow fever patients when their course was radically shifted by their encounter with H. E. Durham (1868–1945) and Walter Myers (1872–1901), who had been sent by the University of Liverpool to study yellow fever in Brazil and had stopped in Havana. The British scientists visited Finlay and were impressed with his ideas and his work.

Although the board had no instructions to look into Finlay's work, on August 1, 1900, they paid him a visit. He received them cordially, gave them reprints of his papers, explained his views, and gave them a valuable gift: a porcelain dish with eggs of the specific mosquito that he had discovered to be the culprit. On the next day, Walter Reed returned to the United States for a vacation with his family. Lazear, the only member of the board who had any knowledge of entomology, hatched the eggs, kept the mosquitoes in individual fastened test tubes, and took them to bite patients with yellow fever; he chose patients with mild cases or those already recovering.

When Lazear's first attempts to inoculate volunteers, including himself, yielded no positive results, he decided to have the mosquitoes fill themselves with the blood of severe cases. Carroll volunteered to be bitten and suffered through a severe case of the fever. Lazear inoculated himself and died on September 25, 1900, after developing a severe case of yellow fever. In letters from the United States, Reed expressed doubts about the mosquito hypothesis, but after returning to Havana and reading Lazear's notebook, he apparently became very excited. He returned to the United States, and on October 23, at a meeting of the American Public Health Association in Indianapolis, declared to the world, exclusively on the basis of Lazear's notes, that the mosquito was the intermediate agent of yellow fever.

After returning to Havana, Reed, with the help of Carroll and Agramonte, staged a controlled experiment that proved without doubt that Finlay had been right. Leonard Wood (1840–1927), military governor of Cuba and a physician himself, ordered a gala banquet held in honor of Finlay at which he stated, "The confirmation of Dr. Finlay's doctrine is the greatest step forward made by Medicine since Jenner's discovery of the vaccination." Agramonte later said, "Thanks to the firmly rooted conviction of a good and modest man, thanks to his unswerving purpose in proclaiming and defending what he knew was right, to his wonderful power of observation and his ability for logical deduction we have found the ounce of prevention necessary in this dreadful disease." Major William Gorgas* proceeded to implement, with *Stegomyia* squads, the measures long recommended by Finlay: isolation, fumigation, and elimination of stagnant water. Within six months, the last case of yellow fever was registered in Havana, where the disease had been endemic for over two hundred years. In a letter to Reed, Gorgas said of Finlay, "I think that he is an old trump as modest as he is kindly and true. His reasoning for selecting the Stegomyia as the bearer of yellow fever is the best piece of logical thinking found in Medicine anywhere." Gorgas went on to implement the same measures and make possible the completion of the Panama Canal.

In 1902 the Republic of Cuba was proclaimed, and Finlay was appointed director of sanitation in the Ministry of Health. In 1905, Nobel Laureate Ronald

Ross (1857–1932) nominated Finlay for the Nobel Prize in Physiology or Medicine. Ross stated that the experimental demonstration would not have been possible but for the previous thoughts and research of Finlay who placed in the hands of the U.S. Army Board the eggs of "the very mosquitoes with which their success was obtained." Colonel John W. Ross (1868–1920), medical director of the U.S. Navy, added, "I have for a long time felt that there is no one who so richly deserves the Nobel Prize as Dr. Finlay in recognition of his brilliant and beneficent service to science and humanity." Nobel Laureate Alphonse Laveran (1845–1922) nominated Finlay for several years in succession, without success. Finlay died in his home in Havana August 20, 1915. In 1933 the French Academy of Medicine celebrated the centennial of his birth, and the city of Paris gave his name to one of its streets.

BIBLIOGRAPHY

Letters and other documents related to the work of Carlos Finlay are held in the Hench Yellow Fever Collection, Manuscripts Division, Claude Moore, Library, University of Virginia, Charlottesville, Virginia. Letters concerning the nomination of Finlay for a Nobel Prize are held in the confidential dossiers of the Nobel Committee for Physiology or Medicine, Stockholm, Sweden. For an account of the special decision of the Nobel Assembly to make documents available to the author, see Juan A. del Regato (1987).

Writings by Carlos Juan Finlay

Abstract. *Proceedings of the International Sanitary Conference*. Washington, D.C.: Government Printing Office, 1881.
"The Mosquito Hypothetically Considered as the Agent of Transmission of Yellow Fever Poison." (Abstract and translation by R. Matas.) *New Orleans Medical and Surgical Journal* 9 (1882): 601–616.
"Yellow Fever: Its Transmission by Means of the Culex Mosquito." *American Journal of Medical Sciences* 92 (1886): 395–400.
"Inoculation for Yellow Fever by Means of Contaminated Mosquitoes." *American Journal of Medical Sciences* 102 (1891): 264–268.
"A Plausible Method of Vaccination against Yellow Fever." *Philadelphia Medical Journal* 1 (1898): 1123–1124.

Writings about Carlos Juan Finlay and Related Topics

Del Regato, Juan A. "Carlos Finlay and the Nobel Prize of Physiology or Medicine." *Pharos* 50 (1987): 5–9.
Matas, R. "Mis recuerdos de Carlos Finlay." *Gaceta Medica Centroamericana* 1 (1943): 75–77.
Reed, W., J. Carroll, and J. W. Lazear. "The Etiology of Yellow Fever. A Preliminary Note." *Philadelphia Medical Journal* 6 (1900): 790–796.
Sternberg, G. M. "Doctor Finlay's Mosquito Inoculations." *American Medical Sciences* 52 (1891): 627–630.

————. "Doctor Finlay's Mosquito Inoculations." *Annali di Medicina Navale (Roma)* 3 (1897): 819–942.

Wood, L. *Civil Report of the Military Government of Cuba during the intervention of the United States of America.* Vol. 4. Washington, D.C.: U.S. Government Press, 1901.

Juan A. del Regato

THOMAS FRANCIS, JR.
(1900–1969)

Thomas Francis, Jr., physician, epidemiologist, pioneering virologist, and director of the 1954 evaluation of the Salk poliomyelitis vaccine, was born in Gas City, Indiana, July 15, 1900, one of five children of a Welsh immigrant family. His father, Thomas Francis, was a devout Methodist employed in the tin mills and active as a lay preacher on Sundays; his mother, Elizabeth Anne Cadogan Francis, had been a missionary captain in the Salvation Army. The family moved several times during Tommy's earliest years, returning briefly to Wales and then to Indiana, before settling in New Castle, Pennsylvania, where the boy grew up. The Francis children remembered their home as happy, although their parents were very strict. Aside from church activities, the family's favorite recreation was group singing; Tommy had a good voice and enjoyed singing with friends throughout his life.

A good student and avid reader, Francis was encouraged to pursue a medical career by the family physician, Dr. William Womer, and by his sister Mildred's husband, Dr. Edgar McGuire. After receiving his B.S. from Allegheny College in Meadville, Pennsylvania, he was accepted at Yale Medical School. Here he became the protégé of Dr. Francis Blake, chair of internal medicine, who had been recently recruited by Dean Milton Winternitz to introduce the Johns Hopkins model—full-time medical faculty and training in laboratory research—to Yale (Paul 1970: 248). Francis remained at Yale for seven years, earning his M.D. in 1924, completing a two-year residency at New Haven Hospital, and then teaching for a year in Blake's department. In 1928, Blake recommended young Dr. Francis to Dr. Rufus Cole, director of Rockefeller Hospital, for a position on the Clinical Pneumonia Service, working under Dr. Oswald T. Avery.

At the Rockefeller, junior staff were expected to be poor, celibate, and hard working. Avery gave his staff great independence and little direction. In this "fly or flop" laboratory where only self-starters succeeded, Tommy Francis thrived, developing his skills in bacteriological and virological research, while carrying major responsibilities for patient care (MacLeod 1970: 226). His first major project, with William Tillett, demonstrated that certain polysaccharides attached to the pneumococcus bacillus acted as antigens, triggering antibody production in humans; previously, only proteins had been identified as antigens. But Francis soon became fascinated by the influenza virus.

Virology was a new and mystifying field; little was known about any virus, except that they were so small they could not be seen under a standard microscope and passed through the finest laboratory filters. Some scientists thought they were minute bacteria or bacterial toxins. Viruses had been implicated in deadly diseases; the polio epidemic of 1916 and the influenza pandemic of 1918 were fresh in American minds. But little was known about the specific viruses involved or how they were transmitted.

In 1933, Patrick Laidlaw, Wilson Smith, and Christopher Andrewes announced the isolation of the first influenza virus in England. Within a year, Francis had confirmed their work by isolating a virus (PR-8) from the saliva of victims of a Puerto Rican flu epidemic and successfully infecting ferrets and mice with the disease. He was recruited in 1936 to join the International Health Division of the Rockefeller Foundation and was given his own laboratory to work on influenza virus. Between 1936 and 1938, he demonstrated that the Puerto Rican virus, the English virus, and a third isolated from Philadelphia patients were immunologically alike; that is, infection with one established immunity against the others. This group was dubbed the Type A strain.

Now in his late thirties, Francis had earned recognition as an authority on influenza and as a skilled laboratory virologist. He had also earned the right to a less spartan and single-minded existence. He had married Dorothy Packard Otton in 1937, and in 1938 he left the Rockefeller for the position of professor and chair of bacteriology at New York University (NYU) School of Medicine. He continued his research and in 1940 announced the isolation of a new influenza virus, designated Type B, which was immunologically distinct from Type A virus.

He was not to stay long at NYU. The newly established (1938) National Foundation for Infantile Paralysis had decided to create and fund a new laboratory dedicated to virus research at the University of Michigan, and its Scientific Research Committee was searching for a director. Several names had been proposed and rejected for various reasons, when Thomas Rivers, who had succeeded Cole at the Rockefeller Hospital, suggested Tommy Francis. Having been assured that he would have freedom to develop the laboratory as he saw fit and would not be limited to polio research, Francis accepted and was appointed professor of epidemiology in the Michigan School of Public Health in 1940.

This appointment began his long association with the National Foundation, which continued to fund the virology laboratory throughout the 1940s. It also introduced Francis to epidemiological fieldwork, an essential part of virus research. Within a year, he and his staff had begun tracing the dissemination of polio in community outbreaks and investigating the incidence among family members of victims (Benison 1967: 261). He also began a program to train young researchers; one of the first of these was Jonas Salk, who worked with Francis from 1942 to 1947.

The National Foundation had encouraged him to continue his influenza research, and events soon made it imperative. By late 1940, the Department of War anticipated large-scale mobilizations in the event of U.S. entry into the war in Europe and was dreading a recurrence of the 1918 pandemic. On February 19, 1941, Francis was appointed a member of the newly formed Armed Forces Epidemiological Board and director of the Commission on Influenza. As with his work for the National Foundation, this assignment involved both laboratory research and field epidemiology. Francis and the other commission members advised the military on troop housing, sanitation, and infection control measures and set up a monitoring network of "watch laboratories" to assist in the early detection of possible epidemics, a system later copied by the World Health Organization. They investigated outbreaks of hepatitis and acute respiratory disease, as well as influenza. Francis himself traveled to both the European and Pacific theaters to monitor and advise on suspected outbreaks (Griffin 1970: 253–254; Davenport, Lennette, and Meiklejohn 1970: 267–270).

His chief accomplishment, however, was the development of an effective dead-virus vaccine. Francis and his Michigan colleagues, including Salk, inactivated cultures of both A and B influenza with formalin; the preparation, administered in saline solution, safely triggered antibody responses, which then remained active to ward off live infection. The vaccine, developed in the fall of 1942, was tested at several universities, then on selected military units. By 1945, it had been shown to be effective against both strains of influenza and was administered to the entire army.

Francis's achievements during the war solidified his reputation among the academic medical elite. The Influenza Commission had accomplished most of the long list of tasks he had outlined in 1941, a success attributed to his disciplined leadership and attention to detail, exemplified by "the little brown notebook" he constantly carried (Davenport, Lennette, and Meiklejohn 1970: 267–270; Wegman 1970: 232). His forthright approach sometimes antagonized colleagues, but it also gained him respect. Above all, he was highly regarded as a scientist, and many of his dicta became virological axioms: his insistence that disease had to be studied as it naturally occurred in humans (MacLeod 1970: 227); his "Doctrine of Original Antigenic Sin," that "primary infection in childhood is determinative for subsequent antibody responses and immunity"; and his "concept of the use of only the essential immunizing antigens" in prophylactic vaccines (Davenport, Lennette, and Meiklejohn 1970: 272).

Francis and his family, now including his daughter Mary Jane and son Thomas III, called "T," were happily and permanently settled in Ann Arbor. In 1947, he was appointed Henry Sewall Professor of Epidemiology at the University of Michigan and received the prestigious Lasker Award for his influenza work. But the greatest challenge of his career lay just ahead.

As a National Foundation grantee, he served on its scientific advisory committees, overseeing the painstaking process of differentiating the three strains of polio virus and discussing the problems of vaccine development. He was present at the January 23, 1953, meeting of the Immunization Committee when Jonas Salk, now at the University of Pittsburgh, presented the results of his trial of an inactivated virus polio vaccine on 161 children. Although Salk's work was promising, many members of the committee urged that the foundation proceed with caution. Several members, including John Enders of Harvard and Albert Sabin* of Cincinnati, thought that only an attenuated vaccine, containing a weak, but live, variant strain of the virus, on the Jennerian model (Edward Jenner's use of the mild cowpox virus to provide protection from the virulent smallpox virus), would ensure the lasting immunity needed to protect the world's children from polio.

Basil O'Connor, president of the National Foundation, and Thomas Rivers, its chief virological adviser, however, decided to plan immediately for a large-scale field trial of Salk's vaccine. More than 57,000 people had been stricken with polio in 1952 and 2,500 had died; the victims, their families, and the foundation's thousands of volunteers were clamoring for some kind of action. By the fall of 1953, preparations were well under way for a field trial in the spring, but O'Connor and Rivers knew that the massive project would have to be carried out and the results evaluated by a scientist whose independence would be unquestioned and whose authority would be sufficient to outweigh the expected criticism. For a second time, the foundation sought out Tommy Francis.

Francis was intrigued by the challenge, then spent two months negotiating his own terms before he accepted the job on February 9, 1954. He insisted on complete independence, ensured by an open-ended, no-strings grant awarded to the University of Michigan to establish the Vaccine Evaluation Center. Equally significant, he was adamant that a major part of the field trial follow the model of the randomized, blinded clinical trial, in which half the children would be injected with a placebo. Many at the foundation had qualms about the "injected control" plan, fearing parent opposition and press criticism; they preferred an "observed control," in which the controls for the vaccinated children would be the nonvaccinated children in other school grades.

Francis won his point. When the field trial began on April 26, 1954, the observed control plan was employed in thirty-three states; 221,998 second graders were vaccinated, and the remainder of the children in the first, second, and third grades were observed for signs of polio. In eleven states, however, all children in the first three grades whose parents had agreed to participation received injections: 200,745 were given vaccine and 201,229 placebo. Although he gave equal attention and energy to supervising both parts of the trial, Francis always considered the placebo control states the only valid test of the vaccine.

While the actual vaccinations were carried out by National Foundation volunteers over a period of six weeks, the Vaccine Evaluation Center, under Francis's constant personal direction, took nearly a year to collect and analyze more than 144 million separate pieces of data, including vaccination records, blood antibody titers, hospital records on polio victims and possible victims, and muscle evaluations to determine the extent of paralysis. The statistical staff was recruited from the Bureau of the Census, and their expertise and dedication proved essential. The Summary Report was not finished until April 9, 1955; three days later, on April 12, Francis was able to announce that the Salk vaccine was safe and highly effective (80–90 percent) against paralytic poliomyelitis.

Salk became an instant public hero and the focus of a glare of publicity; the vaccine was immediately licensed by the Public Health Service. The National

Foundation, although financially overextended, pledged to fund inoculations for all first and second graders. Only a short time after the mass vaccinations began, on April 25, one vaccinated child fell ill with polio. As more cases were reported, Surgeon General Leonard Scheele withdrew all vaccine from the market and recruited a Technical Advisory Committee to consider the next steps. Enders and Sabin again urged caution, more testing, even waiting for the development of an attenuated vaccine. Francis argued vehemently against the proposal "to remove a product that has been proved safe and effective, and substitute for it an unknown . . . which Dr. Sabin thinks might be better, but for which the proof is not yet available" (Benison 1967: 558). His voice proved decisive. The Salk vaccine, under additional safeguards, was released to the waiting children. Although the virologists continued to argue over the merits of the vaccine, by the end of 1956, over 75 percent of children ages five to twelve had been vaccinated, and the incidence of polio had begun to drop dramatically.

Thomas Francis continued to champion the inactivated vaccine on the Technical Advisory Committee and in public fora, but it was Salk who bore the burden of both scientific criticism and public adulation. Francis finished the final report on the field trials in 1957 and was then able to turn his attention to other projects. He made major contributions to the Armed Forces Epidemiology Board, on which he served until his death in 1969, and the Atomic Bomb Casualty Commission (1955–1969), for which he helped to plan the complex procedures of evaluating the effects of radiation on the survivors of Hiroshima and Nagasaki. The latter led to his service on the U.S.-Japan Cooperative Medical Sciences Program (1965–1969).

In his home state, he launched an ambitious public health study in 1959 in Tecumseh, Michigan, an attempt to create "a community laboratory" that would study epidemiology in the light of local history, geography, and culture; this project was ongoing at his death (Wegman 1970: 231). He was active in campus life, participating in the first Vietnam War teach-in at the university. In July 1968, he was one of the first to alert U.S. authorities to the Hong Kong flu epidemic and participated in the preparation of an effective vaccine against this new strain, applying the principles he had developed earlier in his career.

Francis remained active as a teacher, researcher, and administrator until his final illness. He died at University Hospital in Ann Arbor on October 1, 1969, of complications following abdominal surgery.

BIBLIOGRAPHY

The Thomas Francis, Jr., Papers have been deposited at the Bentley Historical Library, University of Michigan. The collection documents his professional and public life, and his interactions with colleagues, very fully; there are also a few personal items. Other useful sources include Saul Benison's masterly oral history with Thomas Rivers (Benison 1967) and several of the articles contributed by colleagues to the Thomas Francis, Jr., Memorial Festschrift and published in *Archives of Environmental Health* (September

1970). Several good popular books on the Salk vaccine trials discuss Francis's crucial role; the most recent, Jane Smith's *Patenting the Sun* (1990), makes good use of the Francis Papers. A solid scholarly account of the trials is still needed. Francis himself authored 261 articles; a very small selection is listed here.

Writings by Thomas Francis, Jr.

"Epidemiology of Influenza." *Journal of the American Medical Association*, (May 1, 1943, pp. 4–8.

(with John A. Napier, Robert B. Voight, et al.). *Evaluation of the 1954 Field Trial of Poliomyelitis Vaccine: Final Report*. Ann Arbor, MI: University of Michigan, 1957.

(with F. H. Epstein). "Studies of a Total Community: Tecumseh, Michigan." *Milbank Memorial Fund Quarterly* 43 (spring 1965): 333–342.

Writings about Thomas Francis, Jr., and Related Topics

Benison, Saul. *Tom Rivers: Reflections on a Life in Medicine and Science*. Cambridge, MA: MIT Press, 1967.

Cannan, R. Keith. "Contribution to the Work of the Atomic Bomb Casualty Commission (ABCC)." In Colin M. MacLeod, ed., *Archives of Environmental Health* 21 (September 1970): 263–266.

Davenport, Fred M., Edwin H. Lennette, and Gordon N. Meiklejohn. "Origins and Development of the Commission on Influenza." In Colin M. MacLeod, ed., *Archives of Environmental Health* 21 (September 1970): 267–272.

Griffin, Herschel E. "Thomas Francis, Jr., MD, Epidemiologist to the Military." In Colin M. MacLeod, ed., *Archives of Environmental Health* 21 (September 1970): 252–255.

MacLeod, Colin M. "Thomas Francis, Jr., MD, 1900–1969." In Colin M. MacLeod, ed., *Archives of Environmental Health* 21 (September 1970): 226–229.

———, ed. "The Thomas Francis, Jr., Memorial Festschrift." *Archives of Environmental Health* 21 (September 1970).

Paul, John R. "Thomas Francis, Jr., MD, as a Clinician." In Colin M. MacLeod, ed., *Archives of Environmental Health* 21 (September 1970): 247–251.

Smith, Jane S. *Patenting the Sun: Polio and the Salk Vaccine*. New York: William Morrow, 1990.

Wegman, Myron E. "Thomas Francis, Jr.: An Appreciation." In Colin M. MacLeod, ed., *Archives of Environmental Health* 21 (September 1970): 230–233.

Marcia Meldrum

SOLOMON CARTER FULLER
(1872–1953)

Solomon Carter Fuller, born on August 11, 1872, was a pioneering African American pathologist and psychiatrist. He was born in Monrovia, Liberia, to Solomon Fuller and Anna Ursula James. His father was a wealthy coffee planter and government official, and his mother was the daughter of Mr. and Mrs. Benjamin Van Renseler James, who were both medical doctors and missionaries. His grandfather, John Lewis Fuller, was a former slave who had purchased his and his wife's freedom and emigrated from the United States to Liberia soon after its founding in the early nineteenth century.

Solomon Carter Fuller reversed his grandfather's journey and emigrated to the United States in 1889, where he entered Livingstone College in Salisbury, North Carolina. Fuller was the only African among the student body, which was otherwise entirely made up of African Americans. As a senior, he was named class speaker and graduated with honors, receiving his A.B. in 1893. He then enrolled in the medical program at the Long Island College Hospital, Brooklyn, New York; after a year he transferred to Boston University Medical School, at that time a homeopathic institution. As such, it was open to both women and African American students. In addition, Boston University had a close relationship with Westborough State Hospital, the only state-supported homeopathic hospital for the insane. The Boston University Medical School Catalogue in the 1890s promised prospective students summer jobs as attendants at Westborough, so it was not surprising that upon receiving his M.D. in 1897, Fuller was immediately appointed as an intern at Westborough. Two years later, in 1899, Dr. Fuller was promoted to the position of pathologist at Westborough, the first African American to hold such a position in the United States.

In that same year, Fuller was also appointed as instructor in pathology at Boston University, the first of several positions he held there. In 1909, he became an instructor and in 1914 a lecturer in neurology. He steadily advanced in rank, becoming successively associate professor of neuropathology (1919) and associate professor of neurology (1921). In 1933, he retired, retaining the title of emeritus professor of neurology.

Although Boston University, like many other sectarian institutions, had admitted women and African Americans as students from its inception and had given Fuller the opportunity to become the first African American professor at a predominantly white medical school, Fuller found himself discriminated against as a faculty member. According to Robert Hayden and Jacqueline Harris (1976), for many years Fuller was not an official faculty member, and his salary was always smaller than those of his white colleagues of similar rank. Fuller's retirement was provoked when, after he had been fulfilling the duties of chairman of the Department of Neurology for five years, a white colleague was both given the official position and promoted to full professor, a title Fuller would never hold. Although he retired rather than publicly protest this discrimination, Fuller was justifiably resentful of this treatment, noting, "With the sort of work that I have done, I might have gone further and reached a higher plane had it not been for my color" (Hayden and Harris 1976: 21–22).

In addition to serving as pathologist at Westborough State Hospital for twenty-two years and as a consultant for twenty-three years, Fuller was a visiting neurologist at the Massachusetts Memorial Hospital and a consultant at the Framingham Marlborough Hospital, the Massachusetts General Hospital, and the Allentown, Pennsylvania, State Hospital. Fuller also pursued advanced studies in 1904–1905 while visiting Germany. He studied there, under Professors Emil Kraepelin and Alois Alzheimer, at both the Psychiatric Clinic and the Pathological Institute of the University of Munich. According to Hayden and Harris, during his trip, he called unannounced upon Paul Erlich—later the winner of the Nobel Prize in Physiology or Medicine (1908)—and spent an enjoyable afternoon talking with him. In 1909, Fuller also participated in the reception held for Sigmund Freud at Clark University, Worcester, Massachusetts.

As might be expected of a student of Dr. Alzheimer, Fuller's best-known research was on the disease named for his teacher. He translated several of Alzheimer's works and in a paper published in 1911 reported on the ninth known case of Alzheimer's disease. In the paper, he questioned whether the observed plaques and neurofibrillar changes in the case were significant, and he suggested that something other than arteriosclerosis, as was then generally believed, was responsible for the disease. Modern research has since confirmed Fuller's doubts.

Fuller's most important contribution to the medical profession was his encouragement of younger African American medical students and psychiatrists, both personally and through his own example. For instance, Dr. George Branche, chief of the Psychiatric Service of the Veterans' Administration Hospital at Tuskegee, Alabama, was Fuller's student, and according to the *Journal of the National Medical Association*, Fuller was "instrumental in guiding Dr. Branche to Tuskegee" (Cobb 1954: 371). Another of Fuller's students, Dr. Charles Pinderhughes, became a professor of psychiatry at Boston University and coordinator of residency training at the Veterans' Administration Hospital in Bedford, Massachusetts. It was in appreciation of Fuller's example and teaching that the Society of Black Psychiatrists presented a portrait of Dr. Fuller to the American Psychiatric Society. In 1953, after Fuller's death, a newly constructed community health center in Boston was named after Dr. Fuller; it continues in operation today.

In 1909, Fuller married the famous African American sculptor Meta Warrick (better known under her married name, Meta Warrick Fuller). They had three sons. After their marriage, they lived in a house they had constructed in Framingham, Massachusetts. (Meta died in 1968.) During construction of the house, when it became known that the Fullers were African Americans, a neighborhood petition was started to prevent them from moving in. Although some of his friends advised against proceeding, the Fullers persisted, and eventually they won the neighbors' friendship. Both Solomon Carter and Meta Warrick Fuller knew well the sting of discrimination, but they did not let it defeat them. As Dr. Charles Pinderhughes, a former student of Dr. Fuller at Boston University, said, "In an era when the professional development of black people was discouraged and inadequately rewarded, Dr. Fuller persevered until he secured the finest training available" (Anonymous 1973: 48).

BIBLIOGRAPHY

There are no archival sources available on Solomon Carter Fuller, and the majority of his work appeared in medical journals (including homeopathic ones) that are not readily available. Several of his most significant papers, however, are listed below. The most readily available sources on Fuller's life are the essay that appears in Hayden and Harris's *Nine Black American Doctors* (1976) and his obituary in the *Journal of the National Medical Association* ("Solomon Carter Fuller, 1872–1953": 1954). Short essays on Fuller and his wife also appeared in the *Dictionary of American Negro Biography*.

Writings by Solomon Carter Fuller

"A Testimonial to George Smith Adams." *New England Medical Gazette* 57 (1912): 467–486.
"A Study of the Military Plaques Found in Brains of the Aged." *Proceedings of the American Medico-Psychological Association at the Sixty-Seventh Annual Meeting held in Denver, Colorado, June 19–22, 1911* (1911): 109–181, plus 16 plates in eight pages.
"Histopathological Alteration in Cellular Neuroglia and Fibrillary Mesoblastic Components of Cerebral Cortical Interstitium." *Boston Medical and Surgical Journal* 190 (1929): 314–322.

Writings about Solomon Carter Fuller and Related Topics

Anonymous. "BU to Memorialize Noted Black Psychiatrist." *Boston Herald American*, October 8, 1973, p. 48.
Cobb, W. Montague. "Solomon Carter Fuller, 1872–1953." *Journal of the National Medical Association* 46, no. 5 (September 1954): 370–372.
Hayden, Robert. "Fuller, Meta Vaux Warrick." In Rayford W. Logan and Michael R. Winston, eds., *Dictionary of American Negro Biography*, pp. 245–247. New York: W. W. Norton, 1982.
———. "Fuller, Solomon Carter." In Rayford W. Logan and Michael R. Winston, eds., *Dictionary of American Negro Biography*, p. 247. New York: W. W. Norton, 1982.

Hayden, Robert, and Jacqueline Harris. *Nine Black American Doctors.* Reading, Mass.: Addison-Wesley, 1976.

Khan, Tira. "Solomon Carter Fuller: Teacher, Scientist, Perpetual Learner." *South End News*, April 7, 1994, pp. 3–4.

John Potter

JOHN FARQUHAR FULTON
(1899–1960)

John Farquhar Fulton, a neurophysiologist who applied laboratory neurophysiology to clinical neurology, a medical historian and bibliophile who helped establish the history of science and medicine as an academic discipline in the United States, and an administrator whose energy and talents contributed significantly to the growth of medical research, was born in St. Paul, Minnesota, on November 1, 1899. His father was John Farquhar Fulton, an ophthalmologist, and his mother was Edith Stanley Wheaton. He married Lucia Pickering Wheatland on September 29, 1923, in Oxford, England. They had no children.

Fulton spent one year at the University of Minnesota (1917–1918) and then transferred to Harvard College, from which he received the bachelor of science degree, magna cum laude, in 1921. From 1921 to 1925 he studied neurophysiology with Sir Charles Sherrington at Magdalen College, Oxford, first as a Rhodes scholar (1921–1923) and then as a Christopher Welch scholar (1923–1925). Oxford awarded him a bachelor of arts degree with first-class honors in 1923 and the master of arts and doctor of philosophy (D. Phil.) degrees in 1925. In 1926, his first book, *Muscular Contraction and the Reflex Control of Movement*, based on his research in Sherrington's laboratory, was published. He returned to Harvard University in 1925 and took his M.D. degree in 1927, after which he was a neurosurgical associate under Harvey Cushing at the Peter Bent Brigham Hospital in Boston.

Fulton was highly endowed with many qualities: not only an omnivorous reader, but also a phenomenal memory; not only catholic interests, but also insight; never selfish, but always generous. Above all, he approached his work—his life—with abundant zest. A surgical case from his time with Cushing illustrates these qualities. In September 1927 a patient who had a hemangioma of the left occipital lobe was admitted to Cushing's service. There was an easily audible bruit in the back of his head, and the patient had noticed that it grew louder when he concentrated on something while looking at it. The case intrigued Fulton, and on October 1, 1927, he noted excitedly in his diary that the increased volume suggested "that the activity in given portions of the brain stimulate[s] and increase[s] blood supply." Qualitative statements, however, are hardly useful in physiology. How could he obtain a quantitative and graphical readout of the noisier bruit? Fulton placed a telephone receiver that was connected to a Einthoven string galvanometer over the patient's shaved scalp and measured the changes in the bruit's intensity—"electrophonograms," he called them—while the patient performed various visual activities. Within a year he published the results. He concluded that mental activity does affect cerebral blood flow, a finding that is now at the center of much neurological research and is studied with far more refined tools. As is typical of Fulton's publications, his introductory literature review not only surveyed current references but also examined older work, and thereby placed the research in a wider perspective.

Fulton's insightful research and meticulous technique endeared him to Cushing, who urged him to pursue a clinical career as a neurosurgeon. Physiology, however, intrigued him more, and a Magdalen College fellowship lured him back to Oxford for two years of additional study (1928–1930). His book, his growing list of publications, and his association with Sherrington and Cushing brought him to the attention of the Yale University School of Medicine. In 1930 they offered him the Sterling Professorship of Physiology; a year later he assumed the chairmanship of the Department of Physiology, an office he held until 1951.

The twenty years during which Fulton directed Yale's laboratory of physiology can be divided roughly into two periods. At first, he and his associates, especially Margaret Kennard and Ted Ruch, concentrated mainly on the nature of the cortical control of muscular contraction and autonomic representation in the cortex; with Carlyle Jacobsen he studied the relation between the frontal lobes and behavior. To pursue this work, Fulton had had built one of the first primate laboratory facilities. Between 1941 and 1945, military needs spurred the laboratory's research as its focus shifted to aviation medicine, primarily decompression studies. One thread tied together the wide array of research done during all these years. Many of Fulton's papers and books demonstrate that from the start of his tenure, he was eager to discover clinical applications of the laboratory's research. At the time such an interdisciplinary approach was almost unknown, and consequently neurologists and psychiatrists as well as physiologists came to New Haven to work in the laboratory. Hebbel Hoff, who worked with Fulton, described the laboratory's atmosphere as "active, effervescent, and productive" (Hoff 1962: 16).

While the work with Kennard and Ruch earned Fulton honor among his peers, the work with Jacobsen brought him notoriety before the public. The goal of their research was to document the effect in primates of motor and premotor cortical lesions on motor deficits and learning. When their experiments finally included bilateral lesions or ablation of the prefrontal lobes, they noticed a "profound change" in the chimpanzee's behavior. Formerly, it had become violent when it failed some tests during experiments; Fulton, using Pavlov's terminology, called it an "experimental neurosis." After the operation, however, the chimpanzee "offered its usual friendly greeting" but "did not show any excitement, but rather quietly sat. . . . Thus while the animal repeatedly failed and made far greater number of errors than it had previously, it was impossible to evoke even a suggestion of an experimental neurosis" (Fulton and Jacobsen 1935: 113–123). From this report, Antônio Caetano de Abreu Friere Egas Moniz developed the prefrontal lobotomy for the relief of psychotic patients, which earned for Egas Moniz a share of the 1945 Nobel Prize in Medicine or Physiology. Fulton and some of his collaborators continued to work on this topic and wrote extensively on it for both the scientific and popular press.

In addition to research, administration, and teaching, Fulton also wrote the *Physiology of the Nervous System* (1938). Its aim was to help medical students bridge the gap between preclinical and clinical neurology. It was highly successful and was translated into five languages. He was also an editor. From the fourteenth edition in 1942 to the seventeenth in 1955, Fulton was the senior editor of *Howell's Textbook of Physiology*, and from 1938 to 1960 he edited the *Journal of Neurophysiology*, which he had cofounded with J. G. Dusser de Barenne.

After Fulton stepped down from the chairmanship of the Physiology Department and the directorship of its laboratory in 1951, Yale appointed him its first Sterling Professor of the History of Medicine. The shift from physiology to history was not difficult for Fulton; his interest in the history of science and medicine was as old as his interest in physiology. Nor was it an area with which he needed to reacquaint himself, for alongside the steady stream of physiological books and articles that began in the 1920s was an equally steady stream of solid historical work. During the four decades in which he was active, Fulton contributed to both the corpus of historical writing and the development of the history of science and medicine as an academic discipline and profession.

The foundation for Fulton's historical work was his immense library that he had gathered with interest and passion. For example, *Muscular Contraction and the Reflex Control of Movement* (1926) has an extensive historical introduction going back to Aristotle and is illustrated with title pages and frontispieces of incunabula or early modern books. His collection had grown so extensive that when he wrote *Selected Readings in the History of Physiology* (1930), he used resources only from his own collection. Robert Boyle (1627–1691), author of *The Skeptical Chymist*, was a favorite collecting area from which he published ''A Bibliography of the Honourable Robert Boyle'' (1932). His own bibliography of over five hundred entries contains many articles, papers, and exhibition catalogs on the history of medicine. With Elizabeth H. Thomson he wrote a biography (1947) of Benjamin Silliman (1779–1864), Yale's first professor of chemistry. Perhaps his best remembered historical work is *Harvey Cushing* (1946), a biography of his friend and mentor.

Not only neurology, but also, or perhaps especially, book collecting cemented the friendship between Cushing and Fulton. Both were ardent bibliophiles, and their correspondence is filled with stories about their successes or failures with book dealers. During the 1930s, Cushing, with Arnold C. Klebs, his friend and another medical historical bibliophile, persuaded Fulton that the three of them should meld their collections and donate them to Yale University, provided that the university maintain the collection and house it in a ''Historical Medical Library'' at the School of Medicine. Yale agreed, and by the mid-1940s their dream had become a reality. (By then only Fulton remained to see the library.

Cushing had died in 1939, Klebs in 1943.) To this day the library remains one of the finest and most extensive research libraries in the history of medicine, especially its early modern period.

Fulton was also active in the affairs of the nascent History of Science Society and the American Association for the History of Medicine. From 1952 to 1960, he edited the *Journal of the History of Medicine and Allied Sciences*, on whose editorial board he had served since the *Journal*'s inception in 1946.

During the 1950s Fulton laid the foundation for a department of the history of science and medicine at Yale. The library was already in place, and he had obtained some funding for the hiring of faculty and the admission of graduate students. This, after the Johns Hopkins University's Institute for the History of Medicine and Harvard University's Department of the History of Science, would be the third such graduate and undergraduate program in the United States. Unfortunately, Fulton died before the department was fully established in 1961.

Fulton's numerous institutional and government activities are difficult to categorize. He served, for example, on the board of trustees of the Institute for Advanced Studies and the Osler Library at McGill University. He was a member of the National Research Council and in 1940 was a liaison to the British Medical Research Council. He gave generously of his time and energy during World War II. For the National Research Council he chaired the committee on historical records (1940–1946), was associate editor of *War Medicine* (1941–1945), and chaired the editorial board of the *Medical History of the War* (1940–1945). He also served on numerous Yale University committees.

In addition to these multifaceted professional activities and membership in several clubs, he garnered many honors. Chief among them are the James Bowdoin Premium of Harvard University (in 1920 and 1921), with Kennard and Jacobsen the Bronze Medal of the American Medical Society (1939), the George Sarton Medal of the History of Science Society (1958), the President's Certificate of Merit (1948), Honorary Officer of the Civil Division of the Most Excellent Order of the British Empire (1948), officer in the French Legion of Honor (1959), fellow of the Royal College of Physicians (1953), and honorary fellow of the Royal College of Medicine (1954). He was awarded honorary degrees from American and European universities and was invited to deliver many distinguished lectureships.

The last years of his life were marked by severe ill health. After a brief illness, he died on May 29, 1960, at his home in Hamden, Connecticut.

BIBLIOGRAPHY

Yale University is the repository of John Fulton's papers. The Manuscript and Archives Division of the Sterling Memorial Library contains his correspondence. To say that John Fulton was a voluminous correspondent is an understatement. He believed that every communication deserved an answer. Even as a medical student he bought an early version of a dictaphone and generated enough material to keep one—sometimes two—secretaries busy. Add to this his habit of not discarding much, and one can imagine the size and scope of the archive. Yale also houses the papers of Lucia Wheatland Fulton, Harvey Cushing, Madeline Earle Stanton, and Elizabeth H. Thomson. Stanton and Thomson worked for many years in the Historical Medical Library and in the Department of the History of Science and Medicine at Yale. Their long association with and devotion to John Fulton make their papers a useful ancillary archive. The Medical Historical Library in the Cushing-Whitney Medical Library in the School of Medicine have additional Harvey Cushing material and the original manuscripts of John Fulton's forty-six-volume diary, which he kept from the early 1920s until nearly his death. Because Fulton's observations were always remarkably frank, even though he knew the diary might become public, many scholars have mined his diary for information on a wide number of topics.

An unsigned entry in the *National Cyclopedia of American Biography* (53:9–11) gives the full list of Fulton's club memberships and honors; see also Elizabeth H. Thomson, "Fulton, John Farquhar Fulton" in *Dictionary of American Biography* 126: 222–224. Whitfield J. Bell, Jr., edited the "John Fulton Number" of the *Journal of the History of Medicine and Allied Sciences* (1962). It contains Thomas Rogers Forbes, "John Farquhar Fulton," Arnold Muirhead, "John Fulton—Book Collector, Humanist, and Friend," Hebbel E. Hoff, "John Fulton's Contributions to Neurology," William LeFanu, "John Fulton's Historical and Bibliographical Work," and Madeline Earle Stanton and Elizabeth H. Thomson, "Bibliography of John Farquhar Fulton, 1921–1962."

Writings by John Farquhar Fulton

Physiological Writings

Muscular Contraction and the Reflex Control of Movement. Baltimore: Williams and Wilkins, 1926.

Selected Readings in the History of Physiology. Springfield, IL: C. C. Thomas, 1930.

(With C. F. Jacobsen). "The Functions of the Frontal Lobes, a Comparative Study in Monkeys, Chimpanzees and Man." *Advances in Modern Biology, Moscow* 4 (1935): 113–123.

Physiology of the Nervous System. New York: Oxford University Press, 1938.

"The Surgical Approach to Mental Disorder." *McGill Medical Journal* 1 (1948): 133–145.

The Frontal Lobes. Research Publications, Association for Research in Nervous and Mental Disease, vol. 27. Baltimore: William and Wilkins, 1948.

A Textbook of Physiology. Originally by William H. Howell, M.D. 16th ed. Philadelphia and London: W. B. Saunders Co., 1949.

Frontal Lobotomy and Affective Behavior. A Neurophysiological Analysis. Thomas W. Salmon Memorial Lectures. New York: W. W. Norton & Co., 1951.

The Frontal Lobes and Human Behavior. Sherrington Lectures. Liverpool: University Press, 1952.

(Edited with Ted Ruch). *Medical Physiology and Biophysics.* 18th ed. Philadelphia: W. B. Saunders Co., 1960.

Historical Writings

"A Bibliography of the Honourable Robert Boyle." *Proceedings of the Oxford Biblio-graphical Society* 3 (1932): 1–172.

"Robert Boyle and His Influence on Thought in the Seventeenth Century." *Isis* 18 (1932): 77–102.

"Science in the Clinic as Exemplified by the Life and Work of Joseph Babinski." *Journal of Nervous and Mental Disorders* 1 (1933): 5–80.

Harvey Cushing, a Biography. Springfield, IL: Charles C. Thomas, 1946.

(with Elizabeth H. Thomson). *Benjamin Silliman, 1779–1864, Pathfinder in American Science.* New York: Schuman's, 1947.

"George Sarton and the History of Medicine." *Isis* 48 (1957) 311–314.

Writings about John Farquhar Fulton

Hoff, Hebbel E. "John Fulton's Contributions to Neurology." *Journal of the History of Medicine and Allied Sciences* 17 (1962): 16–37.

Stanton, Madeline Earle Stanton, and Elizabeth H. Thomson. "Bibliography of John Farquhar Fulton, 1921–1962." *Journal of the History of Medicine and Allied Sciences* 17 (1962): 51–71.

Thomas P. Gariepy

JOSEPH GOLDBERGER
(1874–1929)

Joseph Goldberger, physician and epidemiologist in the U.S. Public Health Service, discovered pellagra to be a dietary deficiency whose prevention and cure existed in fresh meat and vegetables. Throughout his career, Goldberger brilliantly combined sharp observation and common sense with science to fight epidemics and trace the cause of numerous disorders. However, as the battle over pellagra would reveal, Goldberger was a far better medical scientist than social reformer.

Goldberger was born on July 16, 1874, in Giralt, Hungary, then part of the Austro-Hungarian Empire. His parents, Samuel and Sarah Gutman Goldberger, were sheepherders who emigrated to the United States with seven-year-old Joseph and three older children after sickness devastated their flock. Here they had three more children and ran a Lower East Side grocery store on Manhattan's Pitt Street.

For two years, Goldberger pursued a degree in engineering at the City College of New York. Then, in 1892, his career plans changed abruptly. A neighborhood friend, Patrick Murray, later the chief surgeon of the New York City Police Department, invited Goldberger to a lecture at Bellevue by physiologist Dr. Austin Flint, Jr. Entranced by the intricate engineering of the human body, Goldberger transferred to medical school, receiving his M.D. from Bellevue in 1895.

Two years of private medical practice in Wilkes-Barre, Pennsylvania, left shy, young Dr. Goldberger unprosperous and intellectually unfulfilled, except for two papers he prepared for the Luzerne County Medical Society: one on the uses of saline solution and the other on alcoholism. In 1899, he took and passed the entrance examination for the U.S. Marine Hospital Service commissioned corps (later the U.S. Public Health Service, or PHS). Appointed assistant surgeon July 25, 1899, at an annual salary of $1,600, Goldberger's initial post was as medical examiner of immigrants being processed at the Barge Office in lower Manhattan, a temporary facility while the scorched Ellis Island was being rebuilt. However, he was soon reassigned to posts that more rigorously tested his talents.

Between 1902 and 1906, Goldberger fought epidemics. He battled yellow fever in Mexico, Puerto Rico, Mississippi, and Louisiana, in the process contracting the disease himself. Tenacious and clever, Goldberger quickly became one of the service's most respected physicians and skilled epidemiologists. On July 27, 1904, he was promoted to the rank of passed assistant surgeon.

Yellow fever duty in Louisiana and friendship with PHS colleague Farrar Richardson led to an introduction to Richardson's cousin, Mary Farrar. She was the daughter of a wealthy, Episcopalian New Orleans family and grandniece of

Varina Davis, wife of the Confederacy's president. When Joseph asked for Mary's hand in marriage, her father, Edgar Farrar, demurred. Indeed, both families objected on religious grounds, but Edgar Farrar was especially suspicious of this impoverished northerner—an immigrant Jew seeking his daughter's hand. He launched an investigation, writing letters to all who might know of Goldberger or his family, including the surgeon general, Dr. Walter Wyman. In his response, Wyman praised Goldberger as having "commended himself very highly, both to those under whom he has immediately served and to the Bureau. He is considered one of the most promising of the young men connected with the Hygienic Laboratory of this Service" (Wyman to Edgar Farrar, December 30, 1905). On April 20, 1906, Edgar Farrar paid the deputy recorder of Orleans Parish $1.00 to register the marriage of his daughter to Dr. Joseph Goldberger. The couple eventually had four children: Farrar, Joseph, Benjamin, and Mary.

Even before they married, Joseph and Mary decided that traditional religion would not play a central role in their lives. Instead, reason, humanitarianism, research, and science would be the points on their compass. Goldberger shared with Mary his belief that science was the most reasonable evidence of an "Infinite Intelligence" in the universe. He wrote to her, "The truest priest of this 'Infinite Intelligence' is . . . the patient, open-minded, honest worker in science. It is the latter who is striving with infinite pains to learn something" (Goldberger to Mary Farrar, letter fragments, 1906).

With science as his adopted faith, Goldberger immersed himself in the business of fighting disease and relieving suffering. Shortly after his marriage, Goldberger was assigned to the Hygienic Laboratory in Washington to study typhoid fever. The next year, he was sent to Texas after an outbreak of dengue fever. Again, he contracted what he studied. Then it was back to Mexico to battle typhus in Mexico City where, for the third time, Goldberger's health was compromised by the microbes he fought.

During this period, Goldberger made several important epidemiological advances, which he published for his peers. In 1909, he unscrambled the puzzle of Schamberg's disease, characterized by dramatic skin eruptions somewhat like smallpox and intense, debilitating itching. He traced the ailment to an acarine mite, a wheat-infesting creature that hid in the straw mattresses common among poor urban dwellers. Goldberger and Dr. Jay F. Schamberg visited some of the victims' dwellings and ascertained that all slept on straw mats. To test his hypothesis, Goldberger tried self-experimentation, thrusting his arm between two of the mats and keeping it there for an hour. Colleagues volunteered to sleep on the mats. The next day all observed widespread eruptions over their bodies. Goldberger's arm had an itchy red rash. After isolating the mite, Goldberger again used human volunteers to show that the mite, and not some other characteristic of the straw, was responsible for the symptoms. To the sides of his volunteers, Goldberger taped watch crystals under which he capped the mites. Rashes appeared the next day. An admiring Schamberg wrote to Goldberger, "The method employed by you to determine the specificity of the little mite is certainly ingenious, and the result appears practically conclusive'' (Shamberg to Joseph Goldberger, June 19, 1909).

In 1911, Goldberger collaborated with John F. Anderson on a study of Brill's disease, demonstrating that it was identical to typhus and that typhus was transmissible by head lice as well as body lice. In his work on measles, also done with Anderson, Goldberger learned that the disease could be transmitted to monkeys by a germ small enough to pass through a filter and that the filterable virus could be detected in a victim's buccal and nasal secretions.

In 1912, Goldberger was promoted to the rank of surgeon. The following year, he was sent to Detroit to study diphtheria. It was there that he was contacted by the surgeon general in 1914 and reassigned to head the investigation of pellagra. Pellagra, first identified among Spanish peasants in 1735 by Don Gasper Casal, a court physician, was known in Spain as *mal de la rosa*, a skin disease that Casal thought might be a kind of leprosy. In the United States, pellagra was not conclusively identified until 1907. Here, it was considered the disease of the four Ds: dermatitis, diarrhea, dementia, and death. By 1912, South Carolina alone reported 30,000 cases, with a mortality rate of 40 percent. Increasingly known as the ''scourge of the South,'' pellagra prevalence stirred southern congressmen to request that the surgeon general launch an investigation.

Goldberger's pencilings in the margins of state public health reports from Illinois and southern states as well as in essays of Italian physician Cesare Lombroso suggest that even before he headed South, this seasoned investigator of germ diseases speculated that dietary deficiency and not a microbe was at the root of the disorder. Perusing a 1909 report from the Illinois State Board of Health, Goldberger underlined the observation that staff in public institutions did not get pellagra and that health officials thought that improving patients' diets—particularly adding milk—might help.

Goldberger turned from reports to patients. Observation of pellagrins in mental hospitals, orphanages, and cotton mill towns confirmed his suspicions. Struck by the population's monotonous, largely corn-based diets, Goldberger noted that inmates of these institutions often contracted pellagra, while staff, who had access to fresh meats, eggs, and milk, did not contract the disease. He had never known germs to make such social distinctions.

Anxious to test dietary modification in human subjects as a cure for pellagra, Goldberger wrote to Surgeon General Rupert Blue, ''While confident of the accuracy of our observations and of the justice of our inferences, there is nevertheless grave doubt in my mind as to their general acceptance without some practical test or demonstration of the correctness of the corollary, namely, that no pellagra develops in those who consume a mixed, well balanced diet'' (Goldberger to Rupert Blue, September 4, 1914). Shipments of federal food to two pellagra-ridden Mississippi orphanages seemed to confirm Goldberger's hypothesis. All the children recovered.

At the Georgia State Asylum at Milledgeville, Goldberger and his assistant,

Dr. George Wheeler, isolated thirty-six white female pellagrins in a separate ward and thirty-six female African American pellagrins in another ward. The physicians then altered the diets of both groups, adding fresh milk, eggs, meat, and vegetables. A control group of thirty-two nonpellagrous women—seventeen black and fifteen white—continued on their normal diet. Fifteen of this control group developed symptoms of pellagra, whereas the seventy-two pellagrous women on the new diet recovered fully.

These practical demonstrations did not lead to general acceptance of his theory that pellagra was triggered by inadequate diet. Many physicians remained unconvinced, suggesting that bodies made healthier were generally more disease resistant. Some claimed that coincidence rather than cure explained the recovery of those who thrived on Goldberger's diet. Critics insisted that a pellagra germ was present, albeit elusive.

Aware that he needed to demonstrate the existence of a particular substance, the absence of which induced pellagra, Goldberger set out to produce pellagra in robust, vital bodies through dietary modification. With the assistance of Mississippi's governor Earl Brewer, Goldberger fed a corn-based diet to eleven prisoners at Rankin State Prison Farm in early 1915. The healthy inmates were offered pardons in exchange for participating. Six of the eleven eventually showed pellagra lesions. Interestingly, whereas late-twentieth-century critics speculate about whether Goldberger obtained informed consent of his subjects, though he appears to have done so by the standards of his era, southerners at the time were primarily critical of Brewer for agreeing to reward hardened convicts with release.

Goldberger's final experiment to persuade critics was to try to transmit the illness from pellagrins to healthy volunteers as though it were a germ disease. Fourteen friends turned out for what Goldberger termed his "filth parties," to which the doctor added himself and his wife. On April 26, 1916, Goldberger injected five cubic centimeters of a pellagrin's blood into Wheeler's shoulder. Wheeler, in turn, shot six milliliters into Goldberger's shoulder. Then they swabbed out the secretions from a patient's nose and throat and applied the swabs to their own. Other secretions were ingested in pills. No one got pellagra.

Encouraged, Goldberger continued feeding experiments at the Public Health Service's pellagra hospital in Spartanburg, South Carolina, and at the Georgia State Asylum at Milledgeville in an attempt to determine exactly which nutrient was missing from pellagrins' diets. Epidemiological studies in South Carolina mill villages conducted with statistician Edgar Sydenstricker provided unprecedented statistical detail on diet, illness, housing, sanitary conditions, and economic status where pellagra was prevalent. Except for a brief reassignment during World War I to study influenza, Goldberger would devote the rest of his life to pellagra studies.

Most physicians acknowledged that Goldberger's bold experiments had established pellagra as a nutritional deficiency rather than a germ disease. He was even nominated for the Nobel Prize. But many southerners, especially those congressmen who had first appealed to the surgeon general for help, remained adamantly opposed to Goldberger's findings. Pellagra as a dietary deficiency logically became a disease of poverty; the diagnosis stood as a scathing indictment of a region scrambling for political parity and anxious to seem economically dynamic to outside investors.

Goldberger was outspoken in his criticism of the southern economy. As cotton prices plummeted in the early 1920s, Goldberger blasted sharecropping and an agricultural system that impoverished families and militated against growing diversified food crops. Likewise, he attacked mill owners for paying such low wages that workers were unable to afford a balanced diet. South Carolina congressman Jimmy Byrnes took his protests all the way to the desk of President Warren G. Harding in the summer of 1921, but the president stood by the Public Health Service.

By 1925, Goldberger had learned that consuming small amounts of dried yeast could prevent pellagra as easily as milk, meat, and vegetables. He continued to speak of a pellagra-preventive, or P-P, factor, which he now speculated might be associated with vitamin B. Discovering that black tongue disease was the canine equivalent of pellagra, he worked with dogs as well as rats at the Hygienic Laboratory to isolate the nutritional factor at the root of pellagra. Meanwhile, his assistants continued to monitor the diets of humans at the Milledgeville asylum. Always, Goldberger remained cautious in his claims, never exceeding what he could precisely demonstrate.

Creative and precise in the laboratory and in the field, Goldberger nonetheless was wildly impatient with those who ignored his pellagrin demonstrations. To a man who embraced rational inquiry as his personal religion, it was unfathomable that southern business leaders, politicians, and even physicians could dispute hard scientific evidence and continue to argue a germ theory of pellagra. Never was he able to understand or even partially appreciate the impulses that motivated his opponents.

When cotton prices again declined in 1926, followed by the Mississippi flood of 1927, Goldberger repeated his public criticism of the South. Pulling no punches, Goldberger and Sydenstricker wrote, "The economic status of this population is bound up in the tenant system, which, in turn, is involved in single-crop agricultural production and the speculative character of agricultural finance as it is practiced in this area, the seasonal fluctuation in income of the tenant . . . and other factors of an economic nature" (*Public Health Reports*, November 4, 1927). According to Goldberger, husband of the grandniece of the Confederacy's first lady, science could not readily undo the damage of history and human greed in the South.

In 1928, Goldberger fell gravely ill. Speaking in public for the last time, he reminded his listeners that medical science alone could never remedy social conditions, adding that "the problem of pellagra is in the main a problem of poverty" (*Journal of the American Dietetic Association*, March 1929). He died of hypernephroma, a rare form of cancer, on January 17, 1929. He was cremated and his ashes sprinkled over the Potomac River as Rabbi Abram Simon of the Washington Hebrew Congregation chanted the Kaddish. Not long afterward, niacin was identified as the pellagra preventive factor. In 1937, researchers working with Conrad A. Elvehjem discovered that a deficiency of nicotinic acid caused black tongue in dogs. Dr. Tom Spies used nicotinic acid to treat pellagra patients in Cincinnati and Alabama. Subsequently, researchers at Tulane University learned that the amino acid tryptophan was a precursor to niacin. Recommended daily allowances were developed, and today pellagra has all but vanished, with rare outbreaks reported in parts of Africa and India.

Dr. Joseph Goldberger's epidemiology skillfully combined pathbreaking medical experimentation with acute observation of social conditions. As such, his work has become emblematic of modern public health in the United States. Likewise, Goldberger's efforts provoked a classic collision between medical science and social resistance. For this reason, his life continues to be of compelling interest to both historians and contemporary health practitioners alike.

BIBLIOGRAPHY

There are major collections of Joseph Goldberger's papers in the Southern History Collection at the University of North Carolina (UNC), Chapel Hill, and in the Goldberger/ Sebrell Collection at the Vanderbilt University Medical Archives. The former includes the extensive correspondence of Joseph and Mary Goldberger that spanned their marriage. Other major sources are the papers in Record Group (RG) 90 of the U.S. National Archives and the smaller collection at the National Library of Medicine in Bethesda. The latter includes a set of state public health reports on pellagra with Goldberger's marginal notes and underlinings. Direct quotations in this text are from the following manuscripts: Wyman, Walter to Edgar Farrar, December 30, 1905, Box 1, Folder 4, Goldberger Papers, UNC; Joseph Goldberger to Mary Farrar, letter fragments, 1906, Box 1, Folder 6, Goldberger Papers, UNC; Jay F. Shamberg to Joseph Goldberger, June 19, 1909, Box 1, Folder 9, Goldberger Papers, UNC; Joseph Goldberger to Rupert Blue, September 4, 1914, RG 90, National Archives. See also Joseph Goldberger and Edgar Sydenstricker, "Pellagra in the Mississippi Flood Area," *Public Health Reports*, November 4, 1927, pp. 2706–2725. Reprint 1187, quotation on p. 18; and Joseph Goldberger, "Pellagra," *Journal of the American Dietetic Association* 4 (1929): 227. Goldberger spoke to the association on October 31, 1928.

Writings by Joseph Goldberger

Joseph Goldberger was a prodigious writer. Most of his work was published in *Public Health Reports*. Especially important pieces on pellagra are readily available in the collection edited by Milton Terris. See also the collections edited by Richard V. Kasius and by Kenneth J. Carpenter.

Goldberger on Pellagra. Edited by Milton Terris. Baton Rouge: Louisiana State University Press, 1964. (This collection includes a bibliography of pellagra publications by Goldberger and collaborators such as Edgar Sydenstricker and George Wheeler.)

Writings about Joseph Goldberger and Related Topics

Beardsley, Edward H. *A History of Neglect: Health Care for Blacks and Mill Workers in the Twentieth-Century South.* Knoxville, TN: University of Tennessee Press, 1987.

Carpenter, Kenneth J., ed. *Pellagra.* Stroudsburg, PA: Hutchinson Ross Publishing Company, 1981.

Cobb, Mary Katherine. "An Epidemic of Pride: Pellagra and the Culture of the American South." *Anthropologica* 34 (1992): 89–103.

De Kruif, Paul. *Hunger Fighters.* New York: Harcourt, Brace and Co., 1928. (De Kruif* included a chapter on Goldberger, whom he had met and interviewed. It is written in the author's typically breezy style, with ample literary license.)

Elmore, Joann G., and Alavan R. Feinstein. "Joseph Goldberger: An Unsung Hero of American Clinical Epidemiology." *Annals of Internal Medicine* 121 (September 1994): 372–375.

Etheridge, Elizabeth. *The Butterfly Caste: A Social History of Pellagra in the South.* Westport, CT: Greenwood Press, 1972.

———. "Pellagra: An Unappreciated Reminder of Southern Distinctiveness." In Todd L. Savitt and James Harvey Young, eds., *Disease and Distinctiveness in the American South*, pp. 100–119. Knoxville, TN: University of Tennessee Press, 1988.

Kasius, Richard V. *The Challenge of Facts, Selected Public Health Papers of Edgar Sydenstricker.* New York: Prodist, 1974.

Oshinsky, David M. *"Worse Than Slavery:" Parchman Farm and the Ordeal of Jim Crow Justice.* New York: Free Press, 1996.

Parson, Robert P. *Trail to Light, a Biography of Joseph Goldberger.* Indianapolis: Bobbs-Merrill, 1943. (Currently the only full-length biography of Goldberger, this book lacks footnotes or endnotes and contains a variety of errors and exaggerations. It was written by a navy physician with the encouragement of Mary Farrar Goldberger.)

Roe, Daphne A. *A Plague of Corn: The Social History of Pellagra.* Ithaca, NY: Cornell University Press, 1973.

Rosenberg, Charles. "Joseph Goldberger." In Charles Coulston Gillespie, ed., *Dictionary of Scientific Biography*, pp. 451–453. New York: Charles Scribner's Sons, 1972.

Schultz, Myron G. "Joseph Goldberger and Pellagra." *American Journal of Tropical Medicine and Hygiene* 26 (1977): 1088–1092.

Ward, Jr., Thomas G. "The Campaign Against Pellagra in Upstate South Carolina." In Peter Becker, ed., *Proceedings of the South Carolina Historical Association*, pp. 15–23. Columbia: University of South Carolina Press, 1994.

Alan M. Kraut

WILLIAM CRAWFORD GORGAS
(1854–1920)

William Crawford Gorgas, military physician and renowned public health advocate, was born October 3, 1854, in Toulminville, Alabama, the first of six children of Amelia Gayle and U.S. Army captain Josiah Gorgas. On his mother's side, he was the grandson of John Gayle, once governor of Alabama, representative to Congress, and federal judge. His paternal grandparents were Joseph Gorgas and Sophia Atkinson of Meyerstown, Pennsylvania. Captain Gorgas, who had moved his family to Augusta, Maine, and then to Charleston, South Carolina, considered his first child bright, serious, and tolerably mischievous. In April 1861, young Willie and his mother heard the guns of Fort Sumter starting the Civil War. Captain Gorgas made the painful decision to resign from the federal army and join the Confederacy. Jefferson Davis appointed him a brigadier in charge of the Confederate ordnance. The family moved to Richmond, Virginia, capital of the Confederacy, for the duration of the war. William attended the Mistress Mumford Academy, but he was not a very good student. A fire at the arsenal forced the family to move; Brigadier Gorgas went south to Confederate headquarters, while his wife and children lived with relatives in Baltimore, Maryland.

After the war, Josiah Gorgas invested his savings in a blast furnace to make pig iron, but the business did not prosper, and he gladly accepted the presidency of the University of the South in Sewanee, Tennessee, where William Gorgas became a dedicated, award-winning student and a fine athlete. Gorgas, who had always hoped to become an army officer like his father, was greatly disappointed when, in 1875, his application to West Point was rejected. Humbly, Josiah Gorgas made an appeal to his schoolmate and former enemy, President Grant, but the gesture was not successful. After considerable divagation, William accepted his father's suggestion to study law. He went to New Orleans as a guest of his uncle, Thomas Gayne, and diligently applied himself to the study of contracts, torts, and jurisprudence. After one year he admitted that he was not cut out for the law and returned home. The town's physician, Hiram Bartholomew, pointed out that the medical corps provided access to the army, and he offered financial assistance.

In 1876, Gorgas went to New York and registered at the Bellevue Hospital Medical School. The medical profession soon enthralled him and gave him plenty of opportunities for his natural altruism. In August 1878, Memphis, Tennessee, was struck by an appalling yellow fever epidemic. Gorgas and six of his classmates obtained permission to offer their services, but they were turned away by a citizens' committee at the edge of town, because they were not "acclimated" and would only add their names to the grim list of dead physicians in the city. In his last year of school, Gorgas was privileged to have the opportunity to study the nascent science of bacteriology with William Welch (1850–1934). In June 1879 Gorgas received his M.D. degree, and, with some help from his uncle, managed to serve a one-year unpaid internship at Bellevue.

In June 1880, Gorgas passed his examinations and was offered a commission as lieutenant in the U.S. Army Medical Corps. During his first assignment, in southwest Texas, he served at several forts along the Mexican border. During the summer of 1882, while he was at Fort Brown, yellow fever broke out in Matamoros just south of the Rio Grande; eventually cases occurred in Brownsville and in the fort. Disregarding orders, Gorgas deliberately walked into the restricted, "infected" areas of the garrison and performed an autopsy on a yellow fever victim; he was arrested and ordered to move to the "contaminated" area. Within a short time he, as well as others in the "safe" area, including the commander of the fort, came down with the fever. While recovering, Gorgas met frequently with another convalescent, Marie Cook Doughty, the commander's sister-in-law. Eventually they were married and moved to Fort Randall in North Dakota, where Gorgas was promoted to captain. Their first child was born there, but the baby boy lived for only a few hours.

In 1888, Gorgas was transferred to Fort Barrancas near Pensacola, Florida. Yellow fever had developed in Florida, but Gorgas was now immune. For the first time, he was responsible for making administrative decisions that might quell the spread of the disease, which was generally thought to be spread by miasmas, that is, contaminated air. Marie, attended by her mother-in-law in Tuscaloosa, delivered a baby girl in 1890. In 1892, Gorgas was temporarily assigned to the office of the adjutant surgeon general in New York. Six months later the country was at war, and Gorgas was at work outfitting the hospital ship *Relief* in which he left in June 1898 for Siboney, east of Santiago, Cuba. There he found numerous unattended, wounded soldiers and even more suffering from yellow fever. The medical authorities, including Gorgas, decided to burn the straw-thatched *bohíos* in the village of Siboney. A yellow fever hospital, consisting of army tents for about eight hundred patients, was erected two miles away. While directing the hospital, Gorgas received his promotion to major.

Gorgas contracted malaria and was hospitalized at Camp Wikoff in Montauk, Long Island. Marie was amazed at his loss of weight and even more so at his depressed spirits. After a short time he regained confidence and enlisted to be sent back to Cuba, where he was put in charge of Military Hospital Number One in Havana. General Leonard Wood, governor of Cuba, appointed Gorgas chief of sanitation for the city of Havana. With the wholehearted cooperation of its citizens, Gorgas undertook radical measures for cleaning and disinfecting the city's streets, alleys, and yards. It was said that he made Havana one of the cleanest cities in the world. Paradoxically, yellow fever increased and was worse in the cleanest quarters. Gorgas met, almost daily, with Dr. Carlos Finlay,* who argued that sanitation efforts should focus on the destruction of mosquito breeding sites. As he admitted later, Gorgas did not accept Finlay's concepts, but, unlike most others, he came to appreciate his wisdom and depth of knowledge. In the summer of 1900, a U.S. Army board, with Walter Reed as chairman, was appointed to verify claims of a bacterial cause of yellow fever; this theory was promptly disproved.

To test Finlay's mosquito theory, two members of the board submitted to bites by infected mosquitoes; both developed the disease, and one of them, Jesse W. Lazear, died, indicating that the mosquito was the intermediate agent of yellow fever. A grant, made available by General Wood, permitted members of the board to stage a well-planned, controlled experiment with human volunteers that proved Finlay right. Gorgas immediately put Finlay's preventive measures into practice. Any reported case of yellow fever was rapidly transported in a screened ambulance and placed in a screened room, thus eliminating a source of infected blood for mosquitoes, and the patient's house was fumigated. Gorgas's *Stegomyia* Brigades, named for the yellow fever mosquito, invaded all sections of the city, draining pools and gutters, eliminating flower pots in homes and cemeteries, covering cisterns, and eliminating the waters in which the culprit laid its eggs.

Six months later, the last case of yellow fever in Havana, where the disease had been endemic for over two hundred years, was recorded. When Gorgas was reproached by Reed for giving much of the credit to Finlay, Gorgas wrote back that Finlay was "an old trump, as modest and kindly as he is true. His reasoning for selecting the Stegomyia is the best piece of logical reasoning to be found in medicine."

Gorgas, who had been rewarded for his work in Cuba with a promotion to the rank of colonel, realized that his experience could be valuable in overcoming the major obstacle to the construction of the Panama Canal, and he brought this idea to the attention of the surgeon general, George M. Sternberg. The French attempt to build the canal had failed—not because of any lack of engineering skills but because of the remarkable mortality among the officers and workers caused by yellow fever and malaria, estimated at twenty thousand in eight years. In March 1904, Gorgas was appointed chief sanitary officer for the Panama Canal Zone. He took along five capable and dedicated associates. However, their work was obstructed by bureaucratic red tape and the ignorance of the commissioners. The Sanitary Department's requests for large amounts of disinfectants and wire screens, as well as the number of field servants who were employed, were considered excessive. Nevertheless, the fight against *Stegomyia*, the yellow fever mosquito, was successful. By the fall of 1906, no cases of yellow fever were reported. However, *Anopheles*, the malarial mosquito, presented great difficulties. Gorgas's associate Joseph L. Le Prince successfully attacked the mosquito in the swamps, marshes, and underbrush. The Sanitary Department was responsible for more than fifty square miles divided into twenty-five districts, as well as two major hospitals outside the zone—one in

Colón on the Caribbean coast and another in Panama City (Ancón) on the Pacific coast—and several emergency hospitals. In operating these hospitals, Gorgas was greatly assisted by John W. Ross of the U.S. Navy, Henry Rose Carter of the U.S. Public Health Service, and Louis A. LaGarde, U.S. Army. Gorgas and his wife lived in Panama for ten years.

In 1907, Gorgas was appointed a member of the Isthmian Canal Commission, and President Roosevelt praised his work in a message to Congress. In 1908, Gorgas was elected president of the American Medical Association. When his work in Panama was coming to an end, he was asked to go to Rhodesia to give his advice about malaria and pneumonia in diamond mine workers. Upon his return to the United States, he was awarded a doctor of science degree by Oxford University. In 1914, President Wilson appointed him surgeon general of the U.S. Army with the rank of brigadier general. One year later he was promoted to major general by a special act of Congress. The Health Board of the Rockefeller Foundation appointed him chief of a special Yellow Fever Commission charged to study and provide advice about the eradication of all remaining foci of yellow fever in South America. Traveling to several countries and Caribbean islands, Gorgas, Juan Guiteras, and Henry Carter were successful in suggesting the necessary measures.

Anticipating the entrance of the United States into World War I, Gorgas reorganized and reinforced the U.S. Army Medical Corps. In 1920, he received the Harbin Medal at the International Congress of Hygiene in Brussels. Upon his return, he suffered a paralytic stroke and was hospitalized in London. King George V visited him in the hospital and presented him with the insignia of Knight Commander of the Order of Saint Michael and Saint George. General Gorgas died peacefully on July 4, 1920; he was transported to Washington and interred at Arlington National Cemetery.

BIBLIOGRAPHY

Philip Showalter Hench (1896–1965), Nobel Laureate, professor of medicine, University of Minnesota, and chief of rheumatology at the Mayo Clinic, collected the letters and other memorabilia of Jesse Lazear, including his field microscope. Although Hench felt that his collection should not be entrusted to the University of Virginia, the alma mater of Walter Reed, his wife and brother-in-law did just that after his untimely death. The Hench Yellow Fever Collection is located in the Manuscript Division of the Claude Moore Library, University of Virginia, Charlottesville, Virginia. Reed's letter of January 31, 1902, to Gorgas is held in the Denver Medical Society Library. The reply by Gorgas to Reed, dated February 6, 1902, is held by the Gorgas Collection, Graduate Library, University of Alabama, Tuscaloosa, Alabama.

Writings by William Crawford Gorgas

Sanitation in Panama. New York: Appleton and Co., 1918.

Writings about William Crawford Gorgas and Related Topics

Gorgas, Marie Doughty, and B. J. Hendrick. *William Crawford Gorgas. His Life and Work*. Philadelphia: Lea and Febiger, 1924.
Lampson, R. *Death Loses a Pair of Wings. The Epic of William Gorgas and the Conquest of Yellow Fever*. New York: Charles Scribner and Sons, 1939.

Juan A. del Regato

LEONARD GREENBURG
(1893–1991)

Leonard Greenburg, born in New York City, received a civil engineering degree from Columbia University in 1915, a Ph.D. in public health from Yale University in 1923, and an M.D. from Yale University Medical School in 1930. He considered himself an industrial hygienist; today he might be called an environmental engineer. During his long career, one that spanned over forty years, he made major contributions to industrial hygiene and to the health and safety of working men and women. Greenburg's career began during the early stages of the development of the field of industrial hygiene. He brought the skills of both physician and engineer to bear on the public health problems of industrial hygiene and air pollution.

In 1918, Greenburg became one of the first engineers in the U.S. Public Health Service (PHS). Soon after, he received his commission and became one of the first engineers to be a commissioned officer in the PHS. Greenburg later headed the New Haven Health Department. He directed the Division of Industrial Hygiene in the New York State Labor Department (1935–1952), became the first commissioner of New York City Air Pollution Control (1952–1960), and was professor of preventive medicine and community health at Albert Einstein College of Medicine (1960–1969).

Greenburg is best known as co-inventor of the Greenburg-Smith impinger, an instrument designed to measure dust in air, which has been utilized by industrial hygienists for over forty years. In a 1988 interview, Greenburg explained how he had come to invent the impinger:

Shortly after I began [as an engineer in the Public Health Service] we found that the method we were using for counting industrial dust did not check with the method used by the United States Bureau of Mines. So Winslow and I wrote a letter to the Director of the Bureau of Mines. They were using a method they had gotten from South Africa called the sugar tube method. This sugar tube method consisted of sampling the air through a layer of granulated sugar, then dissolving it in hot water, and getting the dust that way and counting it. Their results did not correspond with ours at all. I never made any pretense that ours was any good because it wasn't, but I didn't know anything about theirs. We used a method devised by a fellow named George T. Palmer, who was in the public health field. Ours was a very inefficient way of washing the dust out of the air. So we wrote to a fellow named Arnold Fieldner, who was director of the Bureau of Mines station in Pittsburgh, and we suggested that we do a cooperative study. I went to Pittsburgh and spent three or four months. They assigned a young fellow to work with me whose name was George Smith. Smith was one of those precocious young men. He was a brilliant guy. He had a terrific fund of knowledge and he was a pleasure to work with. And while we were working together on these instruments, we also used another one that came from the Heating and Ventilating Society which used filter paper. I got the idea for the impinger. George says let's try it out. The station was remarkable. There were facilities for doing everything. And we tried it out, and we arrived at the answer. It was the impinger. And that was good in these days and I think it is still good. . . . It gained wide acceptance at that time because it was useful. (Corn 1989: 157–158)

In a 1952 lecture, Greenburg also recalled inventing the impinger: "The problem of appraising the degree of hazard of the dusty environment developed into extensive studies and eventuated in a joint study by the Bureau of Mines and the Public Health Service in the summer of 1922. From this emerged the development of the impinger dust sampling instrument. With all its shortcomings it has served as a useful tool" (Greenburg 1952: 95–104). By the 1930s, the study of dust, including sampling of airborne dust, statistical aspects of particle size, design of dust control systems, and the development of principles of industrial ventilation, had been stimulated by the problems associated with industrial dust, which had become a major occupational health concern.

When Greenburg began industrial hygiene work in 1916, both industrial hygiene and occupational health were considered part of the field of public health. Soon after graduating from Columbia University, Greenburg moved to New Haven to work as an industrial engineer. Here he met C. A. E. Winslow, professor of public health at Yale, who was interested in occupational health. Winslow greatly influenced Greenburg's career; he guided Greenburg's Ph.D. studies and his dissertation. A close bond developed between the two men, and they worked together for many years. Winslow introduced Greenburg to Anthony Lanza, a young physician in the PHS. Lanza brought Greenburg into the PHS as one of its first engineers. While in the PHS, Greenburg together with Winslow, conducted numerous investigations into health conditions in local industries. Their results appeared in *Public Health Reports*, published by the PHS.

One of Greenburg's early assignments after he received his Ph.D. was to investigate sanitary conditions on Ellis Island. He also studied the ventilation of the Capitol Building in Washington, D.C. The PHS reassigned Greenburg to Yale to earn an M.D., which he completed in 1930. In 1932, Greenburg became associate director of the John B. Pierce Laboratory of Hygiene in New Haven. There he studied physiological requirements for ventilation in enclosed spaces and served as health commissioner for the city of New Haven.

Greenburg began his career at the beginning of a transition period in occupational health. In the United States, official interest in industrial accidents and occupational diseases, as well as efforts to understand and control them, began in the first decade of the twentieth century (Corn 1992: 1–22). Hazards to health and safety were many—primitive in nature and large in magnitude. Occupational diseases long known but little understood, such as silicosis, plumbism, phosphorus poisoning, and mercurialism, occurred frequently in workplaces that lacked adequate ventilation and sanitary facilities. Statistical information as to the extent of occupational disease in the United States and scientific studies of factory conditions were minimal and inadequate. Indeed, the first American text-books on occupational health had only recently appeared.

A few notable exceptions did exist. For example, when Greenburg began working for the PHS in 1916, Crystal Eastman had already investigated accidents in Allegheny County, Pennsylvania, for the Russell Sage Foundation (Eastman 1916). Eastman sought indications of responsibility for the material loss and privation experienced by injured workers and their families and concluded from her study that workers were not responsible for accidents. She discovered that in one year (1906–1907) in one county (Allegheny), industrial accidents had caused the deaths of 526 men. Their survivors usually received little or no compensation. Eastman sought enactment of workmen's compensation laws. Alice Hamilton conducted a survey of industrial disease in Illinois in 1910, the first survey of its kind in the United States. She pioneered the fields of occupational medicine and industrial toxicology, helped document the extent of occupational disease in the United States, and became assistant professor of industrial medicine at Harvard University. Frederick Hoffman, the author of *Industrial Accident Statistics* (1915), a publication of the U.S. Department of Labor, documented, as far as possible for the time, industrial accident statistics. Hoffman himself noted the lack of trustworthy industrial accident statistics due to the absence of uniform requirements for reporting in the various states (Hoffman 1915).

The few agencies of the federal government concerned with occupational safety and health, though often only in a peripheral manner, included the Department of Labor (established in 1913), the Bureau of Mines (established in 1910), the Children's Bureau (established in 1912), and the Office of Industrial Hygiene and Sanitation (established in 1914 and later called the Division of Occupational Health in the PHS). Nevertheless, protection of industrial workers' health and safety was considered the responsibility of state and local governments, although prior to 1935 only five state health departments conducted sustained industrial hygiene activity. Massachusetts and New York State had industrial hygiene units in their state labor departments.

The American Association of Labor Legislation (founded in 1906) conducted investigations, held conferences, published reports, and drafted bills to secure enactment of progressive standards into law. Organizations such as the National Council for Industrial Safety, the Industrial Hygiene section of the American Public Health Association, and the American Association of Industrial Physicians and Surgeons were organized in 1913, 1914, and 1916, respectively. In 1918, Harvard University began to offer instruction in industrial hygiene. In this setting, Greenburg participated with a small group in the development of the new discipline of industrial hygiene. The work was new and exciting and the need for remedial action great.

By 1935, when Greenburg became director of the Division of Industrial Hygiene in the New York State Labor Department, his early work and education had prepared him well for the job. In the same year, the newly enacted Social

Security Act allocated funds to the PHS for research and grants-in-aid to states for public health work, including industrial hygiene. Social security funds were given to the states by the PHS. In an effort to channel these funds, the PHS inaugurated a program to develop industrial hygiene in health departments in the states. The money caused a burst of activity. By 1936, seventeen industrial hygiene units existed in the states, and by 1938, the number rose to twenty-six. The 1936 budget of $100,000 climbed to nearly $750,000 in 1938. The New York State effort, under Greenburg's direction, contained the largest number of workers (over 5 million, with almost 2 million of them in mining and manufacturing industries). New York State employed the largest number of personnel in industrial hygiene: seven physicians, seven engineers, twelve technicians, and seven clerical. It also had the largest budget: $118,614 (Bloomfield 1938).

Frances Perkins, the state industrial commissioner, who later became secretary of labor in Franklin D. Roosevelt's cabinet, founded the Division of Industrial Hygiene in New York State in 1924. Under Greenburg's leadership, the division flourished. His staff of leading occupational health professionals (chemists, physicians, and engineers) included Leonard Goldwater, Arthur Stern, William Harris, Theodore Hatch, and Joseph Dalla Valle.

Before Greenburg became director of the New York State Division of Industrial Hygiene, it had no regular program of plant surveys and evaluations by industrial hygienists. Under Greenburg, the division organized and conducted field studies and engineering activities, which included writing codes for the regulation of hazardous work conditions in industry. There was widespread concern over dust hazards in industries such as foundries, stone crushing, glass manufacturing, potteries, other ceramic plants, mining, quarrying, tunneling, and building foundation construction. The division carried out a program of dust control, environmental monitoring, and medical surveillance. Under Greenburg, an able administrator, the New York State Division of Industrial Hygiene made great strides. While serving as director of the Division of Industrial Hygiene, Greenburg worked on a number of committees of the International Labor Organization, the World Health Organization, the American Public Health Association, the American Conference of Governmental Industrial Hygienists, and the American Industrial Hygiene Association.

A major shift in emphasis in industrial hygiene had begun in the late 1920s and continued into the 1930s. During its early days, industrial hygiene focused on industrial medicine. Industrial hygiene in the 1930s stressed the nonmedical contributions of the physical sciences and engineering to occupational health. Greenburg was involved in the changes that occurred in the practice of industrial hygiene and occupational medicine that began in the 1930s. For example, in the 1930s and 1940s industrial hygiene and occupational medicine professionals developed the concept of dose response, which implied measurement of dose and response and the relation between them. It is still understood that a systematic dose-response relation between the severity of exposure to the hazard and the degree of response in the population exposed exists and that a decrease in the level of exposure corresponds with a gradual decline in the risk of injury. The risk becomes negligible when the exposure falls below a certain acceptable level. Analysis and measurement of environmental factors are implied in the dose-response concept. A major stride in environmental analysis was made when Greenburg and G. W. Smith combined the principle of collecting dust by impingement with a water-washing or bubbling method to construct the impinger for use in environmental analysis. The impinger, which took dust out of a measured amount of air so that dust particles could be counted, remained the standard dust collection method for over forty years.

The corollary to measuring airborne hazards (dust) and analyzing environmental factors in the workplace was determining the concentration of a material that would not cause injury—in other words, determining the concentrations at which individuals were exposed but not injured, a process that implies the existence of a standard. Greenburg chaired the Committee on Technical Standards for the American Conference of Governmental Industrial Hygienists in 1941 when that committee was divided into two subcommittees: one on technical standards and the other on threshold limits. What we now refer to as TLVs (threshold limit values) were begun and developed by the threshold limits subcommittee, later called the TLV Committee. The TLVs became the basis to provide a standard for workplace conditions pertaining to airborne toxic materials when no other guidelines existed. Thus, two of the most important contributions Greenburg made were in the field of instrumentation and measurement, which made it possible to quantitate contaminants in air, and in the early development of standards based on quantitative dust studies.

In 1952, Greenburg became the first commissioner of New York City Air Pollution Control. He was appointed by Mayor Vincent Impelliteri and twice reappointed by Mayor Robert Wagner. As commissioner, Greenburg built a laboratory for air pollution control and set up the first systematic air sampling program directed by Morris Jacob. As the first commissioner, Greenburg began the difficult task of developing priorities, educating the public, obtaining data, and developing compliance codes and the means to enforce them. Commissioner Greenburg warned New Yorkers of impending environmental dangers, such as increasing air pollution.

Greenburg spent his last nine working years as professor of preventive medicine and community health at Albert Einstein College. Throughout his career, Greenburg had been a leader in industrial hygiene, air pollution, and public health practice. He was also active in the two industrial hygiene professional organizations, the American Conference of Governmental Industrial Hygienists and the American Industrial Hygiene Association, organized in 1938 and 1939, respectively. In the late 1930s, Greenburg was a member of the Konicide Club. Its membership included practically everyone with a research interest in silicosis and dust hazards. The Konicide Club disbanded with the founding of the American Industrial Hygiene Association. In 1952, Greenburg received the American Industrial Hygiene Association's most prestigious award, the Cummings Award.

By the time Greenburg retired in 1969, after forty-three active years as an occupational and environmental health professional, a great deal had occurred, and he had been a participant in bringing about this change. Both occupational medicine and industrial hygiene became recognized professional endeavors, and the need for air pollution control accepted and acted upon. Occupational and environmental health activities were also accepted as responsibilities of the federal government. The scientific underpinnings for occupational safety and health had been well developed. Most important, during Greenburg's lifetime, the concept of risk to health and safety associated with both the occupational and non-occupational environment had undergone profound change. The idea that prevention and control can minimize and in some cases even eliminate risk replaced the old idea that accidents and diseases are unavoidable by-products of work. In 1970, one year after Greenburg retired, the U.S. Congress passed the Occupational Safety and Health Act and the National Environmental Protection Act, and it organized the Environmental Protection Agency. It is fair to say that Leonard Greenburg's work was in many ways responsible for these changes.

BIBLIOGRAPHY

Writings by Leonard Greenburg

"Cummings Memorial Address." *Industrial Hygiene Quarterly* 13, no. 2 (June 1952): 95–104.

Writings about Leonard Greenburg and Related Topics

Bloomfield, J. J. "Development of Industrial Hygiene in the United States." *American Journal of Public Health* 28 (December 1938): 1388–1397.
Corn, Jacqueline. *Protecting the Health of Workers: The American Conference of Governmental Industrial Hygienists 1938–1988.* Cincinnati, OH: ACGIH, 1989.
———. *Response to Occupational Health Hazards.* New York: Van Nostrand Reinhold, 1992. (For a discussion of the transition period in occupational health in the United States, see chapter 1.)
Eastman, Crystal. *Work Accidents and the Law.* The Pittsburgh Survey. New York: Russell Sage Foundation, 1916.
Hamilton, Alice. *Exploring the Dangerous Trades.* Boston: Little, Brown, 1943.
Hoffman, Frederick. *Industrial Accident Statistics.* U.S. Department of Labor Bulletin 157. Washington, D.C.: Government Printing Office, 1915.

Jacqueline Karnell Corn

CORDELIA AGNES GREENE
(1831–1905)

Cordelia Agnes Greene, pioneer woman physician and health spa entrepreneur, was born in Lyons, New York, on July 5, 1831, the first child of Dr. Jabez Greene and his wife, Phila Cook Greene. Dr. Jabez Greene was never identified as M.D. in the literature, suggesting that his professional claims probably came about through apprenticeship only. Although both parents came from a long line of New England Quakers, they married ''out-of-meeting'' and later attended Methodist and then Presbyterian churches. But they did instill Quaker values in their children.

Cordelia was a frisky, stout child, occasionally subject to moodiness, who enjoyed the outdoor life and natural beauty of the region surrounding her family's farm. Her father served as a trustee of the Lyons public school, and Cordelia attended and worked diligently at her studies to maintain his favor. At sixteen she received a teacher's certificate from the county and taught school for several sessions. The family finally settled on a farm in Castile, New York, when Cordelia was eighteen.

Jabez Greene bought and renovated a tavern in Castile to set up a water cure sanitarium. Patterned on Vincent Priesnitz's water cure sanitarium in Austria, the facility drew cold, clear spring water from the nearby stream, which was carried to reservoirs on top of the building and then ran through a series of pipes to spray down on the clients for a variety of prescribed therapeutic baths. Exercise rooms contained India rubber balls, hoops, a melodeon, and other amenities for physical movement. The surrounding grounds were landscaped and made inviting for brisk walks and outdoor games.

When the sanitarium was opened in 1850, Cordelia was her father's chief assistant. She discovered that she loved nursing and caring for the sick. When she read in the newspaper that a woman had received a diploma from a New York State medical school, she questioned her father if she might do the same thing. He had no objections and thought she was especially suited to such a plan, although he warned her, ''It may be a pleasant thing to study medicine, but it is quite another thing to practice it.'' It is unclear why the Greenes did not consider a sectarian medical school such as Central Medical College in nearby Rochester. Other women closely aligned to the leading hydropathists, such as Rachel Brooks Gleason, wife of Dr. Silas Gleason of the famous Glen Haven Water Cure, were being welcomed as students at these institutions. Greene's avoidance of the sectarian schools is especially curious when it becomes clear later that Greene did not intend to reject the therapeutics she had learned from her father. In retrospect, it can be seen that in her own practice, she expanded on her early experience, adopting an eclectic mix of hydropathy, regular medicine, and religious zeal to develop her unique style.

Jabez Greene continued to support his daughter's plan, but his indebtedness left him with little financial encouragement to offer her. Using the money she earned from nursing at the family spa for her tuition, Greene spent one full session in 1854 at the Female Medical College of Pennsylvania (FMCP) in Philadelphia. She completed her second and concluding session at the Cleveland Medical College (CMC), the medical department of Western Reserve College in Cleveland, where her enrollment was assisted by her father's friend Henry Foster, M.D. Dr. Foster, a graduate of CMC (1848), was a hydropathist and the founder and proprietor of the Clifton Springs Water Cure. He persuaded Dr. T. T. Seelye, influential proprietor of the Cleveland Water Cure, to invite Greene to live and work at his establishment as a hydropathist while earning money toward her CMC tuition. That no objection by the faculty of the regular medical school or by her peers was ever raised regarding Greene's close association with and practice of hydropathy is testimony to her intelligence, skill, and keen sense for negotiation.

As the 1855–1856 session began at CMC, for the first time anywhere, four women, including Cordelia Greene, sat in classrooms with dozens of men for the formal study of regular medicine. One classmate recalled that some of the male students had delivered a petition to the faculty asking for the removal of the women from their classes. However, a sympathetic and supportive dean with a commitment to reform held firm, and the session proceeded without profound difficulties. The four women formed a study group, and engaged in friendly competition with their thirty-eight male classmates that produced an unusually high proportion of commendable graduation theses from this class. Greene graduated with honors.

In her graduation thesis on treating prolapsed uterus, Greene strongly advocated preventive measures, clearly and boldly proposing that avoidance of the social causes, rather than medical intervention, was the best remediation of this painful condition. She called for "radical reform in dress . . . employment for the daughters of opulence . . . a better physiological education among women, the faithful discharge of the duties devolving upon all Mothers; to teach their children early, the principles of chastity and of pure morality." In a scathing tone she insisted that such social issues were as much the province of the true physician as were "those means more properly considered as curative" (Greene 1856: 11, 12).

None of the early women medical students appeared more vulnerable to censure than Greene, because she was associated with hydropathy, one of the reformist irregular approaches to health care and actually earning her tuition money through employment at a water cure establishment. Nonetheless, Greene's practice of hydropathy drew no penalty from the faculty. They may have been impressed with her self-confidence and knowledge, even as she challenged them in her essay to consider preventive measures to be as curative as interventive therapeutics. However, the faculty had already agreed that no more women would be admitted following the graduation of the group of four. A change in leadership was imminent in the faculty and in the policies of the new leadership. By quietly graduating the last four women and accepting applications from no others, the aged leaders—the old guard of the founding faculty of the CMC—could draw this experiment to an end without drawing needless attention to its hapless conclusion.

Inspired by the hydropathic work of her father and the success of Elizabeth Blackwell in attaining a medical degree, Greene sought a medical degree to further the healing work she had begun at her father's side. Her regular medical education only added to the storehouse of therapeutics, common sense, and evangelical enthusiasm from which she developed her own "art of keeping well." The popular health reforms that Greene advocated were prompted not only as an alternative to the harsh therapeutics engaged in by regular physicians but as a response to the changing mores and standards of the new middle class. Assigned to the "sphere of domesticity," women were denied their former roles in the economy of the family. Men assumed new kinds of professional, managerial, or unregulated industrial wage-earning jobs. Urban areas were soot laden, overcrowded, and rampant with disease. The signs and symptoms of stress-related maladies became common. Many members of the new middle class could now afford to indulge in the pursuit of health by visiting spas located in bucolic settings, which offered rest, diet, exercise, medical treatment, and distance from urban tensions.

After her graduation in 1856, Greene returned for a short time to her father's water cure spa but soon became assistant physician at Dr. Foster's Clifton Springs Sanitarium, which he had established in 1848 in a pastoral setting southeast of Rochester on the Canandaigua River. Mineral waters were utilized for treatment internally and externally, in concert with the prescribed drugs in use at the time. Greene practiced there for six years on a staff of two women and three men while also caring for her mother, until she died of a lingering illness in 1858.

When Jabez Greene died in 1864, Greene's family and the townspeople urged her to "come home." Although reluctant to accept such a challenge, after much praying and pondering, Greene agreed to return. At the age of thirty-five, Dr. Cordelia Greene became the proprietor and medical director of an established sanitarium for women and children. She began with one patient, but eventually twelve were in residence, and Greene was confident enough to invest in major improvements in the facilities.

Greene's therapeutic methods drew on a keen talent for diagnosis; uncommon common sense; regular and hydropathic therapeutics using water stored in a reservoir at the top of the building and let down for treatment with a vengeance; regimens of exercise, gymnastics, and diet; daily hygiene; enthusiastic spiritual and moral codes, including the work ethic; inculcation of self-mastery and loyalty in the patient; and, above all, deep breathing. Letters from grateful female patients reveal that Greene recognized that their symptoms of malaise and invalidism were often related less to disease than to their habitual use of the morphine, opium, and alcohol-based concoctions prescribed by regular physicians. The granddaughter of an ardent temperance pioneer, Greene waged an unrelenting campaign against an unacknowledged epidemic of addiction among women. Drawing on all of the resources of her training and personality, Greene developed a holistic program that was more than eclectic. Her inherent understanding of human nature spilled over into her methodology, and she became mother, teacher, and trusted counselor to each of her patients. Persistent questions about sexuality and family relationships led her to publish an extensive "marriage manual" in 1885, which offered advice about love, marriage, and parenting, as well as the evils of sexual overindulgence, onanism, and prostitution.

Greene's successful methods, coupled with her excellent business and administrative skills, drew an extensive clientele, and the Castile Sanitarium became widely known throughout the eastern and northeastern United States. At the height of its popularity, the spa employed a staff of eighteen people, including "reliable nurses, cooks and house-girls." Sunnycrest, a three-story house at the top of a nearby hill, served as a residence for the nurses. Over the years Greene's sanitarium became the rest haven and getaway for many major temperance and woman's rights reformers, including Mary Livermore, Anna Gordon, Elizabeth Gordon, Susan B. Anthony, Rev. Anna H. Shaw, and Alice Gordon Gulick. To these strong women, Greene became fondly known as "St. Cordelia."

If full and total control of a thriving sanitarium was not enough, the indefatigable Dr. Greene bought and maintained a large home, which she named Brookside, across the street from the sanitarium, adopted six children, and cared for an enfeebled uncle. Greene was the prototype "supermom," career woman, and business executive. Edward Greene, the youngest child, adopted in 1873 at age two and the only one to pursue medicine, recalled later that a "kind governess" helped Cordelia bring the lively nursery of children through the kindergarten stage and then assisted with tutoring them in school lessons. All the children took piano lessons and helped with the gardens. The boys were sent for instruction in the manly art of carpentry, and taught to fish and swim. There was a constant stream of visitors at Brookside, including many women reformers and William Pryor Letchworth, president of the New York State Board of Charities, who was a neighbor.

Of all the pioneer women medical graduates, Cordelia Greene became by far the wealthiest from the practice of medicine. She maintained a relationship with the women physicians who had been her classmates at the CMC and donated funds for their causes when she could. Her widely renowned business enterprise made her the largest taxpayer in the region. Her success and benevolence brought local comments that ranged from high praise—"Doctor Greene is the Queen of Castile, and the best of all is, she doesn't know it"—to disgruntlement that things might be better if "a woman didn't run the town" (Gordon 1925). In 1896 Kate Clark, a patient at the sanitarium, organized the Cordelia Greene Library Building Association among patients and many of Castile's leading women. Greene herself, long desiring that a free loan library be available for the children of the town, donated the land across from the sanitarium for this purpose and then funded the formal landscaping. A cornerstone was laid on August 11, 1902, and, when the fireproof building was completed, she donated a $15,000 endowment for its operating expenses and the purchase of books (Weiss and Kemble 1967).

During the last fifteen years of her life, Greene began to take time to travel with her companion, Elizabeth Gordon. In 1891, they sailed to Acapulco by way of the Panama Canal, followed by a voyage up the Pacific Coast. In 1896, Greene and her niece, Dr. Mary Greene, visited Cordelia's daughter Marguerite, who was teaching music at the Kamehameha mission school in Hawaii. Her last trip was in the winter of 1904–1905. Accompanied by Elizabeth Gordon, she traveled to Philadelphia to attend the convention of the National Woman's Christian Temperance Union. Greene became ill in New York City after visiting former patients in Washington, D.C., and underwent surgery at Presbyterian Hospital. She died there on January 28, 1905, surrounded by friends and several of her children. Greene was brought back to Castile for a memorial service. The local newspaper issued a special edition in her memory, reprinting testimonials and telegrams from colleagues, former students, patients, and friends from all over the country. She was buried in the Castile Cemetery near the markers of her parents and her adopted baby daughter Louise. Later, a massive boulder from the village of Pike was placed over her grave, and a bronze plaque was attached to the stone.

Demonstrating how far women physicians had progressed in one lifetime, Cordelia Greene was a member, at the time of her death, of the American Medical Association, the New York State Medical Association, the Wyoming County Medical Society, and the Physicians' League of Buffalo. Because of her exclusive clientele and position within the community, neither Greene's gender nor her novel methods appear to have hampered her progress within the profession. There is no evidence that she endured any harassment once she secured her position as owner and medical director of the Castile Sanitarium. Her sanitarium remained in operation under the direction of Dr. Mary Greene until 1954. The main structure, built as a tavern in 1831, was used by the Greene family as a health facility for over one hundred years.

BIBLIOGRAPHY

Cordelia Greene can best be known through her own writings and publications, including the marriage manual she published in 1885 and her overview of her own work, published posthumously (1906). Greene's friend, Dr. Elizabeth Gordon, published a testimonial work (1925) that contains biographical as well as autobiographical memoirs of

Greene's life and work. Readers can become familiar with general information about the dozens of water cure spas that were established in America during the nineteenth century by referring to the work of Weiss and Kemble (1967). Donegan's more recent work (1986) analyzes the popularity of water spas for women clients and how health reform was a major component of the widespread reform movement at midcentury.

Writings by Cordelia Agnes Greene

"Thesis on Prolapsus Uteri, and Other Malpositions of the Abdominal and Pelvic Viscera." Unpublished thesis, 1856. Allen Memorial Library Archives, Cleveland, Ohio.

Build Well: The Basis of Individual Home and National Elevation. Boston: D. Lothrop and Company, 1885.

The Art of Keeping Well. New York: Dodd, Mead, 1906.

Writings about Cordelia Agnes Greene and Related Topics

Donegan, Jane B. *Hydropathic Highway to Heaven: Women and the Water Cure in Antebellum America.* Westport, CT: Greenwood Press, 1986.

Gordon, Elizabeth R. *The Story of the Life and Work of Cordelia A. Greene, M.D.* Castile, NY: Castilian, 1925.

Weiss, Harry B., and Howard R. Kemble. *The Great American Water-Cure Craze: A History of Hydropathy in the United States.* Trenton, NJ: Past Times Press, 1967.

Linda Lehmann Goldstein

MADHUSUDAN GUPTA
(1800?–1856)

Madhusudan Gupta was a Bengali *vaidya* (a man of the medical caste) who played a critical role in the introduction of "Western" (British) medicine into Southeast Asia. Information about his life is often sketchy and even contradictory, but an examination of his life and times, with special reference to formal medical teaching in Calcutta, in the province of Bengal, British India, provides considerable insight into the development of medicine in nineteenth-century India. In 1690, the (British) East India Company established a "factory" (trading post) in Bengal, in the village of Calcutta. The British presence increased rapidly, until conflict between local rulers and the British became inevitable. In 1757, the British overcame the nawab or king of Bengal and in effect established their own political regime. By the early nineteenth century, Britain controlled large areas of the Indian subcontinent.

There were three organized medical systems in use in British Bengal in the mid-nineteenth century. The native population was largely treated by the *Hakims* of the *Unani* (*Tibbi* or Greco-Arabic or Muslim) system, or by the *vaidyas*, practitioners of Ayurveda (the Sanskrit or Hindu system). The resident English and the army personnel were treated by British doctors trained in Western medicine in the British schools. However, the British doctors always needed "native" doctors as assistants, apothecaries, and dressers.

The difference among the three medical systems was mainly in the stress on anatomy in the Western system and the almost complete disinterest in practical anatomy in the other two. All three systems were based on a humoral theory of disease and primarily employed empirically based treatments with nonspecific herbal remedies. In 1814, the Court of Directors of the East India Company in London encouraged its employees to investigate the values of native herbs, and a "Native Medical Institution" was established in 1822 to teach "native" doctors both indigenous and European medicine.

In the earlier years of the East India Company there were strong Orientalist feelings among the British rulers. The official policy was to encourage knowledge of Sanskrit and Arabic and disseminate Western thoughts through these media. The Calcutta Maddrassah—the first government school in Bengal—was established in 1781, to train students in Arabic law. Its students had the option of studying medicine during their seven-year course. The teaching was in Arabic and the course materials based largely on Arabic texts. However, attempts were made to introduce elements of Western medicine by using two books translated from English into Arabic by the principal of the Maddrassah.

The Sanskrit College, first planned in 1821, formally opened on January 1, 1824, with forty-nine stipendiary pupils. After general studies in Sanskrit, students were encouraged to pursue specialized branches of Hindu Science, such as law (*Report* 1831: 6–9) One lecturer in anatomy and a "pundit" (a person learned in Sanskrit) trained in Ayurvedic medicine were appointed. A small hospital for sick Hindus was established to help train students.

Madhusudan Gupta was to become one of the most outstanding students of medicine at the Sanskrit College. The details of his early life are surprisingly unclear. He was probably born in 1800 (generally only the rich recorded details of births). He was born into a *vaidya* family in the village of Baidyabati (literally home of the B(v)aidyas) in Bengal. He apparently left home at an early age and traveled to Calcutta on his own to study at the Sanskrit College, presumably as a stipendiary student. In 1826, he joined the *Vaidyak sreni*, or medical section of the college, and did exceedingly well. In 1830, when the professor resigned because of ill health, the college authorities appointed Gupta, who was still a student, as a replacement, despite the opposition of other students. During his tenure at the Sanskrit College, Gupta translated two English medical texts into Bengali.

By 1835 the educational climate had changed considerably. A resolution by the government in 1835 stated, "All funds appropriated for the purpose of education would be best employed in English education alone." In 1839, this was changed somewhat so that some support was provided to native education also, although the emphasis would be on European institutions. In 1835 the government directed that a new institution be established to teach medical science on European principles in the English language. Dr. J. Mountford Bramley was selected as the first superintendent on February 1, 1835; his title was later changed to principal. Dr. H. H. Goodeve was appointed as his assistant on February 9, 1835. Madhusudan Gupta was appointed on March 17, 1835, as a demonstrator of anatomy, the only non-European to be employed as a teacher. The medical sections of the Calcutta Madrassah, the Sanskrit College, and the Native Medical Institution were all closed.

Initially the main stress in the new college was on anatomy and surgery, but professors for other subjects, such as medicine, midwifery, chemistry, and pharmacy, were also appointed. A course of lectures on anatomy was started on June 1, 1835, with opening addresses by Goodeve and Bramley. Lectures on osteology were given three times weekly until the end of September. According to the report for 1836, osteology was taught entirely from human bones. After the lectures, the students were encouraged to observe and examine the bones. An extended course of lectures in anatomy began in October 1835 after the holidays, and they continued until the end of March 1836. The instructors noted no signs of repugnance or superstitious fear of the dead among these students, perhaps because they were already familiar with human cadavers from the local custom of exposing the dead. Many of the students had already witnessed the examination of human bodies in the hospitals they had visited, and some were accustomed to handling and examining diseased structures. Nevertheless, the instructors believed it was appropriate to proceed cautiously while introducing impressionable youths to the practice of human dissection, a subject that still evoked feelings of aversion, even in Europe. Introducing this innovation was done "with due regard to secrecy," to avoid embarrassment or harassment of the students who were embarking on this venture.

Madhusudan Gupta is said to have done the first dissection of a human body at the college on January 10, 1836, although this is uncertain (Bose 1994: 28). According to the official report for 1836, the first human dissection was done on October 28, 1836, when "four of the most intelligent and respectable pupils, at their own solicitation undertook the dissection of the human subject, and in the presence of all the Professors of the College and fourteen of their brother pupils, demonstrated with accuracy and nicety, several of the most important parts of the body . . . since this time dissections have been practiced by all the senior class with one solitary exception."

These four pupils were Umacharan Sett, Rajkumar De, Dwarkanath Gupta, and Nabinchandra Mitra. However, a wooden plaque in the Anatomy Dissection Hall of the Calcutta Medical College lists eleven names (all Hindu except one Christian) as the "first students to study anatomy." It is not clear why only eleven students were named as the first to study anatomy; fifty students were selected for the first class, but at the time it was presumably considered inexpedient to release this information. According to the report for 1836, although it might seem appropriate to call attention to the industry and moral courage of the students who had been pioneers in the study of human anatomy, it was judged to be more prudent to conceal both their names and their anatomical labors. The official report for 1836 does not mention Gupta's dissection in January, nor does it mention Gupta's participation in the dissection in October. He was no longer a student, but he might have been involved as the demonstrator of anatomy.

In 1849, an oil portrait of Gupta was unveiled in the Anatomy Lecture Hall. On this occasion John Drinkwater Bethune, an eminent educator, lauded the contributions of Gupta in the following terms:

I have had the scene described to me. It had needed some time, some exercise of the persuasive art, before Modusuden could bend up his mind to the attempt; but having once taken the resolution, he never flinched or swerved from it. At the appointed hour, scalpel in hand, he followed Dr. Goodeve into the godown where the body lay ready. The other students, deeply interested in what was going forward but strangely agitated with mingled feelings of curiosity and alarm, crowded after them, but durst not enter the building where this fearful deed was to be perpetrated. . . . And when Modusuden's knife, held with a strong and steady hand, made a long and deep incision in the breast, the onlookers-on drew a long grasping breath, like men relieved from the weight of some intolerable suspense. (Kerr Part II 1853: 210)

This poetic description does not give the date of this presumed first dissection, nor did Bethune mention who had reported the incident to him. The exact role

Gupta played in the introduction of human cadaver dissection to Southeast Asia thus remains unclear. There can, however, be no doubt that Gupta was an important person in the introduction and acceptance of anatomical studies in India. Hindus generally believed the dead body to be unclean, and a full bath was needed on touching a corpse. The authorities were obviously concerned about the reaction of the local population to human dissection. Whatever the circumstances were surrounding this first dissection, the practice was enthusiastically accepted. In 1837 sixty bodies were dissected and in 1838 double that number. Human dissection was also regularly practiced in the so-called subordinate schools.

In 1839 a "secondary class," in which instruction was in Hindustani, was opened "for educating native doctors" for employment in the Army and Civil Stations; fifty students, generally from provinces other than Bengal, were selected. This "Military" or "Hindustani" class was reorganized in 1843–1844 and put under the charge of Madhusudan Gupta. In addition to the Hindustani class, a Bengali class was opened in June 1852, also under the guidance of Dr. Gupta. In both classes, human dissection was the medium of anatomy instruction. Gupta's efficiency as a teacher and administrator of these sections was commented on favorably in the various official reports of educational activities in Bengal presidency.

The social and intellectual climate of India at the time undoubtedly helped the quick approval of the study of human anatomy. A large segment of the population was anxious to learn English and even adopt "Western" ways, as manifested by conversion to Christianity and the reckless use of alcohol. Teachers at the Hindu school, the Hare School, and the Scottish Assembly School (from which the students had been recruited) were well known as admirers of British culture. Under the influence of charismatic teachers like Henry DeRozio, they wanted to escape the sluggish streams of the established ritual-ridden native culture and escape into the newer and less restraining "Western" thinking. Even then, it must have needed considerable powers of leadership to guide the first students through the actual act of human dissection. As the only native teacher in the medical college, Gupta's role as a leader was undoubtedly crucial.

Although a teacher of anatomy from the beginning, Gupta's qualification was as a *vaidya*. He rectified this deficiency by successfully taking the examination for the M.B. degree in 1840; the first qualifying examination for this degree in India was held in 1838. Madhusudan Gupta was also active in writing medical books in Bengali and translating medical and pharmaceutical texts from English into Bengali. He apparently also prepared and distributed notes for dissection in Urdu, but there is no evidence that these were ever published. Gupta was thus a pioneer in devising technical medical terms in Sanskrit, Bengali, and possibly Urdu. His style was somewhat stiff, and he often used English words without providing a vernacular equivalent. However, using Bengali as a medium of expression for Western science and medicine was a new enterprise, and Gupta's style was not significantly worse than other Bengali authors of the time.

Gupta was a successful practitioner and a respected member of Bengali society, which further demonstrates the ready acceptance of human dissection by the native population. Whether he practiced "Western" medicine only, or also used Ayurvedic drugs, is not known. His excellence as a physician was well recognized. He was one of the experts called on to comment on the possible need to establish a "fever hospital" in Calcutta and improve the city's sanitation.

Gupta remained with the medical college until his death from diabetic gangrene on November 20, 1856. His death was remarked upon and his career extolled in the native press. In his report for 1856–1857, Dr. T. W. Wilson, principal of the Medical College, wrote: "It is hoped that his countrymen appreciating his example will erect some monument to perpetuate the memory of the victory gained by Mudoosoodun Gooptu over public prejudice, and from which so many of his countrymen now reap the advantage."

That hope has not been fulfilled. The only visible testimony of Gupta's illustrious career is the painting by Mrs. Bellnos, still in the Calcutta Medical College Anatomy lecture theater, and a marble plaque in the anatomy dissection hall that mentions his name as the first person to dissect a cadaver in India.

BIBLIOGRAPHY

The current spelling of Gupta's name has been adopted, but in the past various spellings, such as Muddoosoodan Gooptu, were used. Primary sources for investigating his life and work include the various government reports of the period detailing public education. J. Kerr's two-volume review of the development of public instruction in Bengal is an important collection of information from original sources. Descriptions of the personal achievements of Gupta are scanty. Probably the fullest source is in Bengali (Bagal 1958). The history of the Sanskrit College, also in Bengali, has a short biography of Gupta and gives critical information on the medical section of the college. Some information about Gupta's times can be obtained from Bagal (1947) and the centenary volume of the Calcutta Medical College. Unfortunately, his books are now rare and inaccessible.

Writings about Madhusudan Gupta and Related Topics

Bagal, Jogeshchandra. *William Yeats, John Mack, Madhusudan Gupta.* (In Bengali.) Calcutta: Bangiya Sahitya Parishat. 1958.

———. "Early Years of the Calcutta Medical College (Based on Educational Records)." *Modern Review* 82 (1947): 210–215, 291–297.

Bose, D. M., chief ed. *A Concise History of Science in India.* New Delhi: Indian National Science Academy, 1971.

———. "Madhusudan Gupta." *Indian Journal of the History of Science* 29, (no. 1) (1994): 31–40.

Jaggi, O. P. *Western Medicine in India: Social Impact.* History of Science, Technology, and Medicine in India, vol. 15. Delhi: Atma Ram & Sons, 1980.

Kerr, J. *A Review of Public Instruction in the Bengal Presidency from 1835 to 1851.* Part 1. Calcutta: Printed by J. Thomas, Baptist Mission Press, 1852.

————. *A Review of Public Instruction in the Bengal Presidency from 1835 to 1851.* Part II. London: Wm. H. Allen & Co., 1853.

Mookerji, Radha Kumud. *Ancient Indian Education.* 1947. Reprint. Delhi: Motilal Banarsidass, 1960.

Ramachandra Rao, S. K., ed. *Encyclopaedia of Indian Medicine.* Bombay: Popular Prakashan, 1985.

Report of the General Committee of Public Instruction of the Presidency of Fort William in Bengal, for the Year 1836. Calcutta: Printed at the Baptist Mission Press, Circular Road, 1837.

Report on the Colleges and Schools for Native Education, Under the Superintendence of the General Committee of Public Instruction in Bengal. 1831. Calcutta: From the Bengal Military Orphan Press by G. H. Huttman, 1832.

Report of the Director of Public Instruction for the Year 1856–57. Calcutta: Baptist Mission Press.

Zysk, Kenneth G. "The Evolution of Anatomical Knowledge in Ancient India, with Special Reference to Cross-Cultural Influences." *Journal of the American Oriental Society* 106 (1986): 687–705.

Ranes C. Chakravorty

SAMI IBRAHIM HADDAD
(1890–1957)

Sami Ibrahim Haddad was the first Lebanese to be promoted to the rank of professor of surgery and dean of the Medical School at the American University of Beirut (AUB) and to become a fellow of the American College of Surgeons (1934). He collected over 125 Arabic manuscripts on medicine and wrote extensively on the subjects of surgery, urology, and the history of Arab medicine and Arab hospitals. After his retirement from AUB, he founded the Orient Hospital in Beirut in 1947.

Haddad was born July 3,1890, in Jaffa, Palestine. He died on February 5, 1957, in Beirut. At the funeral, his students carried his coffin to the National Evangelical Church, while the empty hearse trailed behind. In a rare display of respect, the mayor of Beirut and the chief of police sent their respective bands to accompany the funerary march. Haddad's pious and puritanical nature derived from his mother's uncle, Shakir alHaajj Dimyanos, a pillar of the orthodox community and church of Hasbayya. His love of work, perseverance, and determination came from his mother's sister, Suwfiyya, a woman of great energy and endurance. The Haddad family of 'Abeih nurtured many intellectuals, professionals, and businessmen, but none was as eminent as Gregorius Haddad, the saintly patriarch of the Greek Orthodox church of Antioch and the Orient. Sami looked up to him as a role model.

Haddad's preparatory education at the Bishop Gobat School (1901–1905) and the English College (1907–1909) in Jerusalem left an indelible mark on him. His asceticism, honesty, discipline, and austerity most probably derived from his early Scottish high school teachers in Jerusalem, where he earned the Gibbon Memorial Prize in July 1906. Haddad graduated with an M.D. degree from the Syrian Protestant College (SPC) in 1913. Founded in 1866 by American missionaries in Beirut, the SPC was renamed in 1920 as the American University of Beirut. For seven years after graduation (1913–1919), Haddad practiced general medicine and public health, and taught the basic sciences at SPC. In 1919, he was nominated physician in charge of the Mental Disease Hospital at Asfuriyeh. When the U.S. King-Crane Commission (created by President Woodrow Wilson to poll public opinion in Syria, Lebanon, and Palestine) arrived in Beirut, he became its physician and interpreter.

Before Haddad joined the Department of Surgery of the American University of Beirut as adjunct professor of surgery in 1920, he was granted a Rockefeller fellowship. He married Lamia Morcos (1896–1994) from Latakia in 1921; she remained a devoted companion and ideal wife, and helped him raise six children, all of whom went on to successful careers in medicine, engineering, and the arts. True to recent theory about "the westward migration of civilizations," his children eventually emigrated westward.

Together with his wife, Haddad traveled to the United States to be trained in urology at the Johns Hopkins University under Dr. Hugh Hampton Young. After nine years of industrious preparation and indefatigable study (1913–1922), Haddad embarked on the difficult path of teaching and practicing urology and surgery. Stephen B. L. Penrose, Jr., who later became president of AUB, said on the appointment of Dr. Haddad to the faculty: "Dr. Sami Haddad was unexpectedly available, and this 'first-class man in every particular' became a permanent member of the faculty of the College."

Haddad taught thousands of medical students, interns, and residents and operated on thousands of patients. In his spare time, he collected Arabic medical manuscripts and wrote about the history of Arab medicine. He kept abreast of new medical developments through trips to the United States, Austria, Brazil, Australia, Iraq, Qatar, England, France, and Spain. On some trips, he photographed Arabic medical manuscripts and other important documents in the libraries in Paris, London, and Jerusalem.

The first Lebanese to become a member of the International Society of Surgery (1931) and a fellow of the American College of Surgeons (1934), Haddad was also a member of the University Council, the highest advisory body of the AUB (1938–1945). He served as president of the Medical Alumni Association (1927–1929). He led AUB's delegation to the medical congress in Luxor (1934) and to the millennium of Avicenna in Baghdad (1952). In 1941, he became chairman of the Department of Surgery and dean of the Medical School of the AUB. After a heated controversy with the president of AUB about part-time status, he became professor emeritus (1949). Twice, he was awarded the Lebanese Honorary Golden Order of Merit (1954 and 1956).

Haddad was proficient in Arabic and English and learned enough French, German, and Syriac to facilitate his historical research. He was a great collector of stamps, glassware, manuscripts, pottery, Roman and Arabic surgical instruments, antiques, precious stones, and ancient coins. During World War II, he offered his vast collection of cholesterol-rich gallstones to Dr. George Fawaz for his work on the synthesis of testosterone, because his supply of imported cholesterol was rapidly dwindling. Haddad dabbled in photography and painting, and left behind scores of plans and drawings for homes, hospitals, and resorts. He was elected master of the Masonic Peace Lodge Number 908 on five occasions and served as an elder of the National Evangelical church of Beirut.

A prolific writer and historian, he wrote ninety-nine articles on various surgical, urological, and historical subjects; sixty-nine Arabic speeches and radio talks on the history of Arab medicine, Arab hospitals, and health matters; and twelve books. Ten of his books were written in English, including *Notes on Embryology* (unpublished), *Essentials of Urinary and Genital Diseases* (1946), and eight volumes of the *Annual Report of the Orient Hospital (AROH)* (1948–

1955). *The Contributions of the Arabs to the Medical Sciences* (1936) and *The Tradition According to Øumar* (1940) were written in Arabic. Half of his articles were written in English and half in Arabic. His articles on urology dealt with cystoscopy, pyelography, hematuria, genitourinary tuberculosis, renal and ureteral lithiasis, hemangioma of the bladder, calculi, prostatic enlargement, and prostatic cancer. He also published articles on various forms of cancer, hydatid cysts, traumatic aneurysms, perforation of the uterus with injury to the gut, foreign bodies of the abdomen and esophagus, diseases of the gallbladder and their surgical treatment, chest and lung surgery, elephantiasis, appendicitis, blood transfusion, spinal anesthesia, and the art of surgery. His research on the history of medicine resulted in articles on Arab hospitals, Ibn Nafiys (Ibn al-Nafis, the thirteenth-century discoverer of the pulmonary circulation), Hippocrates, Galen, Arab dentistry, cesarean section, medical ethics, medical biographies, and a catalog of the Arabic medical manuscripts he had collected. He also wrote about the history of Arabic script, the medical problems of the Arab countries, and the Mameluke documents concerning the Church of the Nativity in Jerusalem.

Although a genitourinary surgeon, Dr. Haddad was proficient in many other fields of general surgery. He had firsthand knowledge of embryology, anatomy, and physiology, subjects he taught for several years. He introduced to Lebanon, then the medical center of the Near East, newly developed methods of diagnosis and treatment, such as the cystoscope, the pyelogram, the PSP (phenolsulfonphthalein) test, pulmonary collapse surgery in the treatment of pulmonary tuberculosis, laryngectomy for laryngeal cancer, and orchiectomy for cancer of the prostate, and he reintroduced patellectomy for comminuted fractures of the patella. He also devised a new technique of retropubic prostatectomy that preserved the urethra. His ideas about prostatic cancer are almost identical to our present-day concept. In 1956 he said: "Don't worry about cancer of the prostate. . . . Man can have cancer of the prostate and live to be 90 years old. You laugh at me when I say cancer of the prostate is nothing! There are however a few cases of bad cancer of the prostate . . . they need very careful attention."

In addition to his regular surgical work at the hospitals of the American University of Beirut, Haddad had admission privileges to the Saint George Greek Orthodox Hospital, the Makasid Hospital in Beirut, the Hamlin Sanitarium in Shibbaniyyah, the Dahr al-Bashek Sanitarium in Roumieh, and several other private hospitals in Beirut. His patients included presidents, emirs, ministers, deputies, bishops, physicians, and people from all walks of life, from Lebanon, the surrounding countries, and more distant ones. However, he never boasted or mentioned the rich and the famous among his patients; instead, in his lectures he would refer to "my neighbor the grocer" or "my friend the carpenter."

His surgical judgment was sound; years of experience and a brilliant mind made him one of the best diagnosticians of his time. He relied more on sound physical examination and the use of the senses than on technical and laboratory aids. In his surgery, he used the minimum number of instruments and equipment, relying more on dexterity and agility. His surgical skill together with a meticulous concern for detail, a gentle and delicate touch, an experienced eye, and a vast knowledge helped him to obtain consistently good results. In 1944 he secretly operated on himself and resumed his work at the hospital the next day.

Although a Christian by upbringing, he was tolerant of other religions and had many friends who belonged to all creeds. He was fanatically loyal to his friends and defended them and their interests under all circumstances. A handsome man with blue eyes, Haddad maintained a puritanical life-style. Thrifty and frugal, he had a very shrewd business sense, especially in real estate matters. His ambition, eagerness to learn and study, and his prodigious energy knew no limit. Even after retirement, he could not remain idle; in 1947, he founded the Orient Hospital, a fifty-four bed nonprofit institution, and singlehandedly shouldered the responsibility of its varied and intricate work. He was its founder, superintendent, chief of staff, chief surgeon, roentgenologist, record keeper, and editor of its *Annual Report*.

He was a serious-minded teacher who insisted that students understand basic principles. He therefore simplified the subject he was teaching and boiled it down to its essential elements. He considered the operating room a holy sanctuary and insisted on approaching it reverently, never allowing the slightest joke or murmur. He was reluctant to teach new theories or techniques that had not been firmly established. However, he liked to bring forth the philosophical aspects of biology as applied to medicine. He was strongly opposed to smoking and abhorred the then rampant practice of prophylactic penicillin. He used to say: ''Inject it in the mattress; it might be less harmful.'' Several of his students followed in his footsteps and became famous physicians and surgeons; others established their own private hospitals; still others became writers, poets, historians of medicine, ministers, professors, politicians, researchers, and presidents of prestigious medical organizations.

Sick with heart disease the last five years of his life, he continued to work stoically, hiding his physical ailment from his nearest relatives. During his final illness, he performed a five-hour operation on a poor, young shepherd who had been paralyzed by a tumor of the spinal cord. Tragically, a few weeks after his discharge from the hospital, the young man was struck by a truck and died instantly. It was said that the ''high powers above'' sent the truck to seal his fate. A few days later Dr. Haddad died.

The American College of Surgeons transmitted to his bereaved family and friends a memorial plaque tendering their sincere sympathy and their respect to his memory. The eulogy of the Senate of AUB ended in the following words:

Sami Haddad was a self made man with an acquisitive and brilliant mind, a limitless ambition, a strong moral fiber and boundless energy. He will be remembered as a great physician, an unforgettable teacher, a pioneering surgeon, an organizer and administrator of great ability, a prolific writer, an accurate and dedicated historian, a multifaceted collector, a shrewd business man, a devoted friend and a beloved husband and father.

BIBLIOGRAPHY

Writings by Sami Ibrahim Haddad

The Contributions of the Arabs to the Medical Sciences. (In Arabic.) Beirut: Rihani, 1936.
"A Forgotten Chapter in the History of the Circulation of the Blood." *Annals of Surgery* 104 (1936): 1–8.
"A Study of Arab Hospitals in the Light of Present Day Standardization." *Bulletin of the American College of Surgeons* 21 (1936): 173–177.
"Dental Gleanings from Arabian Medicine." *Journal of the American Dental Association* 24 (1937): 944–955.
"Surgical Consideration of Hydatid Disease." *Annals of Surgery* 111 (1940): 597–604.
"Arabian Contributions to Medicine." *Annals of the History of Medicine.* 3d series, 3 (1941): 60–72.
Essentials of Urinary and Genital Diseases. Beirut: American Press, 1946.
Annual Reports of the Orient Hospital. Vols. 1–8, 1948–1955.
"Retropubic Prostatectomy." *Annual Report of the Orient Hospital* 3 (1950): 32–37.
"Thoracoplasty in the Treatment of Pulmonary Tuberculosis." *Annual Report of the Orient Hospital* 3 (1950): 52–62.

Writings about Sami Ibrahim Haddad and Related Topics

Haddad, Farid Sami. Dr. Sami I. Haddad. *Annual Report of the Orient Hospital* 10 (1957): 4–20.

Farid Sami Haddad

WILLIAM HEBERDEN
(1710–1801)

Dr. William Heberden made many contributions to medicine but is remembered by medical students because of a minor clinical observation known as Heberden's nodes. That would have amused him. He had described angina pectoris, delineated chicken pox from smallpox, and contributed to the understanding of many other clinical disorders. More important, he increased the recognition that careful case studies would improve the understanding of disease, and his textbook was one of the most prominent in medicine for a century. He was founder and editor of *Medical Transactions*, an important early medical communication, and he was an important and central figure in changing the direction of medicine in the late eighteenth century.

The pattern of medical practice up to that time was based on empirical methods that intermixed the medical traditions of Europe, Arabic and Jewish medicine, Asia, and a dollop of superstition, folk medicine, and quackery. Heberden was able to approach this with a cool objectivity that allowed him to be more open, critical, and even cynical about the practice of medicine and the nature of illness. In his public lectures he called into question the superstitions and useless remedies that were commonplace in the community, and he exhorted his colleagues to base their approach on careful observation and experience.

Recognizing the limitation of many remedies, he influenced the revision of the *Pharmacopoeia* of the Royal College of Physicians and dispensed to his patients advice that was, as Dr. Samuel Johnson said, more prudential than medical (Murray 1979). As noted by his descendant and biographer Ernest Heberden, he could deliver public lectures on the false ideas about disease and treatment, assist the scholar Jeremiah Markland with the publication of great plays, carry out a lengthy experiment on annual rainfall, support Parliament petitions on religious toleration, assess the accuracy of Thomas Mudge's chronometer by astronomical observation, and assist Benjamin Franklin with the concept of smallpox vaccination for America. He seems a man perfectly suited for the Age of the Enlightenment.

William Heberden was born on August 13, 1710, the second youngest of six children. His father, Richard, did reasonably well as an innkeeper, with some responsibilities in the parish as an overseer to the Vestry of St. Saviors. His brother Thomas became a surgeon and naturalist, and brother John became an attorney. The Heberden children attended the Free Grammar School in Suffolk, an impressive school with an emphasis on the teaching of classics. The family's future looked bright; William was expected to enter the university, and Thomas was already apprenticed to a surgeon. However, the father died suddenly without a will, leaving the future of the two promising brothers uncertain.

Fortunately, a benefactor left money in his will for a needy scholar, and William was awarded seven pounds per annum for his studies at Cambridge, which provided minimal support until he was elected a fellow of his college seven years later. At Cambridge William was a sizar, a student too poor to afford the normal university fees and who in return carried out domestic tasks such as waiter to the hall; he received accommodations, reduced tuition, and a small allowance for food. In November 1725 William was awarded the position of a foundress scholar "for the bell," with responsibility to ring the chapel bell for daily services for a weekly sum of two shillings, plus eight pounds a year. William studied for the degree of bachelor of arts and was influenced not only by the traditional concept of classics and religious studies but the new thinking of Locke and Newton, who recognized the importance of personal observation, experience, and experimentation. William achieved his B.A. in 1728 and while awaiting the time period to take his M.A. he was elected to a St. John's fellowship on April 6, 1731, to study medicine.

In July 1734 he was elected to a medical fellowship and later that year appointed Linacre Lecturer in Physics, providing him with an increased stipend but without additional responsibility. Although his brother Thomas had qualified as a liveryman of the Guild of Barber-Surgeons, William planned to become a physician, which had a higher status than that of surgeon. Medical training in England in that era was both depressing and arduous. The medical faculty was described as "small and generally despised" (E. Heberden 1989). Serious students often went off to Leyden to be taught by Hermann Boerhaave or to Edinburgh to hear the anatomy lectures of Alexander Munro, *primus*. Heberden coupled his training at Cambridge with some experience at a hospital in London, probably St. Thomas's in Southwark. Although a doctor of medicine normally required seven years' standing from the degree of M.A., Heberden asked the senate to accept his five years as adequate for the practice of medicine and for an examination by the Regis Professor of Medicine. His request was granted on April 27, 1737, and the next summer he was examined and found competent. In the years following his doctorate, he taught at the university and enjoyed the college life. He joined conversation groups at the coffee houses, and his friends and acquaintances were the intellectual life of Cambridge.

One of his earliest writings was a contribution to a multiauthored fictional work based on letters at the time of the Peloponnesian War. Heberden wrote about Hippocrates, showing his contribution to the advancement of physic as an art. But he also pointed out defects in Hippocrates's writings and noted that his reputation was somewhat overblown. Heberden acknowledged that medicine in his age was also in a state of infancy and could be advanced only by careful and accurate observation. He thought that physicians were confined by the times in which they lived and by their own human frailties, and that they could not escape personal responsibility by referring to some ancient authority. Although the book achieved only minor recognition, Heberden's contribution increased his reputation and provided him an entree into other circles.

He next outlined and designed a course of thirty-one lectures on materia medica, to which he brought an objective view of various treatments, and he interspersed the discussion with relevant literature and history. To deliver such a lecture course demanded broad reading, a large collection of chemicals, specimens, herbs, and, most important, a habit of careful examination of the effects of these remedies on various conditions.

In 1741 he produced a brief work, *An Introduction to the Study of Physic*, to assist students in understanding the steps to become a physician and the many books to read. In his preface, he indicated that previous books of this sort were now out of date, and he expected that the experience of medicine would eventually replace his version. In the first chapter, "Of Introductory Books," he indicates that the physician must be a scholar, reading Greek and Latin as well as one or two modern languages, and should have some familiarity with geography, chronology, history, logic, metaphysics, ethics, mathematics, and natural philosophy. He recommended dissection to learn the lessons of anatomy, and he warned against systems of medicine, as the proponents of systems often bent facts to fit their theories. Again he emphasized the importance of personal observation, and he complimented Thomas Sydenham and Hermann Boerhaave for their powers of objective observation. To complete his recommendations for students, he cataloged 114 books mentioned in the text.

The Royal College of Physicians had the responsibility for producing editions of the *London Pharmacopoeia*, and Heberden argued strenuously for many revisions to this work. For his efforts, the college elected him a fellow of the college. Soon after, Heberden encouraged the college to produce a botanical garden, comparable to that at Oxford and at Chelsea, a recommendation that initially was unheeded. Fifteen years later a garden was begun, with acknowledgment of Heberden's original idea and encouragement.

At this point in his career, further advancement at Cambridge seemed unlikely. Although he had been a resident of Cambridge for twenty-four years, he decided to move to London and was given letters of recommendation by a number of prominent physicians, including Sir Richard Mead. Medical practice was very competitive in London, and there was one physician for every 850 people, not unlike today. Heberden was confident, however, because of his reputation, his membership in the established Church of England, his M.D. degree from Cambridge, and his fellowship in the Royal College of Physicians.

An important opportunity came from Sir Edward Holse, who was about to retire and offered his practice to Heberden. He passed the offer through another physician, however, who, seeing an opportunity for himself, told Holse that Heberden was not interested. Holse discovered the deception and wrote directly to Heberden. On moving to London in 1748, Heberden became a member of the Club of the Royal Philosophers, a dining club that met at the Mitre Tavern on Fleet Street.

To marry at Cambridge would have meant relinquishing his fellowship, but in London he was free to pursue married life. He bought a good home and married Elizabeth, the daughter of John Martin, a banker. Shortly after his marriage he developed a brief acute illness with "unsightly swelling to the limbs, followed by a fit of the gout." Elizabeth later gave birth to a son, John, who died shortly after birth. A second son was born the next year; two months later Elizabeth died, probably of an infection acquired in childbirth. In 1760 Heberden married again; three of the seven children born to his second wife died in infancy.

Heberden had many prominent patients, including the novelist Samuel Richardson, Dr. Herring, the archbishop of Canterbury, Dr. Samuel Johnson, Benjamin Franklin, Josiah Wedgwood, Thomas Gainsborough, and George III. Richardson suffered from a marked tremor that prevented him from using a pen; Heberden suggested that he employ an amanuensis.

Heberden was somewhat cynical about popular treatments of the day, including the upper-class penchant for taking the waters at such spas as Bath and Leamington. He thought they had some limited use, but the same effect could be obtained by taking a bath at home or treating a hangover or gastric problems by drinking any clean water. He felt physicians had few effective therapies, but he did write an unpublished essay on opium indicating this praiseworthy drug could bring benefit to any illness (Paulshock 1983).

Heberden studied the bills of mortality for the parishes of London and felt that useful information could be obtained from these, even though they were inaccurate in many ways. Anonymously, he published a substantial volume on the yearly bills of mortality for the London parishes from 1657 to 1758, and in the preface argued that such a register on a national scale would be valuable. He, like others, was appalled by the high percentage of premature deaths and felt that a strong statistical basis for the population, its illnesses and its deaths, would be the groundwork for designing improvements in a healthy life and the treatment of illness. He complained about unhealthy living conditions, pride, poverty, crowded living quarters, the low reputation of married life, and the high consumption of alcoholic spirits. He fostered the practice of inoculation for smallpox and wrote a pamphlet on the topic and supported a resolution on inoculation by the Royal College of Physicians. He wrote to journal editors and others in support of this boon to humanity. In 1760 he developed a medication known as Heberden's ink, an aromatic mixture containing cinchona powder, cloves, colimba root, cardamom, iron filings, peppermint water, and tincture of orange peel. It remained in the *British Pharmacopoeia* until 1890.

A mark of his success was the offer of an appointment as physician to the queen. Surprisingly, Heberden refused the offer and recommended a colleague. When it was suggested that he and his colleague serve jointly, he again refused. He was elected a fellow of the Royal Society on January 25, 1749/50. His first paper, presented in December of that year, was on a huge bladder calculus that had been on view in the library of Trinity College since the reign of Queen Anne. He traced the history of the "Monstrous stone" to the wife of a locksmith in Bury, who developed bladder obstruction after horseback riding and was in great agony until she died. He suggested that a catheter, or an alteration in the position of the patient, would have provided some relief.

As the 1749 Gulstonian lecturer he spoke on ''The History, Nature and Cure of Poisons.'' In his discussion of two classes of poisons, acrimonious or corrosive, and intoxicating, he listed tobacco among the most severe intoxicating poisons. He also warned against opium, then a popular soporific. Although he admitted that he did not fully understand how nerves operate, he constructed a hypothesis about the effect of poisons on the nerves. In 1750 the college invited him to give the Harverian Oration, and ten years later the Croonian lectures. Sadly, these two addresses have been lost. Heberden presented papers on the importance of clean water for London and, on the psychedelic effects of certain mushrooms, and he was the first to delineate clearly the difference between chicken pox and smallpox. He underwrote the printing of a pamphlet about smallpox inoculation that he coauthored with Benjamin Franklin. He privately printed an essay on the popular drugs theriac and mithridate, arguing that they are dangerous poisons. He also wrote about the pulse, colic suffered by watercolor painters who used white and red lead, and the 1775 influenza outbreak in London.

Perhaps his most notable contribution was a paper published in the *Medical Transactions* entitled ''Some Account of the Disorder of the Breast,'' in which he describes clearly the symptom of angina pectoris and gives it that name. But he was unable to observe the autopsy on such a case. (W. Heberden 1802). The condition was for some years referred to as Heberden's angina or Heberden's asthma. A physician responded to Heberden's original publication, outlining his angina with arrhythmia, and offered his body for autopsy, as he predicted correctly his own death. He died soon after, and his autopsy was done within forty-eight hours by John Hunter assisted by a young Edward Jenner. Although Hunter found no cause for death, Jenner later indicated the coronary arteries were not carefully examined. In his Lumleian lecture of 1910, Sir William Osler commented on Heberden's description, referring to him as ''The English Celsus,'' and praised his graphic and complete description of angina pectoris. When he first described angina, Heberden reported on twenty cases, but when he wrote *Commentaries* (1802) he had the experience of one hundred cases.

Although Heberden played an active role in the Royal College of Physicians, he was never president. Perhaps it was because of his sympathy for the rival licentiates of the college, who demanded and occasionally forcefully broke into committee meetings to indicate that they wished to be full voting members of the college. He was a loyal friend of William Hunter (see John Hunter*), and one of the six people who attended Hunter's funeral. Heberden also sympathized with religious dissenters, although he continued to remain a practicing Anglican, and in 1765 was elected as a Gentleman at the Vestry.

Heberden was present at the founding of the Royal Humane Society, initially dedicated to providing relief for persons ''apparently dead from drowning'' but which later expanded its interest to reviving people who apparently died of strangulation, suicide, and noxious fumes. John Fothergill, a friend of Heberden, wrote a paper in 1745 calling attention to the value of mouth-to-mouth resuscitation. John Hunter* also studied the idea of blowing air into the lungs with a set of special bellows and stimulating the action of the heart by electricity. The society adopted other methods as well, including some Dutch ideas that included, in addition to mouth-to-mouth resuscitation, warmth, fumigation with tobacco smoke via the rectum, friction, stimulants, bleeding, and the inducement of vomiting.

Later in his life William was regarded as one of the outstanding physicians of London, and he was consulted by many prominent people, including Thomas Gray, Samuel Richardson, Horace Walpole, and the circle around Dr. Samuel Johnson, including the Thrales, Cowper, and Warburton. Through his involvement as a fellow of the Royal Society, he exchanged ideas with Stephen Hales, Joseph Priestley, Benjamin Franklin, and Edward Jenner. Johnson and Heberden became friends only in the last years of Johnson's life, and their first contact as patient and physician occurred in 1783, when Johnson suffered a stroke. Heberden retired from practice in 1788. One of his last patients was King George III, who was in one of his fits of madness, likely due to porphyria. George III indicated his trust of Heberden but not of Sir George Baker, the royal physician, as Heberden always told him the truth.

Heberden consistently recommended that physicians keep case notes and careful records, and from his own personal cases came his greatest work, *Commentaries on the History and Care of Disease*. He maintained careful notes on all his encounters with patients and reviewed them monthly. Those that seemed worthy were written in a commonplace book, now preserved at the Royal College of Physicians in London as *Index Historias Morborum*. *Commentaries* became the most popular medical text in the early nineteenth century. It was the last major medical text written in Latin. Heberden entrusted the publication of his book to his son William, with instructions not to publish it until after his death. Although *Commentaries* was completed in 1782, Heberden continued to record notes in his "Index" until 1787; it includes over seven thousand cases. Included are discussions of diet, patient care, and specific diseases, including angina pectoris, chicken pox, Heberden's nodes, ringworm (which he recognized as infectious), mental illness, and gout. He noted that while many medications and therapies were useless, novelty had the capacity to work miracles.

Heberden maintained an interest in his university and published an anonymous pamphlet, *Strictures upon the Discipline of the University of Cambridge Addressed to the Senate* (E. Heberden, 1989). He complained about the decline in religious observance, the failure of the faculty to attend church services regularly, the slovenly performance of the services, and the effect of wordly pursuits on the students. He criticized the senate for its failure to reform the system of study and argued that the courses had been so watered down that a degree would have little or no value.

In his mid-eighties Heberden wrote to friends about the qualities of a good retirement and his feelings that not all were equipped for it. He died in his house in Pall Mall on May 17, 1801, at age ninety-one and was buried in the parish church at Windsor (Davidson 1922). He is still remembered for his observation of certain clinical phenomena. Indeed, his keen observations on rheumatism caused the Committee for the Study and Investigation of Rheumatism in 1937 to change its name to the Heberden Society.

BIBLIOGRAPHY

Heberden's "Index Historias Morborum" and other documents are held at the Royal College of Physicians of London.

Writings by William Heberden

Commentaries on the History and Cure of Diseases. London: T. Payne, 1802. Reprint ed., New York: Hafner, 1962.
"Some Account of a Disorder of the Breast." *Medical Transactions of the Royal College of Physicians, London* 2 (1772) 59–67.
"On the Chickenpox." *Medical Transactions of the Royal College of Physicians, London* 1 (1768): 427–436.

Writings about William Heberden and Related Topics

Briggs, W. W., and B. Z. Paulshock. "Lively Lustre, Kindly Dew: William Heberden's 'of Perspiration.' " *Journal of the History of Medicine* 41 (1986): 467–481.
Davidson, P. B. "William Heberden, M.D., F.R.S." *Annals of Medical History* 4 (1922): 336–346.
Hart, F. D. "William Heberden, Edward Jenner, John Hunter and Angina Pectoris." *Journal of Medical Biography* 3 (1979): 56–58.
Heberden, E. *William Heberden: Physician of the Age of Reason.* London: Royal Society of Medicine Series, 1989. (This biography of William Heberden contains a section on his son. It was written by his descendant, Ernest Heberden.)
Lord Cohen of Birkenhead. "The Heberden Oration, 1961. William Heberden." *Annals of the Rheumatic Diseases* 21 (1962): 1–10.
Murray, T. J. "The Medical History of Doctor Samuel Johnson." *Nova Scotia Medical Bulletin* (April 1982). 71–78.
———. "Dr. Samuel Johnson's Movement Disorder." *British Medical Journal* 239, no. 1 (1979): 1610–1614.
Murray, T. J., with E. Heberden. "Dr. Johnson and Dr. Heberden." *Nova Scotia Medical Journal* (April 1989): 59–64.
Paulshock, B. Z. "William Heberden and Opium—Some Relief to All." *New England Journal of Medicine* 308 (1983): 53–55.
Rolleston, H. "The Two Heberdens." *Annals of Medical History* 5 (1933): 409–427, 566–583.

T. J. Murray

JOHN HUNTER
(1728-1793)

John Hunter, a pioneer of scientific surgery, is not as well known as his older brother, William Hunter (1718–1783), but he was also highly praised for his contributions to anatomy, biology, natural history, and pathology. Hunter was born in East Kilbride near Glasgow, Scotland. Spoiled by his indulgent mother, John showed little interest in getting the kind of education then considered appropriate for the sons of country gentlemen; he preferred to ramble through the woods ''looking after birds'-nests, comparing their eggs—number, size, marks, and other peculiarities'' (Paget 1897: 33).

In 1748, John left home to join his brother William, the best anatomist and ''accoucheur'' in London, who also had a private school for teaching anatomy. William recognized his brother's skill in dissection and allowed John to prepare specimens and assist in classroom demonstrations. John spent some time with the great surgeon William Cheselden (1688–1752) at Chelsea Hospital, and, following his death, John joined Percival Pott (1714–1788) as a surgeon's pupil at St. Bartholomew's Hospital. In 1754 Hunter became a surgeon's pupil at St. George's Hospital and two years later was appointed a house surgeon. On July 22, 1771, John Hunter married Ann Home, sister of Everard Home, a distinguished surgeon. It is not known whether William approved of the matrimony, but he did not attend the ceremony. John found fulfillment in his marriage, which allowed him the peace of mind to pursue his work. John and William Hunter had a close relationship until the publication of William's magnificent *The Anatomy of the Human Gravid Uterus* (1774). In the preface, William acknowledged the help he received from John and praised his well-known ''accuracy in anatomical researches.'' John, however, claimed that he had not only carried out the dissections but also made the discovery on the structure of the placenta and its vascular arrangements. Both brothers wrote to the Royal Society attacking each other, but the society refused to mediate this embarrassing dispute.

John Hunter ''found surgery little more than a trade . . . and showed that there were processes of disease which could be studied just as [William] Harvey had studied the processes of nature, and that only by investigating the changes due to disease in the light of a knowledge of the functions of normal tissues and organs could surgery be properly applied'' (Graham 1956: 248). Pursuing the ''ultimate truths of natural function'' Hunter dissected and described more than five hundred species of animals, birds, fishes, and insects. His insightful observations showed how the study of the lower animals could contribute to understanding the human body. Hunter's researches revealed a descriptive and analytical mind, relentless in the pursuit of details. The extraordinary collection of the Hunterian Museum at the Royal College of Surgeons in London, England, is an enduring legacy to Hunter's genius and prodigious labor. Unlike other eighteenth-century museums, Hunter's was "not merely a collection of exhibits but an illustration of his theories, and in particular of the constant adaptation in living things of structure to function. It was, in fact, John Hunter's unwritten book" (Dobson 1968: 5). The most diverse fields are represented in the collection: pathology, geology, and paleontology. When the Company of Surgeons (later the Royal College of Surgeons) acquired the collection in 1799, it consisted of about 14,000 specimens of some 500 different species of animals. Hunter had spent at least £70,000 over the years for the specimens, which at the time of his death represented the "bulk of his fortune." After his death, Parliament voted a sum not exceeding £15,000 for the purchase of the entire collection. Eventually a museum was built to house it.

Hunter's contribution to surgery is not to be found in the form of a single discovery or text but in the many basic scientific principles he formulated through critical thinking and accurate observations. These led to other discoveries that benefited the practice of medicine and surgery. Because of Hunter's expansive scientific outlook and his special ability to unite different disciplines, it is difficult to categorize his contributions to science and medicine. George Quist's (1981) classification is based on ten subject areas: digestive system, reproductive system, circulatory system, nervous system and special senses, musculoskeletal system, metabolism, comparative anatomy, surgery and clinical subjects, geology and paleontology, and natural history in general.

It has been said that the most important development in the establishment of scientific surgery as a field associated with competence and respectability was a change in thinking "from its traditional reliance on empiricism and toward a reliance on scientific principles" (Buckman 1987: 479). Hunter helped to forge this intellectual revolution and established many fundamental surgical principles. Cryopreservation, hemorrhage, electrical stimulation of the heart in resuscitation, inflammation and the suppuration of wounds, organ transplantation, and the nature of cancer are only some of the areas in which John Hunter was a pioneering investigator. Most surgeons and anatomists know of the adductor canal, but they may not be aware that Hunter described it first as a result of his work on the surgical treatment of popliteal aneurysm. From observations made on the growth of deer antlers and blood circulation in the horns, he discovered the concept of a collateral circulation. In December 1785, Hunter operated on a forty-five-year-old coachman for popliteal aneurysm by ligating the artery proximal to the aneurysm to prevent its further expansion and rupture. Because of the rich collateral circulation around the knee joint, he could ligate the artery at a higher level away from the diseased segment. His recommendation to operate on an aneurysm as early as possible, before it becomes larger, is still valid today.

Three of Hunter's books were published during his lifetime: *The Natural History of Human Teeth* (Parts I and II, 1771 and 1778, respectively), *A Treatise on the Venereal Disease* (1786), and *Observations on Certain Parts of the Animal Oeconomy* (1786). After his death, three works were published under his name: *A Treatise on the Blood, Inflammation and Gun-Shot Wounds* (1794), *Observations and Reflections on Geology* (1859), and *Memoranda on Vegetation* (1860). Some of his unpublished manuscripts were plagiarized and later burned by his brother-in-law, Sir Everard Home.

Hunter was elected a fellow of the Royal Society in 1767 and received the membership diploma of the Company of Surgeons a year later. On December 9, 1765, he became surgeon to St. George's Hospital in London, a position he held for twenty-five years. He was appointed surgeon extraordinary to the king in 1776 and elected to membership of the Royal Society of Gothenberg (1781), the Royal Society of Medicine and Royal Academy of Surgery of Paris (1783), and the American Philosophical Society (1787). In 1790, John became surgeon general of the army and inspector of hospitals. He was one of the first directors of the Royal Humane Society and was appointed the first vice president of the Royal Veterinary College in 1781, which he helped to establish.

In 1793, Hunter encountered considerable opposition from his colleagues at St. George's Hospital when he proposed substantive improvements in the surgical training of pupils and the remuneration of surgeons. On October 16, 1793, Hunter attended a committee meeting at the hospital where "one of his colleagues flatly contradicted something he had said." Almost immediately, he was seized by angina and left the room to deal with the pain by himself. He was followed by Dr. Matthew Baille, but after only a few steps, he "groaned and fell into Dr. Robertson's arms, and died" (Paget 1897: 218–219). Hunter was interred in a vault at St. Martin-in-the-Field's Church, near Trafalgar Square in London. In 1859, his remains were transferred to Westminster Abbey. His grave in the north nave is marked by a memorial tablet with the inscription: "The Royal College of Surgeons of England has placed this tablet on the grave of Hunter to record admiration of his genius, as a gifted interpreter of the Divine power and wisdom at work in the laws of organic life, and its grateful veneration for the services to mankind as the founder of scientific surgery." More than two centuries after his death, Hunter's name is kept alive through the Hunterian Society, the Hunterian Museum, and the Hunterian Orations, and his many distinguished disciples have promulgated Hunterian values and traditions. These luminaries included Edward Jenner, Matthew Baillie, Sir William Blizzard, Sir Anthony Carlisle, Charles White, Sir Astley Cooper, Henry Cline, William Hewson, Philip Wright Post, John Morgan, William Shippen, and Philip Syng Physick.

BIBLIOGRAPHY

Stephen Paget wrote one of the best biographies of John Hunter (1897). Sir Everard Home, Hunter's brother-in-law, wrote an intimate account of his life in Hunter's posthumously published work *A Treatise on the Blood, Inflammation, and Gun-Shot Wounds* (1794). Other useful sources of Hunter's life and work were written by Joseph Adam (1817), George Peachey (1924), John Kobler (1960), and George Quist (1981). Hunter's case books of his surgical practice have been published with commentaries by Elizabeth Allen, John Turk, and Reginald Murley (1993).

Writings by John Hunter

A Treatise on the Venereal Disease. 1st ed. London: G. Nichol, 1786.

Observations on Certain Parts of the Animal Oeconomy. London: Longmans, 1786.

A Treatise on the Blood, Inflammation, and Gun-Shot Wounds. London: George Nichol, 1794.

The Works of John Hunter, F.R.S., with Notes. With a Life by Drewry Ottley. Edited by James F. Palmer. 4 vols. London: Longmans, 1835.

Essays and Observations on Natural History, Anatomy, Physiology, Psychology, and Geology. 2 vols. London: John Van Voorst, 1861.

The Case Books of John Hunter F.R.S. Edited by Elizabeth Allen, John Turk, and Reginald Murley. London: Royal Society of Medicine Services Ltd., 1993.

Writings about John Hunter and Related Topics

Adams, Joseph. Memoirs of the Life and Doctrines of the Late John Hunter, Esq. London: J. Callow, 1817.

Brock, H. "The Many Facets of Dr. William Hunter (1718–83)." History of Science 32 (1994): 385–408.

Buckman, Jr., R. F. "The Surgical Principles of John Hunter." Surgery, Gynecology and Obstetrics 164 (1987): 479–484.

Dobson, Jessie. A Guide to the Hunterian Museum. Edinburgh: E. & S. Livingstone Ltd., 1968.

Graham, Harvey. Surgeons All. 2d ed. London: Rich & Cowan, 1956.

Hunter, William. The Anatomy of the Human Gravid Uterus Exhibited in Figures. Birmingham: Joannes Baskerville, 1774.

Kobler, John. The Reluctant Surgeon: The Life of John Hunter. London: Heinemann, 1960.

Le Fanu, William Richard. John Hunter: A List of His Books. London: Royal College of Surgeons of England, 1946.

Oppenheimer, Jane. New Aspects of John and William Hunter. London: Wm. Heinemann, 1946.

Paget, Stephen. John Hunter. Man of Science and Surgeon (1728–1793). London: T. Fisher Unwin, 1897.

Peachey, George Charles. A Memoir of William and John Hunter. Plymouth: William Brendon and Son, 1924.

Perry, M. O. "John Hunter—Triumph and Tragedy." Journal of Vascular Surgery 17 (1993): 7–14.

Quist, George. John Hunter 1728–1793. London: William Heinemann, 1981.

ACKNOWLEDGMENTS

I am indebted to the Royal College of Surgeons of England for access to the outstanding collection in the Hunterian Museum, and to Cambridge University Library for the archival material I have cited. This essay was written at Wolfson College, Cambridge, where I had been a visiting fellow.

T.V.N. Persaud

THOMAS ADEOYE LAMBO
(1923–)

Thomas Adeoye Lambo may be the most influential African medical practitioner in modern history. His importance lies in his energetic attempts to bridge the cultural distance between Western and African medicine, by making the benefits of Western medicine more widely available in Africa and other underdeveloped regions, while trying to ensure that the benefits of traditional medical systems are not lost. Growing up in the last decades of colonial rule in Africa, he developed an approach to medical policy that was in some ways culturally nationalist, but above all pragmatic. Since the 1940s he has been engaged in a creative and tireless effort to improve public health worldwide, especially in developing countries.

Lambo was born in Abeokuta, a town in the tropical southern region of Nigeria. He studied medicine at the University of Birmingham and specialized in psychiatry at the University of London. He assumed authority over Abeokuta's Aro Mental Hospital in 1954, where he remained until 1963, when he moved to the University of Ibadan medical school, serving first as chairman of the Department of Psychiatry and later as dean, ultimately becoming vice chancellor of the university. In 1971, he joined the staff of the World Health Organization, and became its deputy director in 1973. The project that first brought him acclaim involved the organization of the Aro Mental Hospital, the first mental hospital in tropical Africa, a hospital significant less for being first than for an innovative outpatient scheme Lambo developed.

Lambo was shaped by his cultural background, the history of his town, the colonial regime that dominated Nigeria in his youth, his education, and the coming of Nigeria's independence just as he was coming into his own professionally. He developed psychiatric services in Nigeria in ways no Westerner could have, so it will be useful to begin by considering his cultural background first.

Abeokuta lies in a region of tropical West Africa famous for being the home of a group of culturally related peoples referred to collectively as Yoruba. The Yoruba are significant within the African context for being an unusually urbanized society, with developed markets and long-distance trading that long predated colonialism. With regard to medicine, the Yoruba have used a combination of herbal remedies and dynamic ritual, the latter involving a system of divination based on an especially sophisticated oral tradition known as Ifa. Many of these traditions have continued in the New World, since the region was a major source of slaves for the Atlantic slave trade, especially in the nineteenth century, meaning that many people of African descent in the Western Hemisphere can trace at least part of their ancestry to the region.

The occupation of healer in Yoruba societies is highly professionalized, usually passed on from father to son, and more rarely involving mothers and daughters. Well-trained practitioners are stewards of elaborate oral traditions involving divination and herbal remedies. Yoruba medicine recognizes several types of etiology: organic, preternatural, and supernatural. Preternatural causation refers to curse or bewitchment, whereas supernatural causation refers to the actions of deities offended, for example, by the breaking of a taboo. These categories all apply to psychiatric ailments, which are treated through a combination of ritual invocation, consultations with the family members, and herbal medicines. There was thus an inherent eclecticism to Yoruba medicine, and this eclecticism has been the keynote of Lambo's career.

Significant Christian missionary activity began in the region in the 1840s. The missions were important for a number of reasons relevant to Lambo's development. One was that they represented the first significant introduction of Western medicine into Nigeria. Even more important, a highly successful Anglican mission in Abeokuta had a profound influence on the social history of Lambo's home town, creating an unusual density of people with Western education, a legacy represented in the very high numbers of nationally and internationally prominent Nigerians from Abeokuta, including the Nobel Prize–winning novelist Wole Soyinka. Abeokuta was thus growing more culturally hybrid for several generations before Lambo's birth, a process that helps to contextualize Lambo's own experiments in medical hybridization.

Before examining those experiments, one more aspect of their prehistory must be mentioned: the changes brought about by colonial rule. As in other parts of Africa, over the course of the middle decades of the nineteenth century, European missionaries increasingly were followed by European soldiers and traders, incursions that led to the establishment of European governments in Africa. These governments actively hastened economic and social changes, including the growth of wage labor and increased urbanization. Anyone familiar with the social history of madness in Europe, America, or elsewhere will not be surprised to learn that after two or three decades of these changes, Nigeria's growing urban centers appeared to be swarming with lunatics, for whom no one was eager to take responsibility. The colonial state finally did so, but reluctantly and halfheartedly, with a number of custodial institutions—asylums, that is. Nigeria's colonial asylums were overcrowded and unsanitary prison houses, with virtually no attention paid to the therapeutic needs of the patients. A need for reform of the institutions was recognized by the 1920s, but the reform was not accomplished until the 1950s. When reform was achieved, it was contemporary with Nigeria's shift to independence, and the reform was accomplished largely through the initiatives of Nigerians such as Lambo.

The state eventually developed a plan for a curative institution—that is, a mental hospital. The Alake, or king, of Abeokuta was approached by the colonial government in the 1930s to see if Abeokuta could be a possible site. The Alake was enthusiastic, but government inertia delayed the initiative. In the 1940s, the

future architects of psychiatric care in Nigeria—Lambo and his colleagues Tolani Asuni and A. A. Marinho—were in the United Kingdom working on their
medical degrees. Lambo chose medicine for practical reasons—the large number
of vagrant psychotics represented a visible public health problem—but also
found in psychiatry a link to broader humanistic concerns, as Sigmund Freud
did.

In the mid-1950s, plans for Aro were proceeding, but the physical plant was
not completed. Lambo, whose enthusiasm and commitment were becoming legendary, did not wait for the building to be completed, and he began to develop
the outpatient system. His plan was to persuade a number of families near the
Aro site to allow mental patients to live with them in exchange for work, mostly
help in farming, and a lodging fee. The villagers were provided with health
benefits as well, including piped water and a mosquito control team. Lambo's
roots in Abeokuta were crucial in the negotiations that allowed this to take place.
The patients would go to the hospital for treatment in the morning and work
the farms in the afternoon. The hospital's treatment program strongly emphasized interventions that were then state of the art in Western psychiatry: elec-
troconvulsive therapy, psychotropic drugs such as largactil, interactive
psychotherapy, and an expanded occupational therapy program.

But Lambo recognized that he faced a problem deeper than how to house the
patients. By bringing Nigerian lunatics within the orbit of a Western-style hospital, he was conveying already disoriented mental patients into a strange
world—a world that suffered from associations with a colonial government that
was usually neglectful, and brutally coercive at its worst. In order to help the
patients adjust, Lambo traveled across Nigeria and handpicked twelve traditional
healers from different cultural backgrounds to serve as mediators between the
hospital staff and the patients. The healers were culturally close to the patients
and authority figures in their eyes, and thus they functioned to impart an attitude
of trust—an important aspect of any therapeutic situation, and especially critical
in psychiatry. The healers also actively participated in therapy by conducting
religious ceremonies appropriate to the patients' cultures.

The advantages of the Aro village system were several. The plan offered
outpatient care that could help the patients reintegrate into society, in close
proximity to the medical technology of the hospital. It helped prevent complications in the mental disorder brought on by the hospital setting. According to
Asuni, another advantage of the village system was that mental patients were
exposed to "real-life" situations. Patients were therefore less withdrawn, and
the need for contrived occupational therapy was reduced because patients were
occupied with the normal life of the village. The villagers, meanwhile, derived
economic benefit from renting rooms.

In defining himself professionally and situating himself within the field of
psychiatry, Lambo faced a further challenge, of a more intellectual nature. There
was, by the time Lambo completed his medical training, a substantial literature
on mental illness in Africa, most of it written by European psychiatrists. This

literature was not devoid of insights, but just as colonial hospitals often served the interests of the colonists more than the health needs of African subjects, this emerging psychiatric theory, while claiming to diagram the distinctive psychological traits of Africans, better represented the distinctive worldview of the European colonists.

In particular, by the 1950s, colonial literature had developed elaborate theories of the "African mind," theories that represented the codification and rationalization of the stereotypes that were a prominent feature of colonial domination. This process reached its fullest development in the now-notorious writings of J. C. Carothers, a psychiatrist who did most of his work in Kenya. In articles in Britain's leading psychiatric journal, the *Journal of Mental Science*, Carothers elaborated the colonial cliché of the irresponsible African in rich, racist detail. In a bone-chilling comparison, Carothers ultimately concluded that the normal African was comparable to a lobotomized European.

It is important to realize that mainstream psychiatry at this time did not regard Carothers's work as especially reactionary; it did not even regard it as politically biased. His work, though, did inspire a lengthy rebuttal from Lambo, which also appeared in the *Journal of Mental Science*. In his response, Lambo showed that although African value systems might differ from European ones in ways that made the designation of mental pathology problematic, African culture was not monolithic and certainly not based on inherent biological differences. This line of inquiry was pursued in collaboration with a team of researchers from Cornell University in the early 1960s, resulting in a landmark ethnopsychiatric monograph, *Psychiatric Disorder among the Yoruba* (1963).

The pragmatic eclecticism that characterized the Aro innovations remained Lambo's approach as he turned his attention to global problems. In 1977, while Lambo was deputy director, the World Health Organization resolved to encourage governments in the developing world to train and support traditional healers, in particular, recognition of the importance of ethnopharmacological knowledge. Lambo remained a prolific author, publishing in medical journals articles about epidemic disease, sanitation, and social problems, in addition to psychiatry. In 1988, he left the World Health Organization and returned to Nigeria, where he remains active in the promotion of public health.

BIBLIOGRAPHY

Selected Writings by Thomas Adeoye Lambo

"The Role of Cultural Factors in Paranoid Psychoses among the Yoruba Tribe of Nigeria." *Journal of Mental Science* 101, no. 423 (April 1955): 239–266.
African Traditional Beliefs: Concepts of Health and Medical Practice. Ibadan: University of Ibadan, 1963.
(with Alexander Leighton, Charles C. Hughes, Dorothea C. Leighton, Jane M. Murphy,

and David Maclin). *Psychiatric Disorder among the Yoruba*. Ithaca: Cornell University Press, 1963.

"Patterns of Psychiatric Care in Developing Countries." In Ari Kiev, ed., *Magic, Faith, and Healing*. New York: Basic Books, 1964.

"The Village of Aro." *Lancet* 2 (1964): 513–514.

"Psychiatry in the Tropics." *Lancet*, November 27, 1965, pp. 1119–1121.

"Neuro-Psychiatric Syndromes Associated with Human Trypanosomiasis in Tropical Africa." *Acta Psychiatrica Scandinavia* 42, no. 4 (1966): 474–484.

"Protection and Improvement of World's Drinking Water Quality." In J. Tourbier and R. W. Pierson, eds., *Biological Control of Water Pollution*, pp. 23–29. Philadelphia: University of Pennsylvania, 1976.

"Traditional Medicine—A World Survey of Medicinal Plants and Herbs—Introduction." *Journal of Ethnopharmacology* 2, no. 1 (1980): 3–4.

Writings about Thomas Adeoye Lambo and Related Topics

Abimbola, Wande. *Ifa: An Exposition of the Literary Corpus*. Ibadan: Caxton, 1976.

Asuni, Tolani. "Aro Hospital in Perspective." *American Journal of Psychiatry* 124, no. 6 (December 1967): 71–78.

Buckley, Anthony. *Yoruba Medicine*. Oxford: Clarendon, 1985.

Carothers, J. C. *The African Mind in Health and Disease*. Geneva: World Health Organization, 1953.

———. "Frontal Lobe Function and the African." *Journal of Mental Science* 97, no. 406 (January 1951): 12–48.

McCulloch, Jock. *Colonial Psychiatry and the African Mind*. Cambridge: Cambridge University Press, 1995.

Prince, Raymond. "Indigenous Yoruba Psychiatry." In Ari Kiev, ed., *Magic, Faith, and Healing*, pp. 84–120. New York: Basic Books, 1964.

Smith, Robert. *Kingdoms of the Yoruba*. Madison: University of Wisconsin Press, 1988.

Vaughan, Megan. *Curing Their Ills: Colonial Power and African Illness*. Stanford, CA: Stanford University Press, 1991.

ACKNOWLEDGMENTS

I thank Alexander Boroffka, Carole Modis, and Craig Semsel for their assistance in finding citations.

Jonathan Sadowsky

MANUEL MARTÍNEZ BÁEZ
(1894–1987)

Manuel Martínez Báez was a Mexican physician, politician, and humanist who played an important role in science and politics in Mexico from 1935 to 1965, especially in the public health sector. The life of Martínez Báez may be taken as a model of the origin and evolution of the scientist-politician in Mexican elites. The formation and nature of elites plays an important place in the literature of social studies. Martínez Báez gathers in himself the characteristics defined in great detail by the sociologist A. Roderic Camp. Three well-defined factors framed the life and work of Martínez Báez: his family and place of birth, his generation, and the relationships he established in his youth.

Martínez Báez was born on September 2, 1894, in the city of Morelia in the state of Michoacán and died on January 19, 1987, in Mexico City. Ramón Martínez Avilés (1837–1911), his grandfather, originally studied law but finally devoted his life to music. Martínez Avilés was a pianist, violinist, composer, and founder of orchestras. Martínez Báez's father, Manuel Martínez Solórzano (1862–1924), was a physician and naturalist who made important studies of the flora and fauna of Michoacán. He also was the municipal president of Morelia and deputy to the Constitutional Congress of 1917, which wrote the current constitution of the country. As one of the most important physicians in Morelia, he was in charge of the smallpox vaccine.

According to Martínez Báez's brother Antonio (1901–), their father received abundant scientific literature from Europe. He also remembers a picture of J. H. Fabre, the French entomologist, whose book on insects was translated by Martínez Báez years later. Martínez Báez's mother, Francisca Báez de Martínez, who read French and English, was an elementary school teacher, a privileged position, considering the poor situation of Mexican women in the nineteenth century. Thus, as a child Martínez Báez was influenced by biology, medicine, politics, and music. He would continue developing these aspects for the rest of his life. The conjunction of a liberal, tenacious, and scientifically curious father and a well-educated and religious mother formed the feeling of independence and the ethical code that characterized him.

Martínez Báez studied in Morelia, capital of the state of Michoacán, which had had an important place in the history of Mexico since pre-Hispanic times. In the first half of the twentieth century, Morelia produced an important elite, many of whom, such as President Lázaro Cárdenas (1934–1940), controlled significant aspects of Mexican life. Martínez Báez began his studies of medicine at the School of Medicine in Morelia, after entering El Colegio Primitivo y Nacional de San Nicolás de Hidalgo, which was founded by Vasco de Quiroga in the sixteenth century and inspired by the utopian ideology of Sir Thomas

More. This school played an important role in the three big sociopolitical movements in Mexican history: independence (1810), reform (1857), and revolution
(1910). Martínez Báez deeply assimilated this historical tradition, and, having
accepted the rigorous and comprehensive curriculum of El Colegio Primitivo,
he was fluent in English and French. This enabled him to move freely in the
international, political, and scientific world. Some of his schoolmates, such as
Samuel Ramos, Salvador González Herrejón, Daniel Cosío Villegas, and Ignacio
Chávez, later occupied important political positions. Martínez Báez and his
friends were known as the *esprit coupole* of the college. These relationships
played an important role in his life. Without stealing credit from Martínez Báez,
it is appropriate to state that frequently friendship and fidelity are more important
in Mexican public positions than good qualifications and ability.

In 1913 Martínez Báez worked at the Asociación Mexicana de la Cruz Blanca
Neutral (Mexican Association of the Neutral White Cross) as a physician in the
revolution. In 1916 he got his medical degree with a dissertation about typhoid.
In 1920 he participated in the foundation of the military hospital in Morelia.
This military experience helped establish his discipline and obedience.

Martínez Báez worked for two years as a rural physician in the tropical zone
of Michoacán. There he was confronted by health problems that had their origin
in poverty and poor social conditions. Returning to Morelia, he became rector
of the University of Michoacán (1924–1925). He then moved to Mexico City,
where friends from Morelia helped him to get a job and introduced him to new
friends, including Diego Rivera, Antonieta Rivas Mercado, and the daughters
of Justo Sierra and Mariano Azuela. The cultural and social life of Mexico City
fit very well with Martínez Báez's intellectual standards. His first job was as a
lecturer in the service of hygienic education at the Department of Public Health
(he later became the subsecretary of this department) and as assistant professor
in the School of Medicine at the university, where he would become an emeritus
professor and a member of its governing board.

In these positions, Martínez Báez developed a high sense of responsibility
that enabled him to progress and made him give more than what was expected
of him. Thanks to this, he participated in the organization of the Exposición
Ibero-Americana de Sevilla and was sent to Europe in 1929. In Madrid he
admired the Spanish republicans. In Paris he befriended the parasitologist Emile
Brumpt, who came to Mexico in 1932. Thanks to Brumpt, Martínez Báez returned to Paris in 1933 for graduate studies of malaria at the university (1934).
Because of a scholarship from the Rockefeller Foundation, he also studied malaria in Spain and Italy (Instituto Antipalúdico in Navalmoral and Escuela Experimental de la Lucha Antimalárica, Rome). Returning from Europe, his
vocation was completely defined; he dropped clinical medicine and dedicated
himself to teaching and research on parasitology and public health.

The life of Martínez Báez from 1935 to 1965 was rich in all senses. His work
as a physician was carried out during one of the best moments in the history of
Mexico. In this progressive period, the arts and sciences flourished, the political

system became stable, and economic and social projects gradually developed. The old Spanish concept of health care as charity dispensed by the church was transformed by the principle of health care as the duty of the state. Concerning his personal life, Martínez Báez married Aurora Palomo González (1906–1996) from Asturias in Spain, a well-educated, modest, and cultivated woman and an ideal companion. They had three children: José Manuel (1939), Adolfo (1941), and Francisco (1943).

Martínez Báez was important in the period of Mexican history when institutions and programs for public health were established. He began his academic-scientific and scientific-political careers simultaneously, but these fields assumed different importance in his life during different periods. In the period between 1935 and 1940 he participated in the foundation of important organizations such as the Consejo Nacional de Ciencia y Tecnología (1936). In the following years, scientific-political activities predominated; for example, he was the general director of the section of epidemiology of the National Board of Health (1941–1942), vice president of the committee of experts who formulated the Constitution of the World Health Organization (1946), ambassador of Mexico, and permanent delegate to UNESCO in London and Paris (1946–1948). During the 1950s, he devoted more of his energies to his scientific and academic life; he became a member of the Seminar of Mexican Culture (1949) and the National College (1955) and published 115 papers.

Half of his papers are about parasitology and were basically written between the 1950s and the 1960s. About a quarter concern historic-humanistic topics, including many biographical essays, which were published between 1960 and 1970. The rest of his papers are about public health and medical sociology and were mostly written during the last years of his life. Martínez Báez was particularly interested in onchocerciasis, a form of endemic helminthiasis caused by *Onchocerca volvulus*, which exists in southern Mexico and northern regions of Central America. Indeed, his second (1935) and his last (1977) scientific papers are about onchocerciasis. His work was important for better understanding of the parasite and treatment of the disease.

One of Martínez Báez's most important scientific activities was related to the Instituto de Salubridad y Enfermedades Tropicales (ISET, Institute of Health and Tropical Diseases). During the presidency of Lázaro Cárdenas (1934–1940) the Plan Sexenal (a national plan that was to be accomplished in six years), prepared during the last presidential period, was institutionalized. Its goal was to push the country to progress in every sense. Concerning public health, one of the ideas of the plan was to create an institution for research on health problems and tropical diseases. On March 18, 1939, the ISET became active. Martínez Báez was its first director and also the head of the laboratory of pathological anatomy. After that, he rarely left the institute, and many people remember him always at work, looking through his microscope. The ISET was the first institution dedicated to the investigation of health problems in Mexico. Its name was changed to Instituto Nacional de Diagnóstico y Referencia Epidemiológica, Manuel Martínez Báez (Manuel Martínez Báez National Institute for Epidemiological Diagnosis and Reference) in 1989.

Although Martínez Báez's research on onchocerciasis was significant, his most important contribution was to establish the basis for a better understanding of the social, economic, and cultural aspects of tropical diseases. Martínez Báez was very concerned about the incongruence between the reality of Mexican health issues and the way it was portrayed in medical books written by foreigners. He adapted knowledge of tropical diseases emerging from countries without such problems to the countries that really lived with them. Researchers in tropical medicine, colonial medicine, or exotic pathology studied the diseases of warm countries, such as uncinariasis (hookworm), onchocerciasis, leishmaniasis, malaria, and leprosy. Martínez Báez inferred that these diseases engaged outside interest primarily because foreigners feared being infected. Concern for natives suffering from such pathologies emerged only when the workforce, and consequently production, were affected. In his opinion the term *tropical diseases* reflected the particular point of view of foreigners about a different reality, which they needed to know. For him, tropical diseases were the result of the poor situation of public health in the underdeveloped countries, which originated in poverty, ignorance, poor social organization, and an inequitable distribution of wealth. Martínez Báez spoke of these ideas in many papers but especially in his book, *Factores económicos, culturales y sociales en la génesis de las llamadas enfermedades tropicales* (Economic, cultural, and social factors in the generation of the so-called tropical diseases). He thought that it was fundamental to improve the condition of the people to eliminate tropical diseases. According to him, this was possible through science and goodwill. In his works, it is clear that he was convinced that poverty, ignorance, primitive culture, suppression of liberty, and a poor distribution of wealth would diminish considerably. Martínez Báez was a truthful prophet of a scientific and social utopia.

Many people remember Martínez Báez as an honest, intelligent, and well-educated man. He also was intolerant and of strong and difficult character—very demanding of himself and of others. Martínez Báez was an atheist, he was not rich, he never belonged to any political party and never occupied a nationally elected position, but he lived in harmony with his own moral code. He appeared to be tough-minded, but in reality, he was very sensitive. One of his passions was classical music, especially opera. Unfortunately, during the last years of his life, he became deaf. He was an intense reader; he especially admired Marcel Proust and the Spanish writer José Martínez Ruiz, better known as Azorín. In Azorín's literature the flow of time and the influence of the landscape are the principal ideas and in Proust's literature it is the obsession for the search of happiness. Happiness, time, and landscape were obsessive thoughts in Martínez Báez's mind. He did not think that science produces happiness, but it could help resolve existential problems by providing an understanding of self and society.

Martínez Báez also was a humanist. In 1972 he published the book *Pasteur, vida y obra* (Pasteur, life and work). Eight years before his death, he suffered a stroke, and his wife remembered him typing out his last book, *La vida maravillosa de los insectos contada por J. H. Fabre* (The wonderful life of the insects related by J. H. Fabre), with one finger. It seems his frustrated desire was to be an entomologist. Martínez Báez received many distinctions throughout his life, including, from Mexico, the Condecoración Eduardo Liceaga and Condecoración José María Morelos. He was a member of the Colegio Nacional and professor emeritus of the National University of Mexico. He was an honorary member of the Institute of Parasitology at the Faculty of Medicine in the University of Paris, the Panamerican Health Organization, Academy of Medicine, New York, and the Royal Society of Hygiene and Tropical Medicine, London. He was a member of the Committee of Experts of the Economic and Social Board, United Nations Organization. France honored him with Les Palmes Académiques and La Légion d'Honneur, and Cuba made him a Comendador de la Orden de Finlay.

Martínez Báez was always proud of his family, his birthplace, and his friends; he belonged to a select group in every circumstance of his life. During his childhood, he was profoundly influenced by his father and grandfather. During his adolescence, he established important relationships for his future life. In his youth, he had military experience and was confronted by poverty and misery. As an adult, he was part of the group that played an important role in the creation of modern Mexico. His work was important in parasitology, public health, and medical sociology. As a teacher, his students remember his seriousness, knowledge, and modesty. He brought prestige to Mexico in the scientific-diplomatic milieu as an intelligent, honest, well-educated, man with a strong personality. Nobody escapes from his or her genetic constitution or from external influences. Manuel Martínez Báez was privileged in both, and he used them well.

BIBLIOGRAPHY

Writings by Manuel Martínez Báez

Manual de Parasitología Médica. México: La Prensa Médica Mexicana, 1953, 1967.

Factores económicos, culturales y sociales en la génesis de las llamadas enfermedades tropicales (Economic, cultural and social factors in the genesis of the so-called tropical diseases. México: El Colegio Nacional, 1969.

Pasteur, vida y obra (Pasteur, life and work). México: El Colegio Nacional, 1972.

La vida maravillosa de los insectos contada por J. H. Fabre (The wonderful life of the insects related by J. H. Fabre). México: El Colegio Nacional, 1982.

Writings about Manuel Martínez Báez and Related Topics

Biographical Encyclopedia of the World, 693. New York: Institute of Researching Biography, 1946.

Camp, Roderic A. *Mexican Political Biographies, 1935–1975*. Tucson: University of Arizona Press, 1978.

————. *Who's Who in Mexico Today*. Boulder, CO: Westview Press, 1988.

————. *Mexico's Leaders, Their Education and Recruitment*. Tucson: University of Arizona Press, 1980.

Rodríguez de Romo, Ana Cecilia. "Manuel Martínez Báez: Una visión muy personal de las enfermedades tropicales" (Manuel Martínez Báez: A very personal vision of tropical diseases). *Gaceta Médica de México* 129 (1993): 81–87.

————. "Manuel Martínez Báez: Conjunción afortunada de inteligencia e integridad." (Manuel Martínez Báez: A fortunate conjunction of intelligence and integrity). *Universidad Michoacana* 13 (1994): 115–125.

Ana Cecilia Rodriguez de Romo

SILAS WEIR MITCHELL
(1829–1914)

During the latter half of the nineteenth century, Silas Weir Mitchell, or Weir as he preferred being called, was acknowledged as one of the greatest medical figures in America. His physiological and clinical studies, above all those of the nerve lesions incurred by soldiers in the American Civil War (1861–1865), made him world famous. But no less did his fame come from the novels he wrote with situations and character development drawn from his medical experiences.

At the time of his birth in 1829 in Philadelphia, America was a young nation with memories of the Revolutionary War still fresh. The nineteenth century was a period of immense change. At its beginning, travel was by horse, coach, and sailboat; at the end of the century, by rail, automobile, and steamboat. Oil pumped from the earth replaced whale oil, and electricity began to light the night. Messages delivered by sea packet or by messenger at the onset of the century were sent by telegraph, transatlantic cable, and telephone at the end. Hand printing presses were replaced by the rotary press and hand-set type by machine typecasting; paper handmade from rags was replaced by machine-made paper using plentiful wood fiber.

Mitchell was the son of John Kearsley Mitchell, a well-liked physician who taught chemistry at the Franklin Institute and the practice of medicine at Jefferson Medical College in Philadelphia. He was interested in science and was among the first to use ether clinically. His love of literature and poetry was a major influence on his children. In the days before radio and television, reading and discussion were the chief source of intellectual stimulation. John Mitchell would read his poems at the dinner table, encouraging his children to do the same, a habit Weir Mitchell kept up into his old age. There was a useful collection of books at home, and the public library was scoured by young Mitchell. He was, as he said in his autobiography, a timid and shy boy who devoured books to the neglect of his lessons. Timidity and shyness, as we will see, he fully overcame.

His father often invited prominent men to his home, allowing Weir Mitchell to gain an insight into their thinking. Among them was Oliver Wendell Holmes, who was greatly esteemed for the stories he wrote based on his medical experience. Such influences not only stimulated Mitchell's interest in the new developments then taking place in science and medicine but prefigured his impetus for writing novels and the fame he later won as a novelist.

Upon graduation from Jefferson Medical College in 1849, Mitchell attended medical lectures in Paris for a year. At the time, France was at the forefront in medical science, due in large measure to the discoveries being made in the newly developing field of physiology. Mitchell was most impressed by Bernard and his advice to experiment first and then construct hypotheses. Another teacher in France who befriended and influenced him was Charles Robin. He taught microscopy, at the time a new and exciting subject. It is significant that one of Mitchell's prized possessions was a microscope that he purchased in Europe and later used in his first experimental study on uric acid in the urine.

On his return from France in 1851 to take over his ill father's practice, Mitchell, following the precepts of his French teachers, instituted a program of scientific investigation along with his medical practice. As of 1862 he had published thirty-three scientific papers dealing with various aspects of circulation, respiration, muscle, reflex activity, and the effects of various chemical and physical agents on respiration, the nervous system, and muscle. He had a number of collaborators, among them William Hammond, an army surgeon who later became surgeon general of the Union Army during the Civil War. Their study of the effects of two varieties of curare and snake venom received favorable attention from the scientific community in both the United States and Europe.

The Civil War introduced new technology into warfare: telegraphy, the railroad, new guns, and cannon with rifled barrels giving accurate firing. This resulted in enormous ravages, particularly as the outmoded tactics in use by the armies called for closely packed troops to advance toward the enemy in the face of withering and deadly fire. Often enough a minié ball entering the body left with a large exit wound, leaving mangled flesh and shattered bones behind.

Because medical personnel had no knowledge of bacterial infection and how to prevent it at the time, septicemia, pyemia, erysipelas, tetanus, and hospital gangrene were common, and mortality rates were high. Amputation of gunshot-injured, gashed, or mangled limbs was frequently practiced because it was found to save lives. The surgeons worked at homes and farms close to the battlefield, requisitioning them for field hospitals. Ignaz Philipp Semmelweis's studies on cleanliness were little attended to until the introduction by Joseph Lister of antiseptic principles in the treatment of compound fractures in 1867, too late to help in the Civil War.

Following amputation, and whatever care that could be given at the field stations, the patients were removed to cities farther away from the battlefields for nursing. The large number of such patients with lingering pain and disability led to the establishment by John Hammond, then surgeon general of the army, of a special hospital for "stumps and nervous diseases," to which he assigned Mitchell, who was joined by Dr. George R. Morehouse and by Dr. William Wilson Keen as assistant surgeon. Mitchell wrote that the opportunity was unique, and they knew it: "The cases were of amazing interest. At one time there were eighty epileptics and every kind of nerve wound, palsies, choreas, stump disorders" (Mitchell, Morehouse, and Keen 1864). This was followed by Mitchell's monograph published in 1872, in which he added his later clinical experiences and tried to account for their observations on the basis of the newer findings in the anatomy and physiology of the nervous system.

After amputation of a limb, the stump presented particular management and conceptual difficulties. It was often tender to the touch and painful. Some relief could be provided by cooling the stump, injecting morphine, or cutting the nerve above the stump on the basis that an irritation of the nerve end, where a neuroma had formed, was the source of the pain. However, amelioration did not last long, and weeks or months later, an additional transection at a higher level was called for. This too would eventually fail to relieve the pain. Mitchell related this to an ascending neuritis, though some change in the higher central nervous system following the original lesion was suspected.

This was underlined by the illusion that the missing member was still present. The phantom limb phenomenon had been noticed in earlier times but was either unreported or dismissed as a neurosis or hallucination. Aaron Lemos in his thesis of 1798 gave as the earliest mention of the phenomenon that by Ambroise Paré: "For patients, long after the amputation, say they still feel pain in the dead and amputated parts; and complain strongly about this, something worthy of admiration, and almost unbelievable for those, who have no experience with it." The phenomenon received relatively little attention until Mitchell's detailed description of the phenomenon in his Civil War cases and his use of the term *phantom limb*. In the case of an arm amputation, the hand might still be felt to be present, with fingers extended or painfully clenched, the nails digging into the palm or the thumb under or over the fingers, the hand held crossed over the chest or extended forward, but with a curious foreshortening such that the hand appeared to be attached to the elbow. In the case of a lower limb amputation, the foot might appear to be still present, with sensation present on the sole and over the dorsum, with the foot attached to the knee. The phantom limb would generally slowly disappear, only to be reactivated even years later by a blow to the stump or during an illness.

When recourse was had to surgery, the phantom usually recurred later on, as did the pain. Some changed organization of the central nervous system is involved, as had been suggested by Lemos, who attributed the phenomenon to an enduring association of sensations and movements in the brain. Mitchell was to some degree aware of this possibility. He himself had described the phenomenon of "mirror" pain and hyperesthesia, where, following injury to one limb, that on the other side becomes painful and hyperesthetic. This would demand some enduring reorganization in the brain, though peripheral evocation, as from bruising a tender neuroma, can also evoke it. The central aspect appears to be an incorporation of the phantom limb into the body image, into the "neuromatrix."

The influence of the mind to construct the phantom limb was described by Mitchell in a short story published anonymously in 1866, a few years after he completed his book on gunshot wounds. In "The Case of George Dedlow," the protagonist joined the Northern army, where he served as an assistant surgeon, a background enabling him to describe knowledgeably what happened to him. A ball wounded the nerve in his right arm, leaving it insensate and powerless. He describes the agony of the burning pain that followed and the relief afforded by cold water. The arm removed, he was free of the neuralgia and later returned to duty. In another encounter, both thighs were hit and removed under chloroform. On recovery from the anesthesia, Dedlow feels a cramp in his left leg and asks to have it rubbed. He is amazed to hear that it is gone. In his final ordeal, he develops hospital gangrene in his remaining left arm, and it too is removed, leaving him a helpless torso. He was transferred to the Army Hospital for Injuries and Diseases of the Nervous System, a reference to Mitchell's clinic. Dedlow found that nearly all of his fellow patients were conscious for many months afterward of their lost limbs. Dedlow felt acute pain in his missing left hand, particularly the little finger, which was greatly relieved by morphine injections.

A fellow patient seen in the ward by Dr. Neek (with letters transposed, this is Dr. Keen, Mitchell's former collaborator who later achieved fame as one of America's foremost neurosurgeons). The man had been shot in the shoulder and was treated with a "lightnin' battery." This refers to Mitchell's use of electrical stimulation to prevent muscle atrophy from disuse following a nerve section. The patient is represented as a "plain man" who finds spiritual uplift and comfort by his attendance at the New Church. This is the Swedenborg church, whose members followed the teachings of the polymath Emanuel Swedenborg (1688–1771), a mining expert of the Swedish government, philosopher, theologian, and latterly Christian mystic who professed to have held conversations with the souls of the deceased.

Invited to join a session of the church group, Dedlow was carted to what was a séance. When he was asked to call on a departed spirit, the answer rapped out was of two numbers, which, with surprise, he recognized as those of the storage jars in the Army Medical Museum holding his amputated legs. Then Dedlow asks "what no one believe unless he can." The legs appeared to attach themselves to his body, he rose, and he walked on them. But soon they wavered; he sank to the floor and rolled over. The story ends with Dedlow's saying that he is "an unhappy fraction of a man, eager for the day when he will rejoin the lost members of his corporeal family in a happier world." An outpouring of sympathy and offers of help came from the reading public, and Mitchell the popular writer was born.

Mitchell's later neurology practice included many neurotic and hysterical patients, particularly a class of women into whose mind he believed he had a special insight: those "well known to every physician,—nervous women, who, as a rule, are thin and lack blood. Most of them have . . . passed through many hands and been treated in turn for gastric, spinal, or uterine troubles, but who remained at the end as at the beginning, invalids, unable to attend to the duties of life, and sources alike of discomfort to themselves and anxiety to others." This passage says much about the times. The role of women as keeper of the home was unquestioned, the obligations of the workplace for them little recognized, and the social strictures that shaped women's role determining what the doctor saw. Oppenheim has admirably pictured the relation of doctor to the neurotic patient in Victorian England (Oppenheim 1991). The effect of sexual problems masked as physical ailments, a realm probed and developed by Sigmund Freud, was only lightly hinted at by Mitchell. His view of Freud's concepts were that they were "filthy things that should be consigned to the fire."

The therapy Mitchell ordained was, in his own words, not remarkable: rest, systematic feeding, and passive exercise. While the use of rest in medical practice was a received principle in his time, its practice became associated with Mitchell. He prescribed his "rest cure" for such notables as Walt Whitman, Edith Wharton, Charlotte Perkins Gilman, and Virginia Woolf; artists Thomas Eakins and John Singer Sargent; and Victorian literati Edmund Gosse, the Brownings, Swinburne, and the Rossettis, among others.

The basic theory behind the rest cure was that there is a reservoir of nervous energy in the body, which can be exhausted by too much "wear and tear." With rest, the reservoir is restored. Writing about neurasthenia and hysteria in 1884, Mitchell explained that "the rest I like for them is not at all their notion of rest. To lie about half the day, and sew a little and read a little, and be interesting as invalids and excite sympathy, is all very well, but when they are bidden to stay in bed a month, and neither read, write, nor sew, and to have one nurse,—who is not a relative,—then repose becomes for some women a rather bitter medicine, and they are glad enough to accept the order to rise and go about when the doctor issues a mandate which has become pleasantly welcome and eagerly looked for."

Rigorously adhered to, this treatment could be tyrannical. *The Yellow Wallpaper*, written by Gilman, who had been a rest cure patient, is a frightening picture of what strict isolation of the patient could produce. In that story the doctor, Mitchell, thinly disguised, has the patient practically isolated in her room until she has a complete nervous breakdown.

William Osler, who had been helped in his appointment to the University of Pennsylvania by Mitchell and became his lifelong friend, became an archetypical figure of the great physician. Astutely commenting on Mitchell's regimen, Osler noted that the success of the rest treatment was largely the result of a personal factor: the deep faith that people had in the power of a strong man armed with good sense, and with faith in himself, to cure them.

In 1875, thirteen years after the death of his first wife, Mary Elwyn, Mitchell remarried. The forty-five-year-old physician and his socially prominent wife, Mary Cadwalader, moved into her large house at 1524 Walnut Street. Mitchell was elevated to the rank of brahmin in Philadelphian society. There in his office he received patients, friends, and visiting prominent figures, and he wrote his clinical studies and fiction. This inner sanctum contained his rare books, paintings, letters, and curios. Originally, writing novels was a diversion from his full schedule of clinical work and experimental studies, but later he devoted more time to it, and it became a parallel second career, one that brought him considerable fame and income. He wrote some fifteen novels plus twenty-two other literary works, most dealing with historical and psychiatric themes. As of 1894, including his scientific works, he listed 225 publications, but other minor writings increase the number.

His life was rich. Visitors would be served by a butler wearing green silk breeches, the wine was madeira at opulent dinners, closing with cigars and, above all, good talk by eminent figures in literature, medicine, politics, and business. It was said that Mitchell was a proud man. His friend John Shaw Billings* noted that he had much to be proud of. But other terms, less charitable, were used for him, such as *autocrat*, particularly in his later years. Perhaps his character was altered by the rejections he had earlier received from the two medical schools he had earlier petitioned for the chair of physiology. But more so his character was formed by his being a member of the upper class, a situation that in itself could have aroused some to feelings of antipathy. As the sociologist G. W. Domhoff (1986) wrote, "The idea that a relatively fixed group of privileged people might dominate the economy and government goes against the American grain and the founding principles of the country." He defined the upper class in the United States as socially cohesive, the members marked by their social contacts and clubs, education of their children in private schools, their marriages, and family continuity. They are not for the most part idle, preoccupying themselves with finance, business, the law, medicine, scholarship in academia, and writing, while their wives busy themselves by volunteer work or serve as homemakers. Mitchell fits the mold.

When a new building of the College of Physicians of Philadelphia was dedicated in 1909, the great hall was named for Mitchell. At the dedication ceremonies, Andrew Carnegie, a major benefactor, spoke of his friendship and affection for Mitchell, concluding: "Here he sits today—all that can accompany old age he has—honor, love, obedience, troops of friends, and the record you leave behind you." He was the acknowledged nestor of American neurology. Mitchell died in 1914, just short of his eighty-fifth birthday, a life in medical science and practice fulfilled.

Mitchell was honored at the centennial celebration of the American Physiological Society in 1987 (Ochs 1987). In the medal struck for the occasion, he is prominently figured among the other founding fathers of the American Physiological Society: Henry Newall Martin, Henry Pickering Bowditch, Russel H. Chittenden, and John Green Curtis, with Mitchell most likely the leader in bringing the society into being.

Several years ago, while on a trip to the library of the College of Physicians to examine Mitchell's files, I stopped to read the plaque erected to his memory on the front of the large office building that replaced his home at 1524 Walnut Street:

On this spot stood
The House of
S. Weir Mitchell
Physician, Physiologist.

Poet. Man of Letters.
He taught the use of rest for the nervous
He created "Hugh Wynne"
He pictured for us "The Red City" in which
He lived and laboured from 1829 until 1914.

Erected by Franklin Inn of which
he was a founder and first president.

Automobile traffic on the one-way street was choked, in glaring contrast to the tree-lined suburban road it had been in Mitchell's day. This is a paradigm of the changes in mores that make his novels little read today. But although his position as a novelist is now a minor one, his rest cure laid to rest, it was his studies of nerve lesions, his efforts to make medicine scientific, to base it on experimental physiology, and his leadership in founding the professional societies manifesting that spirit to this day, that rightfully make him a great pioneer of American neurology.

BIBLIOGRAPHY

The library of the College of Physicians of Pennsylvania in Philadelphia holds the major collection of materials relating to Mitchell, including letters, diaries, and manuscripts.

Writings by Silas Weir Mitchell

(with J. Morehouse and M. Keen). *Gunshot Wounds and Other Injuries of Nerves*. Philadelphia: Lippincott, 1864.
Wear and Tear, or Hints for the Overworked. Philadelphia: Lippincott, 1871.
Injuries of Nerves and Their Consequences. Philadelphia: Lippincott, 1872. (Reprinted by the American Academy of Neurology with a New Introduction by L. C. McHenry, Jr., New York: Dover, 1965.)
Fat and Blood: An Essay on the Treatment of Certain Forms of Neurasthenia and Hysteria. London: Lippincott, 1884.
Doctor and Patient. Philadelphia: Lippincott, 1888.
A Catalogue of the Scientific and Literary Work of S. Weir Mitchell. Philadelphia: Library of the College of Physicians and Surgeons, Philadelphia, 1894.
The Autobiography of a Quack and Other Stories. New York: Century Co, 1901. ("The Case of George Dedlow," which is in this collection, was originally submitted anonymously to the *Atlantic Monthly* 18 [July 1886]: 1–11. In the Introduction to the 1901 compilation, Mitchell described the original publication of "The Case of Dedlow" and how the spiritualists of the day were pleased by the story.)

Writings about Silas Weir Mitchell and Related Topics

Burr, A. R. *Weir Mitchell: His Life and Letters*. New York: Duffield, 1929. (The best source for Mitchell's autobiography and letters.)

Coco, G. *Vast Sea of Misery*. Gettysburg, PA: Thomas Publications, 1988.

Domhoff, G. W. *Who Rules America Now?* New York: Simon & Schuster, 1986.

Earnest, E. *Weir Mitchell, Novelist and Physician*. Philadelphia: University of Pennsylvania Press, 1950. (The best treatment of Mitchell as novelist.)

Fye, W. B. *The Development of American Physiology*. Baltimore: Johns Hopkins University Press, 1987.

Gilman, C. P. *The Yellow Wallpaper*. New Brunswick, NJ: Rutgers University Press, 1993.

Goldner, J. C. "S. Weir Mitchell: Nerves, Peripheral and Otherwise." *Mayo Clinic Proceedings* 46 (1971): 274–281.

Judd, C. S., Jr. "Osler and Mitchell." *Transactions and Studies of the College of Physicians and Surgeons of Philadelphia* 45 (1977): 99–104.

Levin, K. "S. Weir Mitchell: Investigations and Insights into Neurasthenia and Hysteria." *Transactions and Studies of the College of Physicians and Surgeons of Philadelphia* 38 (1971): 168–173.

Melzack, R. "Phantom Limbs and the Concept of a Neuromatrix." *Trends in Neuroscience* 13 (1990): 88–92.

Mumey, N. *Silas Weir Mitchell: The Versatile Physician (1829–1914)*. Denver: Range Press, 1934.

Ochs, S. "S. Weir Mitchell: Pioneer American Physiologist and Neurologist." *Physiologist* 30 (1987): 80–81.

Oppenheim, J. *"Shattered Nerves": Doctors, Patients and Depression in Victorian England*. New York: Oxford University Press, 1991.

Price, D. B., and N. J. Twombly. *The Phantom Limb: An 18th Century Latin Dissertation Text and Translation, with a Medical-Historical and Linguistic Commentary*. Washington, D.C.: Georgetown University Press, 1972.

———. *The Phantom Limb Phenomenon: A Medical, Folkloric, and Historical Study. Texts and Translations of 10th to 20th Century Accounts of the Miraculous Restoration of Lost Body Parts*. Washington, D.C.: Georgetown University Press, 1978.

Rein, D. *S. Weir Mitchell as a Psychiatric Novelist*. New York: International Universities Press, 1952.

Sunderland, S. *Nerves and Nerve Injuries*. 2d ed. Baltimore: Williams and Wilkins, 1978.

Tucker, B. B. *S. Weir Mitchell*. Boston: Richard G. Badger, 1914.

Walter, R. D. *S. Weir Mitchell, M.D. Neurologist. A Medical Biography*. Springfield, IL: Charles C. Thomas, 1970. (The best source for Mitchell's neurological studies other than those on phantom limb.)

Sidney Ochs

CARLOS MONTEZUMA
(1865?–1923)

Carlos Montezuma, physician, publisher, and activist for American Indian rights, was of Yavapai ancestry. He was born in Arizona to Coluyevah and Thilgeyah, who named him Wassaja. At the time of his birth, the American Southwest was becoming increasingly populated with non-Indian immigrants, whose presence placed a great demand on the natural resources of food, water, and land. This increasing demand produced intense competition, not only between Indians and non-Indians but also among various Indian tribes. Such competition fundamentally shaped Montezuma's life. The growing scarcity of resources helped exacerbate a long-standing conflict between the Yavapais and another tribe, the Pimas. As a young child, Montezuma and his two sisters were captured in a skirmish between the two groups. Although Pima captives traditionally were brought up within the Pima tribe, a harsh drought made this economically unfeasible, and Montezuma was sold to Carlos Gentile, an Italian immigrant and itinerant photographer who gave the young boy the name he would use in the English-speaking world. He never saw his sisters, who were sold to another man, or his parents again.

Gentile traveled widely, and Montezuma grew up and attended school in places such as Chicago, Brooklyn, and Galesburg, Illinois. After Gentile lost his business in a devastating fire, he decided that he could no longer care for Montezuma, and the boy eventually came under the care of a Baptist minister in Urbana, Illinois. Montezuma completed his college preparatory work in Urbana and entered the University of Illinois, where he received his bachelor's degree. He then decided to pursue a career in medicine and became one of the first American Indians to receive the M.D. when he graduated from Chicago Medical College in 1889.

Montezuma began his medical career by opening a private practice in Chicago. It soon foundered due to a lack of patients, however, and Montezuma eventually accepted a position as a physician with the U.S. Office of Indian Affairs (OIA), the government agency responsible for supervising relations with Native American peoples and administering Indian reservations. Between 1889 and 1893 Montezuma served as an OIA doctor at three separate posts: Fort Stevenson in Dakota Territory, the Western Shoshone Indian agency in Nevada, and the Colville Indian Agency in Washington State. His experience serving in the Indian service was crucial in the development of his ideas. He grew disgusted with the ways in which the reservations were administered, the continual lack of vital equipment and supplies, and the treatment of American Indians by agency personnel. At Fort Stevenson, for example, Montezuma came into conflict with the superintendent, who told the commissioner of Indian affairs that

Montezuma was incompetent, disliked by the children for whom he cared, insubordinate, and "filthy." Montezuma responded by noting that conditions for the children at the agency were poor; most were afflicted with chronic eczema due to the poor sanitary conditions in the school bedrooms and bathrooms, and they were not provided with changes of clothing or bedding. The superintendent's charges simply reflected his biased attitudes toward Indian employees.

The conflict between Montezuma and the agency superintendent was rectified when Montezuma was transferred to Western Shoshone. Although conditions there were better, the physician was still hampered by a lack of equipment and supplies, such as fresh smallpox vaccine or a horse that would have allowed him to travel to outlying villages. Similar conditions prevailed at Colville, where Montezuma was transferred in early 1893.

Six months later, Montezuma accepted a fourth position, that of physician at the Carlisle Indian School in Pennsylvania. Here the young doctor came under the mentorship of Richard Henry Pratt, the school's founder and a leading proponent of American Indian assimilation. According to mainstream popular opinion in the late nineteenth and early twentieth centuries, the eventual disappearance of the American Indian race was inevitable. Proponents of this view pointed to the decline in the American Indian population and to continued high rates of tuberculosis mortality on reservations as proof that the race must inevitably become extinct. Pratt was among a group of influential reformers, most of whom were white and lived on the East Coast and who believed that such a potential tragedy could be averted only if American Indians adopted the ways of mainstream society.

The boarding school was designed to be a major instrument in this process. The idea was that if children could be removed from the influences of their families and communities, they could be taught the ways of "civilized" society. The idea, as Pratt himself put it, was to "kill the Indian and save the man." Students at Carlisle and other Indian schools were thus forbidden to speak their native languages, wear traditional clothing, or maintain traditional religious ceremonies and practices. Instead, they were forced to learn English and were subjected to a rigorous program of study which included attention to science, mathematics, and American history and government. Students also received vocational training and instruction in the principles of Christianity. The intent was to sever all connections with traditional tribal cultures.

Montezuma and Pratt had known each other for several years. As a struggling medical student, Montezuma had written to the Carlisle superintendent seeking guidance, and the two had begun what would become a lifelong correspondence. Montezuma had even, at Pratt's invitation, traveled to New York and Philadelphia, where he had provided a kind of example of how education might benefit American Indians by giving speeches to audiences of Indian reformers. At Carlisle, Montezuma experienced none of the problems that had plagued him in his earlier reservation posts, and he became increasingly active in Indian reform circles, giving regular speeches at reform conventions and meetings. These speeches showed the influence of both Pratt and Montezuma's experiences working for the OIA. The reservation, Montezuma argued, was "a demoralizing prison, a barrier to enlightenment, a promoter of idleness, gamblers, paupers, and ruin" (Lake Mohonk Conference 1915: 19). It was only by being allowed to receive the benefits of an education such as that provided at Carlisle that American Indians could realize their talents and become fully functioning members of mainstream American society.

In 1896, Montezuma left Carlisle with the intent of once again establishing a private practice in Chicago. Although he initially experienced the same difficulty attracting patients that he had encountered just after leaving medical school, Montezuma's luck changed after a chance encounter with Dr. Fenton B. Turck, a leading Chicago internist. The two physicians had met when Turck had given a demonstration of his work at Carlisle. When Turck offered Montezuma a position in his clinic, the younger doctor quickly accepted. The senior physician continued to serve as mentor to Montezuma, helping him build up his private practice and become established on the Chicago medical scene. Montezuma would remain in practice in Chicago until shortly before his death in 1923.

Although by this time Montezuma had already achieved recognition through his association with Pratt, his stature as a national Indian leader continued to increase. In Chicago, he continued over the next several years to write and to speak publicly on the topic of Indian affairs, and to criticize not only the reservation system but also the OIA itself. This activity won him growing recognition, and it made him a logical choice to be involved in the creation of a national organization for American Indians. Although Montezuma himself had proposed such an organization as early as 1888, the immediate impetus for it came from Fayette McKenzie, a professor of economics and sociology at Ohio State University. McKenzie had written his Ph.D. dissertation on the condition of American Indians, and he had become convinced that a national-level organization of Indian leaders would be a significant step in improving those conditions. In 1909, McKenzie began corresponding with a number of educated American Indian leaders, including Montezuma, about the possibility of forming such a group. Two years later, McKenzie, Montezuma, and five other prominent American Indian leaders met in Columbus, Ohio, to help plan the organization. They issued a statement declaring that its purpose was to provide educated leadership for American Indians, assess conditions that affected American Indians, and promote the idea of Indian self-help, and they announced plans to organize a national convention.

Six months later, in October 1911, this convention opened its doors. The more than fifty men and women who attended heard numerous speeches, on topics such as "Industrial Organization for the Indian" and "The Philosophy of Indian Education." Participants decided that full voting membership in the organization would be limited to Indians only, although non-Indians could become nonvoting associate members. To separate the group from other non-Indian reform groups, the participants decided to adopt the name Society of American Indians (SAI).

Montezuma, surprisingly, had chosen not to attend the convention. As plans to organize the meeting had taken shape during the previous summer, a conflict had developed over the role to be played by the OIA. Among those invited to the convention were several American Indians who held posts in the OIA. McKenzie himself, meanwhile, agreed to conduct the OIA's national Indian census. These developments were troubling to Montezuma, who was unwilling to compromise at all in his belief that the Indian Bureau should be abolished, and he feared that such connections to the OIA would threaten the organization's independence.

The following year other members of the SAI persuaded Montezuma to overcome his objections and speak at the group's second annual convention. But the issue of the OIA's role continued to be a source of divisiveness. Although Montezuma remained an active supporter of the group, in its early years he was often critical of it for not going far enough in its criticisms of the Indian Office. Throughout his life, he was uncompromising in his demand that the OIA be abolished. The Indian Office was, he declared in one speech, a "tyrannous institution" that presented "the atrocious spectacle of a Prussian system buckled down upon and burdening the free development of a whole race of people." The agency's original aim, to protect American Indians, had been accomplished, and its continued existence now served merely to perpetuate the "Reservation prison" and to limit any possibility of Indian advancement. "The fact of persistent paternalism of the Government through the Indian Bureau," Montezuma concluded, ". . . is a damnable condition of tutelage that degrades the Indian's manhood and enervates his once strong character" (Montezuma 1919: 11–14).

Although Montezuma continued to participate actively in SAI conferences throughout the 1910s, he remained convinced that the organization would not go far enough in opposing the OIA. This belief led him in 1916 to begin publishing his own newsletter, which he named *Wassaja*. *Wassaja*'s purpose was clear: to bring about the OIA's abolition. It would, Montezuma declared in the first issue, "be published only so long as the Indian Bureau exists. Its sole purpose is Freedom for the Indians through the abolishment [sic] of the Indian Bureau." The paper's masthead—a drawing of an American Indian man pinned underneath a huge log labeled "Indian Bureau"—made the point quite clear.

Although the newsletter struggled financially, it remained one of Montezuma's chief passions until shortly before his death. (He often worked on editorial and production tasks between midnight and 2 A.M., after the details of his medical practice and the events of the day were complete.) Early issues consisted of frequent editorials attacking the OIA, as well as stories discussing OIA malfeasance on particular reservations. The SAI and its leaders also frequently came under attack for what Montezuma saw as an excessive readiness to compromise with the Indian Bureau. These criticisms ended after the SAI voted in 1918 to support the OIA's abolition and after Arthur C. Parker (Seneca), a longtime officer in the organization and target of the editorials in *Wassaja*, was replaced as editor of the SAI's official journal by Zitkala-Sa (Dakota), a close Montezuma ally. Thereafter Montezuma was a consistently strong supporter of the society.

In 1915, during the height of Montezuma's activity with the SAI, the Chicago physician married Marie Keller, a young Romanian-American woman from Chicago. Although archival information about their marriage is scant, it appears as if the couple enjoyed a strong and mutually supportive relationship. Montezuma meanwhile remained active not only in the area of national Indian affairs, but also with issues affecting American Indians in the American Southwest. He had made the first of what would be numerous visits to the region in 1900, when he accompanied the famous Carlisle football team on a southwestern tour. The following year he returned on his own to the community in which he had been born, to reestablish contact with distant relatives and other members of the Yavapai community whom he had known as a child.

In 1903, by executive order, President Theodore Roosevelt created a new reservation for the Yavapais. Government officials believed that the new Fort McDowell reservation, which was located along the Verde River Valley in central Arizona at the site of a former military reserve, could serve as an instrument to help the Yavapais become self-sufficient. Much of the land on the reservation could be irrigated and could therefore be used to help the Yavapais become thriving, independent farmers. But once the reservation had been created, the plan ran into problems. Existing irrigation ditches at Fort McDowell were in poor condition and subject to frequent, costly repairs. Moreover, water in the Southwest was becoming an increasingly precious commodity as more and more non-Indians moved into the area. In recognition of this development, the U.S. Congress in 1902 had passed the Newlands Act, which established the Federal Bureau of Reclamation (BAR) as the agency responsible for irrigation projects in Arizona and elsewhere throughout the West. By 1905, the BAR had entered into plans to construct a reservoir on the nearby Salt River.

OIA officials decided that instead of constructing a new, functioning irrigation system at Fort McDowell, it would be less costly to move the Yavapais to the nearby Salt River reservation, where they would be able to use water made available by the Salt River project. Since such a plan would benefit the Yavapai, the officials reasoned, they should also contribute to its cost, something that would reduce the expense to the government. Finally, moving the Yavapai would free up the waters of the Verde River for reclamation projects that would presumably benefit the residents of nearby Phoenix.

The Yavapai had been promised the land at Fort McDowell, and they were vehemently opposed to the plan. Montezuma became a leader in organizing opposition to the OIA and devoted much of his time to fighting the efforts at removal. He corresponded regularly with Yavapai leaders at Fort McDowell, urging them to reject the proposed relocation plan, and he sent frequent missives to government officials and members of Congress detailing the plan's flaws. One of these congressmen was James Graham, the chair of a special house committee that had been established to investigate the way the Interior Department spent its money. At Graham's invitation, Montezuma and other leaders of the Yavapai expressed their official opposition to the relocation program in 1911 at hearings held by this committee.

During the 1910s, Montezuma's advocacy efforts for the Yavapai expanded to include other Native Americans in the Southwest, such as the Pimas and Maricopas, and he made frequent visits to the region. His efforts to represent the interest of these Indian groups, and his continued staunch opposition to the removal of the Yavapais from Fort McDowell, won him the undivided antagonism of local reservation superintendents. These officials enjoyed nearly unlimited authority during this period. Their power allowed them to restrict the movement of people on and off the reservation, decide who was eligible to receive government rations, restrict traditional dances and ceremonials, and determine whom the Indians might choose to represent their interests. Thus, Montezuma himself had been accepted as a representative of the Yavapais only after much bureaucratic wrangling, and only then under the title of "voluntary charitable worker."

That an Indian man might be more educated than they were and that he would act to challenge their authority was nearly unthinkable to these officials. It was Montezuma, in their view, who bore responsibility for stirring up the Yavapais in opposition to the removal plan. As one local superintendent put it, "That this man can and probably has done much to hinder the work among [the Indians] is unquestionably a fact and that if he is permitted to spread this sort of doctrine without let or hindrance will seriously interfere with law and order, Administrative control and the furtherance of the policies of the Administrative Office along all lines, is also a bare statement of fact" (cited by Iverson 1982: 133).

In spite of this opposition, Montezuma continued to fight against the Indian Bureau until the end of his life, not without cost; it seems clear that his opposition to the OIA played a key role in causing that agency, in the early 1920s, to reject his petition to be allotted land at Fort McDowell. Still, Montezuma continued his crusade. Although the SAI had entered a period of decline (and would hold its last annual conference in the fall of 1923), the pages of *Wassaja* continued to promote the organization and publicize its annual meetings. And Montezuma continued to speak and write against the removal of the Yavapais. His efforts would ultimately prove successful, as the OIA would abandon all plans to transfer the Yavapais to Salt River.

Montezuma continued his activities with the SAI and in the Southwest even after developing active pulmonary tuberculosis in 1922. But his health grew progressively worse, and in December 1922 he returned home to spend his final days at Fort McDowell. Marie Montezuma soon joined him, and he died on January 31, 1923, with his wife at his side.

BIBLIOGRAPHY

The best archival source on Montezuma's life is his collected papers, mainly held by the Wisconsin Historical Society. The University of Arizona and Arizona State University also maintain significant Montezuma holdings, and a comprehensive microfilmed edition of the Montezuma papers is available from Scholarly Resources. Peter Iverson's excellent 1982 biography stands as the authoritative scholarly work on Montezuma. See also Hazel W. Hertzberg (1971) for a discussion of Montezuma's activities with the SAI.

Writings by Carlos Montezuma

"Abolish the Indian Bureau." *American Indian Magazine* 7, no. 1 (1919): 9–20.
Papers. 9 microfilm reels. Washington, D.C.: Scholarly Resources, 1983.

Writings about Carlos Montezuma and Related Topics

Hertzberg, Hazel W. *The Search for an American Indian Identity: Modern Pan-Indian Movements.* Syracuse, NY: Syracuse University Press, 1971.
Hoxie, Frederick. *A Final Promise: The Campaign to Assimilate the Indians, 1880–1920.* Lincoln: University of Nebraska Press, 1984.
Inverson, Peter. *Carlos Montezuma and the Changing World of American Indians.* Albuquerque: University of New Mexico Press. 1982.
Lake Mohonk Conference of Friends of the Indian. *Annual Report.* 1915.

Todd Benson

NAGAYO SENSAI
(1838–1902)

Nagayo Sensai was the founder and administrator of the first Western-style medical and public health institutions of modern Japan. Nagayo Sensai was born to a physician's family in Omura domain, Hizen Province (now Nagasaki Prefecture) in the late Tokugawa period. In 1838, the year of his birth, Japan was an isolated country ruled by feudal lords and a hereditary overlord, the Tokugawa shogun. When Nagayo died in 1902, Japan was a modern nation-state administered in the name of the Meiji emperor by a powerful oligarchy and bureaucracy. This transformation from feudal domains to nation-state was accomplished by young nationalists, many of whom had trained in medicine, who were interested in creating a centralized, bureaucratic state along Western lines. Nagayo Sensai played a major role in establishing Western medicine as state medicine during the period in which the Japanese state was formed.

In the early nineteenth century, most Japanese physicians practiced Chinese-style traditional medicine. However, the region around Nagasaki where Nagayo Sensai was born became a center for Western-style medicine during this period. Japanese physicians from many parts of Japan went to Nagasaki to study Western medicine and science by reading imported European medical books written in Dutch. Such physicians were known as *ranpō-i*, or Dutch-method physicians. Nagayo's grandfather and father were both *ranpō* physicians. His grandfather was a medical pioneer. He advocated the Chinese method of variolation to immunize children against smallpox; however, after cowpox vaccine became available, he endorsed the Western technique of Jennerian vaccination.

Nagayo Sensai's father died when Nagayo was eight. This loss required an acceleration of Nagayo's education, which began with his grandfather as tutor. At age eleven Nagayo was sent to the official domain school to study the Chinese classics. In 1854, he was sent to Tekijuku, Japan's most prestigious private Dutch Studies academy in Osaka. Tekijuku was founded in 1838 by Ogata Kōan, a *ranpō* physician who taught many of Japan's early Meiji leaders. Nagayo remained at Tekijuku for six years and in his final year was ranked first among the school's students. Tekijuku was regarded as a medical school because Ogata Kōan was a practicing physician, but Nagayo claimed it was actually a school where students learned how to read Dutch books. Some of the students were interested in Western artillery and military strategy rather than medicine.

Nagayo Sensai formally succeeded to the family headship when his grandfather died in 1855, but he continued his studies at Tekijuku until 1860. He then returned to western Japan, where he was expected to take up the family medical practice and his hereditary position in the medical hierarchy of Omura domain. However, on the advice of Ogata Kōan, he went instead to Nagasaki, where he began to study Western medicine under the supervision of several Dutch physicians.

Nagasaki was the place to be in the 1860s. The Tokugawa government in Edo, buffeted by both internal and external forces, was rapidly losing its capacity to rule the country. In its final decade of rule, the shogunate opened a medical school and hired Dutch physicians to teach Western-style medicine in Nagasaki. The first of these physicians, Johannes Lidius Catharinus Pompe van Meerdervoort, came to Japan in 1857. A Dutch physician trained in military medicine at Utrecht Medical College in Holland, Pompe was the first of many influential Westerners to come to Nagasaki to teach medicine. Nagayo Sensai was among the first to have the opportunity to attend lectures and see patients in clinics supervised by Western physicians. In spite of many years of studying Dutch, Nagayo at first understood virtually nothing of Pompe's lectures. However, he claimed that Pompe's method of teaching—using graphs and drawings to illustrate diseases, instruments, and medical techniques and very simple language to describe things—made comprehension possible within a short period of time.

Japan's first Western-style hospital, originally called Yōsei-sho and later Seitoku-kan, was established in Nagasaki in the 1860s. In 1868, with the defeat of the shogun's troops by those loyal to the emperor, the shogun's officials fled Nagasaki, and Nagayo Sensai was chosen director of the Hospital. He began to work with Western physicians hired to supervise the practice of hospital medicine. Among these physicians were Antonius Franciscus Bauduin, who taught Nagayo surgical medicine, and Cornelius G. van Mansvelt, who played an important role as Nagayo's adviser during his implementation of medical reform in Nagasaki.

As the new director of the Seitoku-kan, Nagayo quickly initiated major reforms of the medical system. He began with medical education, creating a curriculum that included anatomy, physiology, and pathology. These subjects were taught by dissection and autopsy. On the advice of van Mansvelt, Nagayo also initiated a premedical program that included mathematics, chemistry, physics, botany, and zoology. Students were required to master these basics before they could advance to the medical program. The new curriculum and method of teaching followed a European model that was entirely different from the time-honored way of teaching medicine in Japan, which was to read and memorize the Chinese medical classics. Anton Cornelius Johannes Geertz, a Dutch pharmacist and science teacher, was put in charge of developing a premedical program at the Nagasaki Medical School.

From the beginning of his career, Nagayo Sensai relied on foreign advice and expertise, but he also engaged the cooperation and active assistance of Japan's new political leaders. Some of the most influential of the early Meiji leaders were from western Japan and were in Nagasaki at the end of the Tokugawa period. As a student and young administrator, Nagayo formed close working relationships with several of these men. Inouye Kaoru, a future Meiji statesman, was serving the new government in Nagasaki when Nagayo began his reform of the Nagasaki Medical School. Nagayo successfully appealed to him for funds to buy books and equipment, hire foreign faculty, and provide the school with cadavers of executed criminals for dissection. When Inouye and other Meiji leaders from western Japan moved to Tokyo to take leadership roles in the Meiji government, they were well aware of Nagayo's accomplishments in the area of medical reform.

In 1871 Nagayo was called to Tokyo to undertake the same kinds of reform that he had initiated in Nagasaki. Reluctant to become involved in the still unstable politics of the new capital, he chose instead to join the Iwakura mission, an official government delegation being formed to visit the United States and Europe. As a representative of the Ministry of Education, his assignment was to study medical education in the West. Much of his time was spent in European capitals, visiting medical schools and hospitals, an experience that was a major turning point in his life. It changed the primary focus of his career from medical education to public health. "I heard the words 'sanitary' and 'health' everywhere after I came to Berlin," he wrote, "but I really did not understand those words. What I eventually came to understand was that these words meant not only the protection of the citizens' health, but also referred to an entire administrative system that was organized to protect the public's health. . . . This system operated administratively, through the state, to eliminate threats to life and to improve the nation's welfare" (Nagayo 1902; Ogawa and Sakai 1980: 133–134). This concept reached far beyond the traditional practice of medicine, which focused on the individual relationship between doctor and patient, into the realm of public works. It meant draining swamps and providing proper sewage disposal and clean water systems. It meant documenting the incidence and distribution of disease, developing statistical measurements, and educating the public about proper hygiene. Such activities lay outside the scope of individual physicians. Under Nagayo Sensai's direction, these activities became the public health agenda of the new Meiji government.

When Nagayo returned from Europe in 1872, he was given a position in the Education Ministry and appointed director of the new Bureau of Medical Affairs. In this capacity he wrote a medical code intended to change the teaching and practice of medicine radically in Japan. The code established central government regulations for medical education and practice, and adopted national sanitary regulations for the first time. It also established the general principles for local sanitary administration, testing and licensing physicians, and testing and licensing pharmacists. After the code was approved by the cabinet, responsibility for its implementation within the central bureaucracy of the Meiji state was reallocated. Responsibility for medical education remained with the Ministry of Education, and responsibility for disease prevention was moved to the powerful Home Ministry. A Central Sanitary Bureau was created within the Home Ministry and placed under the administration of Nagayo Sensai as its first director.

The Central Sanitary Bureau was made up of four departments: General Administration, Bureau of Statistics, Bureau of Vaccination, and Bureau for the

Control of Medicine. The Vaccination Bureau was the first to begin operations. A strong advocate of vaccination, Nagayo Sensai wrote and promulgated Japan's compulsory vaccination law. Jennerian vaccination had been in use in Japan since the arrival of cowpox lymph in 1849, and the efforts of committed physicians to spread vaccination had been remarkably successful. Vaccine production, storage, and distribution, however, were beyond the capacity of individual physicians and needed the supervision of a higher coordinating body.

Nagayo Sensai's family had been directly involved in the business of disseminating cowpox lymph in Omura domain; consequently, Nagayo was familiar with these matters. During his visit to Holland with the Iwakura mission, he had gone to the Hague to observe the calf inoculation method used to produce cowpox vaccine. He returned to Japan with the appropriate equipment, and in 1873 he bought a calf and successfully reproduced the Dutch method. With the establishment of the Central Sanitary Bureau, cowpox vaccine production and storage became a public enterprise. Eventually two Vaccination Institutes were set up, one in Tokyo and one in Osaka. Directorships of the Vaccination Bureau remained in the hands of the Japanese, because, unlike other bureaus, there was no need to hire foreign experts.

The Bureau for the Control of Medicines developed differently. Its original purpose was to control the importation of foreign medicines that were entirely unknown in Japan. A foreign expert was needed for this task, and Nagayo hired Anton Geertz, the pharmacist from Holland who had helped him develop the premedical program at Nagasaki Medical School. Geertz set up the Bureau for the Control of Medicine in Tokyo and eventually organized and supervised the work of regional bureaus in Kyoto and the port cities of Osaka, Nagasaki, and Yokohama.

Between 1875 and 1878, Nagayo Sensai served as the president of Tokyo Medical School, which would later become the University of Tokyo Medical School. The Meiji government was simultaneously developing a central bureaucracy and founding imperial universities to train Japanese youth in Western science. The shortage of qualified professionals to fill key positions in these new institutions meant that a few individuals often served in both government and university posts. Nagayo Sensai's extensive experience in medical education in Japan and his contacts with university faculties and government bureaucrats abroad made him a valuable asset in an academic setting that required government support.

The field of public health changed rapidly in the nineteenth century as more rapid dissemination of disease caused worldwide pandemics of cholera and bubonic plague, and as the discovery of the germ theory of disease suggested new ways to control and prevent the spread of disease. As international contacts in the fields of medicine and public health became more important to effective control of disease, Nagayo Sensai continued to emphasize an international role for Japan. He personally represented Japan at the U.S. Centennial Exhibition in

Philadelphia in 1876 and regularly sent Japanese health officials to international sanitary conferences during his tenure as director of the Central Sanitary Bureau.

Nagayo Sensai was a transitional figure who spanned Japan's great Tokugawa-Meiji divide. He had a long and distinguished career as a medical administrator and public servant; however, his early commitment to the practice of Western medicine remained the focus of his life. It was his interest in broadening the concept of Western medicine to include medical education and the new idea of public health, and his ability to adapt his strategies to meet Japan's needs and capabilities, that made him an effective administrator. His policies helped to bring a backward and isolated Japan onto the world scene and laid the foundation for Japan's long-term commitment to Western medicine.

BIBLIOGRAPHY

There is little mention of Nagayo Sensai in English-language publications, the exception being a short entry in the *Kodansha Encyclopedia of Japan* (1983). The main source for details about Nagayo Sensai's life is his autobiography, which was written in his early sixties and published as *Shōkō shishi* (1902) in conjunction with the autobiography of Matsumoto Jun, a Japanese physician-statesman of the same generation. The 1902 joint biographies are available in *Matsumoto Jun jiden to Nagayo Sensai jiden* (1980), edited by Ogawa Teizō and Sakai Shizu, professors of medical history at Juntendo University. Appendixes include Nagayo Sensai's *Kyū Omura han shutō no hanashi* (The story of vaccination in old Omura domain) and a chronology of the main events in Nagayo Sensai's life. *History of Japanese Medicine in the Edo Period* (1991), by Nagayo Sensai's grandson, Nagayo Takeo, introduces many *ranpō* physicians to the English-language reader.

Published documents that shed light on the activities of Nagayo Sensai after he became director of the Central Sanitary Bureau are the *Eisei kyoku nenpō* (Annual reports of the Central Sanitary Bureau), 1877–1900, which were reprinted in 1992. These reports include information by prefecture on physicians, local health authorities, hospitals, and apothecaries, and statistics on acute infectious disease, causes of death, and vaccinations. English translations of the bureau reports are available for the First and Second Annual Report (1877–1879) and the Annual Report of 1903.

Writings by Nagayo Sensai

Ogawa Teizō, and Sakai Shizu. *Matsumoto Jun jiden to Nagayo Sensai jiden* (The autobiographies of Matsumoto Jun and Nagayo Sensai). Tokyo: Heibonsha, 1980.

Writings about Nagayo Sensai and Related Matters

Bowers, John Z. *Western Medical Pioneers in Feudal Japan*. Baltimore: Johns Hopkins University Press, 1970.

Keene, Donald. *The Japanese Discovery of Europe, 1720–1830*. Rev. ed. Stanford, CA: Stanford University Press, 1969.

Kodansha Encyclopedia of Japan. 9 vols. Tokyo: Kodansha, 1983.

Meiji-ki Eisei kyoku nenpō, Dai i-ki (Annual reports of the Central Sanitary Bureau in the Meiji era, first series), *1877–1900*. 7 vols. Tokyo: Hara Shobō, 1992.

Nagayo Takeo. *History of Japanese Medicine in the Edo Period*. Nagoya: University of Nagoya Press, 1991.

Rubinger, Richard. *Private Academies of Tokugawa Japan*. Princeton: Princeton University Press, 1982.

Ann Bowman Jannetta

ROSWELL PARK
(1852–1914)

Roswell Park, physician, surgeon, chairman of surgery at the University of Buffalo, and founder of a cancer research institute, was born in Pomfret, Connecticut, on May 4, 1852. His father, Rev. Roswell Park, D.D., had a multifaceted career as professor of chemistry and natural philosophy at the University of Pennsylvania, writer of poems and textbooks, and founder and first president of Racine College in Wisconsin. His mother, Mary Brewster Park (née Baldwin), a member of an eminent New England family, died when Park was two years old, and the boy spent his childhood in the care of his uncle, Dr. Lewis Williams of Pomfret, Connecticut, who stimulated his interest in medicine and science. Park attended private schools in Pomfret, Racine, and Chicago. He received the bachelor of arts degree from Racine College in 1872 and the master of arts degree in 1875. Thereafter, he studied medicine at the Chicago Medical College and received the M.D. degree in 1876.

Dr. Park began his career as an intern and house physician at Mercy Hospital, Chicago, followed by several years at Chicago's Cook County Hospital. In addition to his clinical work, he taught anatomy at the Women's Medical College of Chicago. In 1880 he was appointed adjunct professor of anatomy at Chicago Medical College. He resigned this position in 1882 to gain experience at clinical and research centers in Berlin, Vienna, and Prague. When he returned to Chicago from Europe, he was appointed lecturer in surgery at Rush Medical College and attending surgeon at Michael Reese Hospital.

During these early years, Park had begun the contributions to medical science that were to bring him international recognition as a master surgeon. Noteworthy among these initial reports on anatomical, infectious, and surgical subjects was one of the earliest papers in the United States on antisepsis in surgery. The paper, published in 1882, was timely. Joseph Lister (1827–1912), whose papers on antisepsis began appearing in 1867, progressively altered operating room techniques as his principles gained acceptance. Lister's operative technique required spraying carbolic acid over the operating field and irrigating wounds with carbolic acid. Prominent American surgeons were far from unanimous about the virtues of the Listerian system. Park proposed a moderate view, endorsing Lister's concepts in general but advocating methods of operative management and wound treatment that were kinder to body tissues than Lister's. Park's recommendations were offered just before antiseptic surgery began to be supplanted in about 1888 by modern aseptic technique with the change to moist heat sterilization.

In 1883, with the retirement of the notable surgeon Dr. Edward Moore, the chair of surgery in the Medical Department of the University of Buffalo became vacant, and Roswell Park was highly recommended by his surgical mentors in Chicago for the appointment. The selection process was remarkably brief, and on June 23, 1883, Park was made professor of surgery at the University of Buffalo. Shortly after, he was designated surgeon in chief to the Buffalo General Hospital.

The next few years were clinically and academically productive. Park was soon viewed by students and physicians as a superb teacher and a skillful surgeon. His publications from 1883 to 1900 reflect a wide range of surgical activities, including the treatment of surgical infections, the use of antiseptic techniques, and some of the earliest reported operations for tumors of the brain, base of the skull, and larynx. His monograph in 1888 on surgery of the brain was one of the first on the subject. Also among his publications in 1883 was an editorial on the treatment of gunshot wounds in which he supplemented his experience with a review of the recommendations of other surgeons derived from the treatment of injuries sustained in warfare, especially in the Russo-Turkish War of 1877. In this editorial, he discussed the management of the abdominal gunshot wound that President Garfield had sustained on July 2, 1881. President Garfield died of infection after a prolonged course of treatment, and Park, who considered the death avoidable, wrote that the president had endured five probings of the wound "without the slightest antiseptic precaution" before he was moved, and "on the second day the bullet hunt was resumed with sounds and bougies and the attendants arrived at a conclusion that was already self-evident, namely—that no vital organs were injured."

Park was impressed by the high incidence of cancer in Buffalo. In 1892, he gave an address to the Medical Society of the State of New York on cancer as a parasitic disease. In the published address, in which he reviewed existing knowledge of the causes of cancer and focused on the earlier work of previous investigators, he wrote, "I have for years had a growing conviction that cancer—and syphilis too—were parasitic diseases, due to either unfamiliar or yet unknown organisms." In his concluding remarks, he expressed his impatience and anxiety about the pace of progress in determining the cause of cancer, stating "My home is in Western New York ... where the death rate from cancer is greater than in any other part of our continent."

In the late nineteenth century, investigators searching for the cause of cancer had divergent views, which centered on whether the disease originated from factors within the body or was caused by an external agent. Some investigators had described inclusion bodies within cancer cells and thought that these represented pathogenic protozoa or yeast. Other scientists attached little importance to these inclusion bodies, noting that a large number of investigators had searched for a specific microbe as a causative agent for cancer, but all had failed to show that cancer was produced by a microorganism introduced from without. Looking at the evidence, Park expressed the conviction that cancer was a parasitic disease, by which he meant an external infectious agent of unknown type.

In 1898, largely as a result of persuasion by Park and Edward H. Butler, publisher of the *Buffalo Evening News*, the New York State legislature provided a $7,500 grant to Park to establish the New York State Pathological Laboratory of the University of Buffalo to investigate the causes, nature, mortality rate, and treatment of cancer. The laboratory was set up in three small rooms in the University's Department of Medicine. Park recruited Dr. Harvey Gaylord, who had received his degree in medicine from the University of Pennsylvania in 1893 and had studied in Germany with Professor Ludwig Aschoff, to join the research effort. Recruitment of additional faculty followed, and Park's research program quickly grew too large for the space. Through the generosity of local citizens, the Gratwick Research Laboratory of the University of Buffalo was built on High Street in 1900–1901. This was the first research institution in the world devoted exclusively to cancer investigations.

In 1901, Park was president of the American Surgical Society, and at its meeting in Baltimore, he lectured on his investigations on the nature of cancer. Recognizing the confusion of thought concerning the cause of cancer, Park held firmly to the belief that cancer was a disease of infectious nature. In 1902, he referred to the cause of cancer as a "virus," in the classical sense of an unknown agent of infection. (The modern meaning of the word *virus* as an obligate intracellular parasite had not yet been established.)

Park was director of the Gratwick Research Laboratory from 1901 to 1904. Because of increases in the staff and research activities, Park appointed Gaylord as the director and remained as chairman of the Advisory Committee. In 1911, the laboratory was renamed the New York State Institute for the Study of Malignant Diseases. Park was appointed for life as the chairman of its board of trustees. A thirty-bed cancer research hospital (the Cary Pavilion) was added to the institute in 1913, thereby adding to the research capacity of the facility. Yearly reports from the institute emphasized research in immunology, chemotherapy, and X-ray therapy; important work reported each year steadily increased the prestige of the growing institute.

During his years in Buffalo, Park was a leader of the local medical community, the foremost surgeon in Buffalo, and an excellent teacher of students and practitioners. Park had married Martha Prudence Durkee in Chicago in 1880. Their home in Buffalo became a social and cultural center. Dr. Park played the piano, composed music, provided leadership in numerous community activities, and supported many efforts directed toward civic growth. His many friends considered him a witty conversationalist and a kind, dignified man with a large measure of self-control. After his wife's death in 1899, Park continued to work and study despite physical disability and recurrent respiratory problems, the sequelae of diphtheria years earlier. When associates urged him to rest more often, he quoted a favorite aphorism: "The future reserves for us repose enough."

He frequently visited and lectured at diverse American and foreign medical centers. Noteworthy was a series of lectures on surgical pathology (the Mutter Lectures) given in 1890–1891, which correlated bacteriology and pathology with surgical disease. He wrote on an astonishing variety of surgical topics, including infections, tumors, trauma, and congenital diseases, as well as three books on surgery, one on the history of medicine, and a collection of essays on nonmedical subjects. He edited the *Weekly Medical Review of Chicago* for two years and the *Medical Press of Western New York* for three years.

Park formed strong personal friendships with other great physicians in American medicine. He was elected to membership in the American Surgical Association in 1885 and later served as its president. He also served a term as president of the Medical Society of the State of New York. He was a member of numerous other American and foreign professional societies, including the American Association of Genitourinary Surgeons, the American Orthopedic Association, the International Society of Surgery, and the German, Italian, and French Surgical Societies. He received honorary degrees from Yale (LL.D.), Harvard (A.M), and Lake Forest University (M.D.).

Dr. Park died in Buffalo on February 17, 1914, after a short attack of syncope. His death was a great loss to the community of Buffalo and to American surgery. Measured against the prominent surgeons of his time, judging from interactions at the meetings of the American Surgical Society and other professional organizations, Park was clearly in the forefront of surgical thought and practice. Publishing 153 reports while in Buffalo (1883–1914), he left a clear trail of his opinions and methods. He was among the first in knowledge of tumors and consistently publicized the fact, long contested, that cancer was steadily increasing. "Dr. Park has done more work and better work than any other person in America in this direction," said Dr. W. W. Keen, a prominent American surgeon, "and his work has not only met with great encouragement and recognition abroad but is recognized as being as good as any done there" (Park 1914: xviii). Park's work and name are perpetuated and memorialized by the Roswell Park Cancer Institute in Buffalo, which continues to investigate the causes and treatment of cancer.

BIBLIOGRAPHY

Writings by Roswell Park

"Editorial." *Physicians' Magazine* (August 1883). (Reprinted in *Selected Papers*, p. 33.)
The Mutter Lectures on Surgical Pathology. Delivered before the College of Physicians of Philadelphia 1890–91. St Louis, MO: Chambers, 1892. (Reprinted from *Annals of Surgery* 13, 14, 15.)
"The Parasitic Theory of the Aetiology of Carcinoma." *New York Medical Journal* March 4, 1893. (Reprinted in *Selected Papers*, p. 130).
A Treatise on Surgery by American Authors. Edited by Roswell Park. Philadelphia: Lea Brothers and Company, 1896. (This is a multiauthored textbook edited by Park, which is representative of surgical thought and practice in the 1890s. The review

of the causes of cancer is particularly noteworthy because of Park's involvement with research in the subject.)

An Epitome of the History of Medicine. Philadelphia: F. A. Davis Co., 1897. (Later editions 1899, 1903.)

An Epitome of the History of Carcinoma. Fourth Annual Report of the New York State Laboratory for the years 1902–1903. James B. Lyon State Printer, 1903.

The Principles and Practice of Modern Surgery. Philadelphia: Lea Brothers and Company, 1907. (This textbook of surgery was one of the most complete and respected one-volume works of its time.)

The Evil Eye, Thanatology and Other Essays. Boston: R. G. Badger, 1912. (This collection of essays features nonmedical subjects, such as superstitions and magical charms, and "The Knights Hospitallers of St. John of Jerusalem." The book also includes essays on the history of medicine and surgery.)

Selected Papers. Surgical and Scientific. Buffalo, NY: Published for subscribers, 1914. (This volume consists of thirty-six papers previously published by Park and selected by his close associates to provide an idea of the wide range of his thought and practice. It contains a complete listing of his 167 articles written during the years 1878 to 1914. It is also valuable for an informative introductory memoir written by Charles A. Stockton, M.D., a well-known internist in Buffalo and close associate of Dr. Park.)

Writings about Roswell Park and Related Topics

McGuire, Edgar R. *Roswell Park*. Chicago: Surgical Publishing Co., 1922.

Mettlin, Curtis, and Gerald Patrick Murphy, eds. *Progress in Cancer Control: Proceedings of the First Conference on Progress in Cancer Control, Held in Buffalo, September 29–30, 1980, Sponsored by the Association of American Cancer Institutes and Roswell Park Memorial Institute*. New York: A. R. Liss, 1981.

Murphy, G. P. "Roswell Park Memorial Institute, Genesis of a Cancer Center." *Oncology* 37, no. 6 (1980): 426–428.

Olson, James Stuart. *The History of Cancer: An Annotated Bibliography*. Westport, CT: Greenwood Press, 1989.

Rather, L. J. *The Genesis of Cancer: A Study in the History of Ideas*. Baltimore: Johns Hopkins University Press, 1978.

Rein, Robert. *Molecular Basis of Cancer: Proceedings of the Conference Held at Roswell Park Memorial Institute, May 30–June 2, 1984*. New York: Liss, 1985.

Shimkin, Michael Boris. *Contrary to Nature: Being an Illustrated Commentary on Some Persons and Events of Historical Importance in the Development of Knowledge Concerning Cancer*. Washington, D.C.: U.S. Department of Health, Education, and Welfare, Public Health Service, National Institutes of Health, 1977.

Andrew A. Gage

THOMAS J. PARRAN, JR.
(1892–1968)

Thomas J. Parran, Jr., the sixth surgeon general (1936–1948) of the U.S. Public Health Service (PHS), remains among the most influential figures in twentieth-century public health in the United States. A brilliant administrator, he worked during an era of unprecedented cooperation between Congress and the executive branch to expand federal involvement in public health. Parran promoted a vision of health services organized regionally and informed by clinical medical re-search, with an active role played by government. He is best remembered for leading a national campaign to eradicate syphilis.

Parran was born on September 28, 1892, and raised near St. Leonard's, Mary-land, on his family's tobacco farm. He was named after a forebear believed to have served George Washington as a physician during the Revolutionary War and would recall that it was expected that he would follow two of his uncles into general practice. He was tutored at home by a relative, attended St. John's College in Annapolis on scholarship (1911), and accumulated enough credits to receive an A.M. (1915). Finances dictated his decision to attend Georgetown (M.D., 1915) and to follow with an internship at Sibley Memorial Hospital in Washington, D.C.

Parran's lifelong interest in research was sparked during medical school. He volunteered for two summers at a health laboratory operated by the District of Columbia, under Dr. Joseph J. Kinyoun, founder of the PHS's Hygienic Lab-oratory (renamed the National Institute of Health in 1930). But Parran was to remain, in his words, "a frustrated researcher." Kinyoun recruited Parran to join a field team of young physicians under the PHS's Dr. Leslie L. Lumsden, building privies and surveying conditions in the South. In March 1917, Parran reported to Okmulgee, Oklahoma, for the first of many assignments in rural sanitation.

After he qualified for a regular PHS commission in September 1917, Parran continued on assignments in rural health services administration, sanitation, and the control of communicable diseases. After a year stationed near Fort Oglethorp in Chattanooga, Tennessee, Parran was assigned to the dam-building project at the Muscle Shoals Nitrate Plant near Florence, Alabama. He handled outbreaks of malaria, smallpox, and venereal diseases and won attention for his contain-ment of the Spanish influenza, which arrived at Muscle Shoals shortly after he did in 1918. Subsequent assignments to the Tri-State Sanitary District (head-quartered in Missouri) and a host of health departments in the Midwest and South taught him, Parran would later recall, about the value of county health departments and how outside experts could leverage local decision making.

Between field assignments, Parran tasted life as an administrator in Washington, D.C. During the summer of 1919, he held a desk job, rating disabilities for the Bureau of War Risk Insurance, which would separate from the PHS in 1922 to become the new Veterans Bureau. In October 1923 Parran joined a group of young medical officers who attended six months of public health course work at the Hygienic Laboratory, receiving the practical equivalent of a master's degree in public health.

At the time that Parran accepted his commission, the PHS was a relatively small, independent agency under Secretary Andrew W. Mellon in the Treasury Department. Its main duties were domestic and international quarantine, sanitation, and a growing roster of laboratory and field research projects. Its leadership cadre, a uniformed but nonmilitary commissioned corps, consisted of about 200 physicians, to be supplemented by a reserve corps instituted in 1918 and a workforce of roughly 2,000 civil service and contract employees.

To Parran, World War I demonstrated how federal dollars and legislation could boost the effectiveness of public health departments. Sanitation activities outside military areas spurred states to hire full-time professional staff, and the Chamberlain-Kahn Act of 1918 crowned a successful wartime campaign to control venereal diseases, funding new programs, including the Division of Venereal Diseases within the PHS.

The division was Parran's first leadership position. When he was appointed chief in September 1926, appropriations for the 1918 act had dwindled considerably. Parran worked to sway public sentiment away from moral condemnation of venereal diseases and toward consideration of syphilis as a medical condition and threat to public health. He took his inspiration from a League of Nations–sponsored study tour to Denmark he had taken in the months immediately preceding his time at the division (1925).

Parran advocated the strengthening of health departments and the sponsorship of clinical medical research, two themes that would define his career. In 1927 he hosted a meeting of health departments where informal agreement was made to treat venereal diseases. The following year, Parran helped found the Committee on Research in Syphilis (1928) and its successor, the Cooperative Clinical Group (1929). The group sponsored comparative studies of syphilis treatments and provided a scientific basis for promoting the use of salvarsan. The PHS provided partial funding of the group's studies and published its findings in the PHS's *Venereal Disease Information.*

Parran's talents in rural health administration would soon lead him temporarily in a new direction. A reform-minded Governor Franklin Delano Roosevelt requested that Parran be loaned to the State of New York. In April 1930 Parran took up his post as state health commissioner of New York.

Parran's primary task was to join Cornell University Medical School president Livingston Farrand in chairing a commission on the reorganization of public health services. In 1931 the Special Health Commission released its recommendations (*Public Health in New York State*, 1932). The recommendations provided a framework that would bolster county health departments in order to replace a messy patchwork of town and village health boards ill equipped to handle an expanded set of Great Depression–era services.

Although few of the commission's recommendations were enacted, Parran's work on syphilis achieved more success. The Columbia Broadcasting System inadvertently launched Parran's campaign after executives censored the phrase "syphilis control" from a talk, leading Parran to cancel his appearance. Newspapers across the nation reprinted the censored speech. At New York City Mayor Fiorello La Guardia's suggestion, Parran led a fact-finding tour to England and Scandinavia in 1935, and in October of that year, New York City's Department of Health established a Bureau of Social Hygiene.

Parran became active in New Deal politics in New York and entered national politics as well. In 1934 recently elected President Roosevelt appointed Parran to the Committee on Economic Security, the group that drafted what would become the Social Security Act of 1935. Parran joined the committee's Science Advisory Board (1934–1935) as a member of a subcommittee on medical research. Guided by Dr. Lewis R. Thompson, chief of the PHS's Division of Scientific Research, and Edgar Sydenstricker of the Milbank Memorial Fund, the group crafted Title 6 of the 1935 act; building on Parran's approach to public health, Title 6 authorized $8 million for public health departments and $2 million for scientific research into disease.

President Roosevelt appointed Parran as surgeon general in the spring of 1936, following the end of Surgeon General Hugh Cummings's term. Parran was sworn in on April 6, 1936.

Parran's syphilis control campaign was in full swing by the fall of 1936. According to historian Allan Brandt (1987) Parran's "scientific, bureaucratic" approach consisted of the following elements: (1) free diagnostic centers, aided by the advent of a simplified Wasserman test; (2) prompt therapy; (3) case finding of contacts; (4) mandatory premarital blood tests; and (5) public education, including the highly acclaimed book he published in 1937, *Shadow on the Land*. Title 6 funds supported drives to identify and treat syphilis, and Parran called a series of national conferences for public health officers. Passage of the National Venereal Disease Control Act of 1938 (the LaFollette-Bulwinkle Act, an amendment of the 1918 act) made funds available for rapid treatment centers that employed the new sulfa drugs, and later, penicillin, to replace arsenicals.

Under Parran's leadership, his close associate and collaborator, Dr. Raymond Vonderlehr, transformed a syphilis control demonstration project in Macon County, Alabama, into an open-ended survey of the disease's effects. The now infamous Tuskegee Study of Syphilis in the Untreated Negro Male intentionally deceived the men enrolled as subjects. During the same time in which Parran and Vonderlehr published *Plain Words About Venereal Disease* (1941), a critique of the slack wartime mobilization against syphilis, Division of Venereal Disease policy actively prevented public health officials from treating the men enrolled in the Tuskegee Study. The shameful and tragic circumstances surrounding the study would continue until it was terminated in 1972.

While Parran is commonly associated with an enormously successful campaign against syphilis, he left his greatest mark on the administration and scope of the PHS. Parran and Dr. Lewis R. Thompson worked skillfully with Congress and, beginning in the 1940s, with philanthropists Albert and Mary Lasker, to expand the federal presence in public health. The PHS became part of the New Deal, joining the new Federal Security Agency in 1939. By the time of Parran's retirement from the PHS in 1948, there were over 17,000 civil service and contract employees and approximately 2,000 commissioned corps officers, the latter distributed across ten professional categories and split about evenly between regular and reserve commissions.

Parran also served as a mentor to a generation of commissioned corps physicians to whom he gave the leeway to create new institutions and programs. They included Robert Felix (National Institute of Mental Health), Herman E. Hilleboe (tuberculosis control), Joseph W. Mountin (Communicable Disease Center), Leonard Scheele (National Cancer Institute, the Clinical Center), Vane M. Hoge (facilities planning), and Louis L. Williams, Jr. (malaria, international health).

The entrance of the United States into World War II (1941) spurred new projects and laid the foundations for postwar expansion. The Community Facilities Act of 1941 (Lanham Act) enrolled PHS officials in regional planning and construction. Extra-cantonment sanitation in the South was expanded into the Malaria Control in War Areas project (1942), the basis for a new Communicable Disease Center in 1946. Mobile public health units were created to track plague outbreaks. Record levels of federal support, through annual emergency health and sanitation appropriations (1941–1944), made possible mass campaigns to screen for tuberculosis and to identify and treat the victims of syphilis.

During the war Surgeon General Parran made the PHS the premiere federal health agency. The National Institute of Health was turned to military projects, especially in the areas of industrial toxicology and vaccines for typhus, yellow fever, and Rocky Mountain spotted fever. One important discovery that resulted, for example, was Dr. John F. Mahoney's demonstration of the efficacy of penicillin against syphilis (1943). Interagency efforts such as the Eight-Point Agreement (1940) on venereal diseases, the U.S. Typhus Commission (1942), and the Interdepartmental Quarantine Commission (1943) featured PHS officials in leadership positions. PHS officers were assigned as liaisons to dozens of federal programs involved in the war effort. New categories of beneficiaries and great numbers of them crowded PHS hospitals and clinics, and inactive reserve officers were employed to staff the Office of Civilian Defense. The PHS entered the arena of labor policy through participation on the War Manpower Commission, administered the Cadet Nurse Corps established by the Nurse Training Act of 1943 (Bolton Act), and provided federal dollars for health professions education.

To accommodate the significant expansion and reorganization of duties, Parran and Thompson set out to rewrite the statutes underlying PHS operations. Their efforts became the Public Health Service Acts of 1943 and 1944. The agency's new four-bureau structure would remain in place until 1967. Wartime also allowed Parran and Thompson to promote clinical medical research. Under pressure from Congress, the duo had drafted what became the National Cancer Act of 1937, with generous provisions on which to base future research authorities. With these authorities written into the 1944 act, Parran and Thompson deftly arranged for the transfer of wartime research contracts from the Office of Scientific Research and Development, creating an extramural grants program for the NIH. Parran laid the groundwork for the creation of new institutes within the NIH and the National Institute for Mental Health.

Parran's stature as surgeon general and his vision of regional coordination of public health propelled him into leadership of international health affairs during the 1940s. His involvement had started in the 1930s with the board of scientific directors of the Rockefeller Foundation's International Health Division and the Pan American Health Organization. In 1943 he began work in the State Department's Office of Foreign Relief and Rehabilitation Operations, subsequently affiliated with the new United Nations (UN). When plans were laid in 1945 and 1946 to formalize the World Health Organization (WHO), Parran, working from the plans of Dr. Louis L. Williams, Jr., engineered the adoption of a decentralized, regional organizational structure based on the model of PHS's district or regional offices. Parran chaired the International Health Conference where WHO's draft constitution was adopted (1946) and led the U.S. delegations to the WHO Interim Committee and the First World Health Assembly (1948). President Truman's decision not to reappoint Parran in the spring of 1948, in favor of Leonard Scheele, reflected Parran's success in crafting a central role for the PHS in clinical research. It may also have been an outcome of public disputes over the issue of national health insurance and differences between Parran and his more outspoken chief, Administrator Oscar R. Ewing of the Farm Security Administration (FSA).

National health insurance was a hotly debated issue that pitted the American Medical Association (AMA) against many public health officials. Parran was an early and vigorous advocate of government schemes to ensure general medical care. As surgeon general, he had loaned Dr. Ralph C. Williams to the FSA to organize health insurance cooperatives in rural areas (1936–1938), hosted the July 1938 National Health Assembly where the elements of the first Wagner-Murray-Dingell bill were laid out, and participated in the Children's Bureau's wartime experiment in care delivery for the families of service members, the Emergency Maternity and Infant Care Act of 1943. But Parran shielded his agency from direct conflict with the AMA by tempering public advocacy for insurance with a focus on creating a regionally organized health services infrastructure or federally supported "system," particularly in rural areas, to be set in place before adding the federal dollars that would fuel consumer demand. The Hospital Survey and Construction Act of 1946 (Hill-Burton Act) was a signal step in this direction. Nevertheless, Parran was attacked by AMA editorialist Morris Fishbein for supporting President Truman's proposed national program. In 1947, Parran became the subject of a red-baiting investigation by a Republican-led Congress.

On October 1, 1948, Parran retired from the PHS to begin a career in academic administration. Paul Mellon, the son of Parran's former chief, Secretary of the Treasury Andrew W. Mellon, had brokered an agreement with the University of Pittsburgh that endowed a new school of public health. Parran served as the school's first dean. Parran made Pittsburgh a proving ground for ideas developed during his tenure at the PHS and during a survey of public health schools he had conducted with Cornell's Dr. Farrand for the Rockefeller Foundation (1939). He recruited the school's first generation of senior faculty and brought with him his deputy surgeon general and veteran international health administrator, Dr. James A. Crabtree, who succeeded him as dean in 1958. Parran facilitated the integration of area institutions into a medical center, including teaching hospitals and the Western State Psychiatric Institute. In the process, Parran challenged and ultimately prevailed over a vocal group of physician-instructors at the university's medical school.

Beyond his tenure as surgeon general, Parran sustained a prominent role in international health. He remained active in the Pan American Sanitary Organization. During the Korean War, he sat on the Rockefeller Foundation's International Development Advisory Board as an adviser to the Point Four technical assistance program, and helped found the Population Council (1953). He led a number of fact-finding missions for the PHS and the WHO, including tours to the Far East (1948), sub-Saharan Africa (1952), Japan (1956), the Soviet Union (1957), and Liberia (1962). Through his association with the Milbank Memorial Fund, he helped to found the national Citizens Committee for WHO (1953).

On his retirement from the University of Pittsburgh in 1958, Parran assumed the presidency of the Avalon Foundation, affiliated with the Mellon family, and became active in the A. W. Mellon Educational and Charitable Trust, which he had served as a trustee since 1955. While at the Avalon, first as president (1958–1961) and later as a trustee and consultant, Parran was involved in awarding grant money in higher education, science, and the arts. He also remained active as an adviser in the area of health policy. Parran continued his work in philanthropy and public health until his death on February 16, 1968, at the Presbyterian University Hospital in Pittsburgh, Pennsylvania. A true statesman of the New Deal, Dr. Parran transformed the PHS, bringing to syphilis and other diseases his deeply held belief in the powers of science and administrative reform to advance public health.

BIBLIOGRAPHY

Among the primary references related to the work of Parran, the following are especially useful: interview with Thomas J. Parran, Jr., M.D., 1962, Box 3, George Rosen Papers, MS.C.203, History of Medicine Division, National Library of Medicine, Bethesda, MD; OPM Folder for Thomas J. Parran, Jr., M.D., Division of Commissioned Personnel, PHS, USDHHS, St. Louis, Missouri.

Writings by Thomas J. Parran

Public Health in New York (State). Albany, NY: State of New York, Department of Health, 1932.

Shadow on the Land: Syphilis. New York: Reynal & Hitchcock, 1937.

(with Raymond A. Vonderlehr). *Plain Words about Venereal Disease*. New York: Reynal & Hitchcock, 1941.

"The U.S. Public Health Service and the Social Security Act." *American Medical Association Bulletin 31*, no. 9 (December 1946): 177–180.

Writings about Thomas J. Parran and Related Topics

Blockstein, Zaga. *Graduate School of Public Health, University of Pittsburgh, 1948–1973*. Pittsburgh, PA: A. W. Mellon Educational & Charitable Trust, 1974.

Brand, Jeanne L. "The United States Public Health Service and International Health, 1945–1950." *Bulletin of the History of Medicine* 63, no. 4 (winter 1989): 579–598.

Brandt, Allan M. *No Magic Bullet: A Social History of Venereal Disease in the United States since 1880*. New York: Oxford University Press, 1987.

Duffy, John. *A History of Public Health in New York City, 1866–1966*. New York: Russell Sage Foundation, 1974.

Fee, Elizabeth, and Barbara Rosenkrantz. "Professional Education for Public Health in the United States." In Elizabeth Fee and Roy M. Acheson, eds., *A History of Education in Public Health*, pp. 230–271. New York: Oxford University Press, 1991.

Fox, Daniel M. "The Politics of the NIH Extramural Program, 1937–1950." *Journal of the History of Medicine and Allied Sciences* 42 (1987): 447–466.

———. *Health Policies, Health Politics: The British and American Experience, 1911–1965*. Princeton, NJ: Princeton University Press, 1986.

Furman, Bess. *A Profile of the United States Public Health Service, 1798–1948*. DHEW Publ. (NIH) 73–369. Washington, DC: U.S. Government Printing Office, 1973.

Galishoff, Stuart. "Parran, Thomas." In Martin Kaufman et al., eds., *Dictionary of American Medical Biography*, 2:580–581. Westport, CT: Greenwood Press, 1984.

Poen, Monte. *Harry S. Truman Versus the Medical Lobby*. Columbia, MO: University of Missouri Press, 1979.

Whitman, Alden. "Dr. Parran Dead; Ex-Health Chief." *New York Times*, February 17, 1968, pp. 1, 29.

Lynne Page Snyder

PHILIPPE PINEL
(1745–1826)

Philippe Pinel was born on April 20, 1745, in Roques (Tarn), France, and died on October 25, 1826, in Paris as physician in chief of Salpêtrière Hospice, professor of internal medicine at the medical faculty, member of the Academy of Sciences, and honorary member of the Academy of Medicine. He is known worldwide as the French champion of humane treatment for the mentally ill, yet he was neither the first nor the only person to replace chains with straitjackets. In France he was famous for his books on nosology, mental illness, and clinical teaching. Pinel exemplifies a comprehensive approach to the patient, considering physical and mental aspects of illness as closely interrelated. This attitude is symbolized by his thirty years of residence at the Salpêtrière where the section for the mentally ill remained part of an all-inclusive institution for old, indigent, ailing, and acutely ill women. As their physician, Pinel was an early representative of psychiatry and comprehensive clinical and geriatric medicine.

Four major epochs are significant in French medicine as well as in Pinel's life. The struggle of science to free itself from the bonds of religion provides the theme for Pinel's adolescence. He grew up in St. Paul Cap-de-Joux, in a region where the revocation of the Edict of Toleration of Protestants in 1685 entailed their forcible conversion, exile, and persecution. Pinel's mother's family in Castres belonged to this group. The boy grew up with a deep commitment to tolerance, combined with conformity to the practices of Catholicism. Religion was taught at the seminary in nearby Lavaur staffed by the fathers of the Christian Doctrine and at the University of Toulouse, bastion of Dominican orthodoxy.

The path toward a good education opened for nine-year-old Philippe with the arrival of a new village schoolmaster, the abbé Jean Pierre Gorsse, in 1754. Trained by the Jesuits at nearby Albi, Gorsse was an excellent Latinist as well as an inspiring teacher. He had been tonsured, probably to be eligible for a prebend or scholarship: the fact that we later find Pinel at nearby Lavaur seminary as a tonsured scholarship student suggests that Gorsse managed to transfer his prebend. The abbé became the Pinels' family friend. When he shed the cassock to marry a local woman, Pinel Sr., then consul at St. Paul, defended him before the shocked villagers and saved his teaching job. Abandoning a career in the church and choosing a secular calling thus became an acceptable alternative for the boy.

The Doctrinaire teachers at Lavaur seminary opened a new view of the world to Pinel. Though good Catholics, they were Gallicans, favoring a French church over subservience to the pope. The rich collection of their books in the "old section" of the Lavaur public library, discovered in 1989, reveals that they favored Latin over Greek and prized teaching in French, emphasizing literature, geography, history, and the sciences; they turned Pinel into a humanist. Once a bachelor of arts, he transferred to the Doctrinaires' College de l'Esquille in Toulouse, where he earned a master's degree in the humanities. Then he spent two and a half years at the Toulouse faculty of theology in quest of a doctorate.

Deep-seated hesitation beset the young scholar during those years (1767–1770). At the theological faculty, he registered seven times in the theology course of the Dominican father Jacques Bourges, the priest who had calmly presided over the torture and execution of Jean Calas in 1762. While thus trying to come to terms with orthodoxy, personified by this awesome churchman, Pinel was also drawn to Jean Baptiste Gardeil, a classicist, physician, mathematician, and corresponding member of the Academy of Sciences, linked in friendship and mutual admiration with d'Alembert, Diderot, and other philosophes. Pinel was studying mathematics with Dr. Gardeil when medicine moved into his private life: his younger brothers, Charles, François, and Louis, came to share his lodgings and begin apprenticeships in surgery. Their presence reminded Philippe of the family's medical tradition. Upon turning twenty-five in April 1770, Pinel opted for medicine.

To reject a religious upbringing in favor of a worldly career was a well-trodden path for young Frenchmen of the Enlightenment. Pinel now renounced all his learning of holy scripture; nowhere in his writings is there so much as a story from the gospels to illustrate an argument. Immediately after earning the M.D. on December 23, 1773, he left for Montpellier. Here the oldest and most distinguished French medical faculty offered courses to attend, and the Hôtel-Dieu St. Eloi housed a fabulous library donated for the use of students by the late dean, Henri Haguenot. The published catalog informs us that it contained 853 medical books, mostly in Latin; the learned allusions in Pinel's later writings tell us that he read most of them. Again, his experience was typical. Students in mid-eighteenth-century Europe acquired medical knowledge largely on their own: in the library, rarely in the hospital (we do not hear of any dissections he might have attended), and often in the botanical garden, which in Montpellier was outstandingly large and rich.

The most significant scholarly preoccupations Pinel took to Paris in 1778 dealt with nosology and vitalism. The classification of diseases was a theme of ubiquitous discussion in Montpellier, where its premier French theorist, Professor François Boissier Sauvages de la Croix, had recently died. In 1785, Pinel would translate *First Lines on the Practice of Physick* by the foremost English nosologist, William Cullen. As for vitalism, this was the explanation for living phenomena favored at Montpellier; the mechanism of René Descartes and Herman Boerhaave seemed as unsatisfactory as the animism of Georg Stahl. Many Montpellerian physicians were materialists who also offered a vitalist explanation for the phenomena of life such as Théophile de Bordeu's research on glands, mucous tissue, or pulse. Pinel, his colleague P. J. G. Cabanis, and his most illustrious student, Xavier Bichat, espoused that position.

Pinel embraced his new profession with dedication and fervor as a calling. He brought to the clinical approach, particularly to the doctor-patient relationship with the mentally ill, a respect and interest for the individual, however humble or poor, that reminds one of the educational philosophy of the Doctrinaires or of the relationship of confessor to believer. Pinel became a dedicated clinician.

The second period of his life exemplifies the existence of hundreds of talented and ambitious young men living on the fringes of Enlightenment activities in Paris. Excluded from the ranks of practicing physicians by a mere provincial diploma, Pinel translated Cullen, reedited, and annotated the works of Giorgio Baglivi, edited the *Gazette de santé*, and composed a long essay, *The Clinical Training of Doctors*. Mainly he studied at the Jardin des Plantes, investigating animal behavior and comparative anatomy, particularly the shape and size of skulls. When, in August 1793, he was appointed "physician of the infirmaries" at Bicêtre Hospice, he perceived the health, illnesses, and behavior of his patients as part of the "natural history of man." His nineteen months' experience on Bicêtre's mental ward (September 11, 1793–April 20, 1795) launched his career and laid the basis for his three books. Pinel spent much time observing each patient and interviewing each repeatedly to collect a case history. He sketched a basic classification (or nosology) of mental illness. His most remarkable formulations were that of "periodic insanity," recurrent attacks interspersed with lucid intervals useful to a skilled therapist, and of "reasoning madness," where a delusion dominated an otherwise rational human being. Pinel made a fundamental presentation to the Natural History Society in Paris on December 11, 1794, explaining his principles of mental illness in a "Memoir on Madness."

Pinel learned practicable management and therapy from Jean Baptiste Pussin and his wife, Marguerite Jubline. Pussin had been governor of the ward for mentally ill men since 1785. He knew from experience which men required close supervision and how to control others with quiet words and firm authority. His wife was a valued helpmate who succeeded in turning scarce rations into edible meals. Pussin's skillful management of the insane and Pinel's formulations coalesced into "moral treatment"—a term that has produced two centuries of misinterpretation. To Pinel it simply meant rational and humane psychologic management, with the hope of cure and eventual discharge.

Pinel's speech of December 1794 helped open a new era in French and modern medicine, and it heralded Pinel's appointment to the faculty of the new Paris Health School. In this third and most creative epoch of his life, he helped fashion a modern medical curriculum based on the natural sciences and on clinical instruction at the sickbed. While composing a new lecture course on internal medicine in 1795, he accepted appointment as physician in chief of Salpêtrière Hospice. In the subsequent seven years he published three books, taught in the academic and clinical settings, and labored to improve the quality of life of the eight thousand old, ailing, senile, or acutely ill women entrusted to his care.

With the backing of his friends Cabanis and Dean Michel Augustin Thouret, who were members of the Paris Hospital Commission, he helped reduce the number of inmates to five thousand by transfers; promote salubrity by removing shacks, partitions, and refuse; renovate the laundry service; and produce more appetizing meals and their punctual distribution in a new refectory. He appreciably raised morale among the hale, while comforting the sick by his frequent presence in the 400-bed infirmary.

The initiative to improve hospital life should be credited to the minister of internal affairs, the physician and successful industrial chemist Jean Antoine Chaptal, Pinel's friend since Montpellier student days. At Chaptal's behest, the prefect of the Seine Department, Nicolas Frochot, chair of the new Paris Hospital Council since 1801, created an innovative, centralized, municipal hospital system. In 1802 the government assigned to Pinel the treatment of all mentally ill women in the Paris region who needed hospitalization at public expense. Newly discovered hospital registers show that between 1802 and 1805, Pinel and an assistant personally examined 1,044 women. We have more than five hundred diagnoses and histories established by Pinel.

To care for these women, Pinel applied his seven-year experience in the Salpêtrière infirmary. He divided the mentally ill into groups of curable and incurable patients, and, for those whom he considered curable, he instituted the residential arrangement essential for their recovery. The sickest ones were strictly supervised; the improved ones were given more liberty and room to exercise, garden, or sew. The greatly improved ones showed their adaptation to a normal social existence by their steady work, their offers to help the servants, and their sociability. In a widely publicized report, Pinel claimed a curability rate of well over half for manic patients. It is significant that he presented this report to the Academy of Sciences; from his election in 1803 until his final illness, he hardly missed a meeting. He wanted to make sure that clinical medicine would be accepted as scientific. The use of mathematical probability to project extravagant percentages of cures later led Pinel into fanciful abstractions that ultimately undermined his prestige.

The year 1811 was a tragic turning point that ushers in the fourth and last period of Pinel's life. He lost both his wife and his collaborator Pussin within three months. This was also the height of Napoleon's empire; ahead lay foolish foreign adventures, defeat, and a period of political turmoil and social ferment. In the medical sciences, the early nineteenth century saw the rise of the anatomopathologic method, when even psychiatrists turned into organicists, looking for lesions in the brain as the causes of mental illness. Pinel never believed that the brain could explain the mind or mental illness; his point of view was to be out of favor for two generations. He was viciously attacked by his student François Broussais, and his own son, the physician Scipion Pinel, depicted him as an irrelevant philanthropist. But it was his professional heir, J. E. D. Esquirol, who effectively shunted his teacher aside, usurping his role at the Salpêtrière and depicting Pinel as a mere figurehead. The image of Pinel the chainbreaker was a fabrication, and it became a myth.

Pinel never publicly answered his critics, whether they attacked his psychologic approach or his mistaken nosologic category of "essential fevers." He spent much time in his country house at Torfou, where he served as mayor for ten years. He was conscious and proud of being a public servant but troubled by the knowledge that he had wrestled with the most intractable problem in modern democratic society: the attempt to provide decent psychiatric care to huge numbers of indigent patients.

Because of Pinel's position and prestige, the new psychiatric specialty emerged in France, during the Consulate, within an official setting. This model stands in contrast to other Western countries where private or local leadership prevailed. As a clinician, Pinel insisted on the psychologic management of the mentally ill. As an academician, he initiated the elaboration of key psychiatric concepts in the *Encylopédie méthodique* and the *Dictionnaire des sciences médicales*, thus educating a wide public. His goal was a comprehensive, humane public medicine that includes psychiatry, a concept recently endorsed by two prominent French psychiatrists, Henri Ey and Henri Baruk. It remains a model.

BIBLIOGRAPHY

The only extant archival sources relating to Pinel are some two dozen letters addressed to his young brothers, several holograph diagnoses, and a few case histories and personal items. No manuscripts have survived (except for two essays), and almost none of his correspondence. Only the first edition of Pinel's *Treatise on Insanity* is available in English, under an unsatisfactory title. Pinel edited the *Gazette de santé* from 1784 to 1790, contributed to the *Journal de physique*, to *La Médecine éclairée par les sciences physiques*, and published seven articles in the *Encyclopédie méthodique* and twenty-five in the *Dictionnaire des sciences médicales*. These played an essential role in defining the concepts and vocabulary of modern psychiatry. His disciple J. E. D. Esquirol continued this task. Reliable secondary material on Pinel in English is scarce. See Chabbert (1974). For a complete bibliography, see Weiner (1990).

Writings by Philippe Pinel

Nosographie philosophique: Méthode de l'analyse appliquée à la médecine. Paris: Brosson, 1798. (Further editions in 1802–1803, 1807, 1810, 1813, 1818.)

Traité médico-philosophique sur l'aliénation mentale ou la manie. Paris: Caille et Ravier, 1800. (2d ed. 1809, translations into German, Spanish, English, and Italian, in that order.)

La médecine clinique rendue plus précise et plus exacte par l'application de l'analyse ou Recueil et résultat d'observations sur les maladies aigües, faites à la Salpêtrière. Paris: Brosson, Gabon, et Cie., 1802. (Further editions in 1804, 1815.)

Writings about Philippe Pinel and Related Topics

Chabbert, Pierre. "Pinel." *Dictionary of Scientific Biography* 10 (1974): 611–614.

Riese, Walther. *The Legacy of Philippe Pinel: An Inquiry into Thought on Mental Alienation.* New York: Springer, 1969.

Weiner, Dora B. *The Clinical Training of Doctors: An Essay of 1793.* Baltimore: Johns Hopkins University Press, 1980.

———. "Mind and Body in the Clinic: Philippe Pinel, Alexander Crichton, Dominique Esquirol and the Birth of Psychiatry." In G. S. Rousseau, ed., *The Languages of Psyche: Mind and Body in Enlightenment Thought*, pp. 331–402. Berkeley: University of California Press, 1990.

———. "The Apprenticeship of Philippe Pinel: A New Document, 'Observations of Citizen Pussin on the Insane.' " *American Journal of Psychiatry* 136 (1979): 1128–1134.

———. "Philippe Pinel's 'Memoir on Madness' of 11 December 1794: A Fundamental Text of Modern Psychiatry." *American Journal of Psychiatry* 149 (1992): 725–732.

———. *The Citizen-Patient in Revolutionary and Imperial Paris.* Baltimore: Johns Hopkins University Press, 1993.

———. "Le Geste de Pinel: History of a Psychiatric Myth." In M. S. Micale and R. Porter, eds., *Discovering the History of Psychiatry*, pp. 232–247. New York: Oxford University Press, 1993.

Dora B. Weiner

NICHOLAS J. PISACANO
(1924–1990)

Nicholas J. Pisacano was one of the key figures in the evolution of the area of medical specialization now known as family practice. Historians have only recently begun to pay attention to the history of family practice in the United States and the individuals who guided the specialty's establishment. Pisacano represents one of the key figures in the development of this field. Born in Philadelphia on June 6, 1924, the son of Joseph and Rae Pisacano, he graduated from Hahnemann Medical College in 1951, completing an internship and residency at Stamford Hospital in Connecticut by 1953. During his first decade of practice, he engaged in general medicine in South Royalton, Vermont (1953–1955), and Philadelphia (1955–1962), before he finally settled in Lexington, Kentucky, for the remainder of his career (1962–1990).

Pisacano's experience at the University of Kentucky defined not only the last twenty-five years of his professional career but also the field of family practice. He became assistant professor of medicine in 1962 and rose to the rank of associate professor three years later. Pisacano also interacted with the College of Arts and Sciences, where in 1966 he became associate professor of biology and assistant dean. His popularity as a faculty member was acknowledged by the University's Favorite Professor Award in 1966 and a Distinguished Teaching Award in 1967. By 1968 Pisacano had assumed the position of assistant vice president of the University of Kentucky Medical Center. Pisacano's position within academe helped to provide family practice with the credibility it sorely needed during its early years. This capacity placed him among professionals who could best influence medical education as well as specialization within American medicine.

Pisacano helped to charter the Advisory Group of the first American Board of Family Practice in 1964. The 1964 board, however, lacked the approval of the Advisory Board for Medical Specialties (ABMS); ABMS did not provide formal endorsement until February 1969. Between 1964 and 1965, Pisacano emerged as one of the leading spokesmen for the establishment of an approved specialty of family practice. Without his leadership, the field might never have developed as it did throughout the 1970s.

One of Pisacano's primary concerns was the future professional position of American family physicians. Unless they enjoyed coequal status with other specialists, Pisacano believed that other specialists would relegate them to second-class standing within American medicine, just as they had done to general practice in the previous decades. Pisacano made some of his most important contributions through his publications. Throughout the 1960s, he published a number of articles that lobbied for the end of general practice and the creation of the new specialty of family practice. General practitioners (GPs), Pisacano wrote in the journal *GP* in 1964, faced professional extinction. Their role no longer commanded great respect within American medicine or, in some urban areas, hospital admitting privileges. Few general practitioners performed surgery any longer, and as a professional group they were aging very quickly. They were, he said, "a dying breed."

Pisacano believed that previous attempts to salvage general practice had been strictly rhetorical. As an alternative, he proposed a separate family practice board, approved and jointly administered by the existing boards: preventive medicine, pediatrics, psychiatry, and internal medicine. He viewed this specialty as unique in the sense that it would require "periodic recertification" to maintain high professional standards. Pisacano blamed the American Academy of General Practice (AAGP) for the majority of general practice's problems. He criticized the academy because it had not supported, and did not plan to support, the creation of a board. The AAGP, he believed, only wished to protect what little professional authority remained for American GPs. In Pisacano's view, that was not much. He even accused academy leadership of substituting dues and certificates for an approved course of residency training.

Pisacano used his academic position to advance the creation of family practice. When he became the first executive director of the approved American Board of Family Practice (ABFP) in March 1969, he became central in the definition of ABFP objectives, selection of its leadership, and certification of its diplomates. The survival of the new specialty depended on such efforts.

Following ABMS approval of the American Board of Family Practice, Pisacano and the board leadership first needed to determine basic examination guidelines. This was not only a matter of who would take the first examination but what would be the cutoff scores for passing and failing. The first board certification examination in family practice took place in late February and early March 1970. Pisacano also had managed to obtain extensive publicity for the first ABFP examination, informally by word of mouth and formally through notices of examination guidelines and dates that appeared in nearly two dozen medical journals in the United States, Canada, and Europe.

Pisacano's efforts attracted praise as well as criticism. Younger physicians tended to support his leadership, viewing board certification as a prerequisite for professional survival. Older physicians considered board certification to be a means of further defining family practice within narrow professional parameters. To some, Pisacano represented not an individual who had led family practice into the 1970s but the one who had masterminded their exclusion from the operating room. Others complained that they could purchase a luxury automobile for little more than the ABFP planned to charge them to sit for the certification examination. They did not need board certification to practice medicine, they said. Pisacano honed his diplomatic skills as the leader of the ABFP. During the first years of examinations, petitions for special consideration flooded the ABFP office in Lexington. Most individuals requested exemption from the board certification exam because of age or previous level of training. As a rule, Pisacano refused preferential treatment for any potential diplomates of the ABFP. To do so, he reasoned, would undermine the credibility of the certification process itself.

Pisacano closely guarded the credibility of the ABFP. To achieve this goal, he consistently maintained the certification guidelines of the board, despite complaints on a variety of fronts. The most vehement complaints came from general practitioners, who saw no need for certification in family practice. They argued that they had practiced for years without it, and they saw no reason to have it now. Others cited what they viewed as the high cost of certification, a price that they were unwilling to pay. Some questioned the need for the three years of residency training and certification in family practice in order to become a fully credentialed diplomate in the field.

Leaders within American medicine generally considered Pisacano an ideal choice as the executive director of the ABFP. Pisacano, many believed, understood American medical education as well as anyone else in the United States. Furthermore, he embodied the academic credibility and leadership skills needed to guide family practice into the last quarter of the twentieth century. Throughout the twenty years that he held this post, he faced several complicated showdowns over the approval of the American Board of Emergency Medicine, Certificates of Added Qualification in geriatrics and sports medicine, and reciprocity agreements with the General Practice Colleges of several other English-speaking countries.

The American Academy of General Practice, founded in 1947, represented one of Pisacano's primary adversaries throughout the 1970s. The AAGP, which changed its official name to the American Academy of Family Physicians early in that decade, had attempted to protect the professional interests of American general practice since the late 1940s, but now, two decades later, the ABFP represented family physicians instead of general practitioners in the United States. The board had pushed the academy aside as the central credentialing organization for American family physicians. It fell to Pisacano to help the ABFP maintain that position. Pisacano led the ABFP from 1969 until his death in 1990. During this period, he expanded the professional authority and parameters of the ABFP and the family physicians that it certified. Full hospital privileges for general practitioners had been a controversial point for several decades, and a similar situation threatened family physicians in the 1970s and 1980s. Despite ongoing criticism from other boards, Pisacano consistently fought for full admitting privileges for diplomates of the ABFP. Hospital governing boards, he believed, did not realize that family physicians were not certified for an indefinite period of time; the ABFP required recertification every six years. Unless family physicians sat for the recertification exam and presented a requisite amount of continuing medical education credits, the ABFP would revoke their certification.

Pisacano's greatest achievements lay in his ability to insulate the ABFP from criticism leveled by other boards. During the early years of the ABFP, he spent considerable time dealing with the leadership of the American Board of Medical Specialties over payment of dues for each newly certified ABFP diplomate. The ABFP paid the fees after Pisacano haggled with the ABMS leadership for many months. Pisacano also helped to internationalize family practice. By the time he died, Pisacano had masterminded alliances between the ABFP and the College of Family Physicians of Canada and the Royal College of General Practitioners of England. Shortly after his death, the ABFP leadership forged additional reciprocal agreements with the Royal Australian College of General Practitioners and the Royal New Zealand College of General Practitioners. In effect, qualified GPs from these countries could sit for the ABFP certification examination, and ABFP diplomates could do the same in those countries.

Pisacano also established agreements for certificates of added qualification (CAQ) in geriatrics and sports medicine. Other boards, Pisacano realized, had established similar CAQs, and he hoped to pursue a similar path with the ABFP. The first of these was a joint certificate between the American Board of Internal Medicine and the ABFP in geriatrics and another with the American Board of Orthopedics in the emerging area of sports medicine. By 1990, plans for fellowship training in both fields were well under way in residency programs across the United States.

In 1989, Pisacano retired from the executive directorship of the ABFP, a position he had held for two decades. His resignation, he explained in October 1989, offered him the chance to spend more time reading the literary classics that he loved. Pisacano died suddenly at his home in March 1990. As the individual whose name had become synonymous with the global success of the American Board of Family Practice, his passing was widely mourned.

BIBLIOGRAPHY

Archival sources on the history of general and family practice sit in files around the country. Most are contained at the American Academy of Family Physicians, Kansas City, Missouri; the American Board of Family Practice, Lexington, Kentucky; the American Medical Association, Chicago, Illinois; and the American College of Physicians, Philadelphia, Pennsylvania.

Writings by Nicholas J. Pisacano

"General Practice: A Eulogy." *GP* 19 (February 1964): pp. 173–179.
"Family Practice." *Journal of the American Medical Association*, June 6, 1980, pp. 2185–2186.
"Certificate of Added Qualifications." *Journal of the American Board of Family Practice* 2 (July–September 1989): 143–144.
"Twenty Years: More Answers Than Questions. Non Amo Te." *Journal of the American Board of Family Practice* 3 (January–March 1990): 63–65.

"American Board of Family Practice Statistics." *Journal of the American Board of Family Practice* 3 (April–June 1990): 137–139.

Writings about Nicholas J. Pisacano and Related Topics

Adams, David P. "The Best of Both Worlds: General Practice in Rural Florida, 1928–1950." *Journal of the Florida Medical Association* 73 (April 1986): 312–316.

————. "Community and Professionalization: GPs and Ear, Nose and Throat Specialists in Cincinnati, 1945–1947." *Bulletin of the History of Medicine* 68 (1994): 664–684.

————. *The American Board of Family Practice, 1969–1994*. In press.

Adams, David P. and Robert J. Fitrakis. "General Practice and Rural Health Reform in Kansas, 1948–1950." *Professional Ethics*, no. 2 (spring–summer 1993): 59–82.

Stoeckle, John, and George Abbott White. *Plain Pictures of Plain Doctoring: Vernacular Expression in New Deal Medicine and Photography, 80 Photographs from the Farm Security Administration*. Cambridge, MA: MIT Press, 1985.

David P. Adams and Alan L. Moore

EUNICE RIVERS
(1899–1986)

Eunice Verdell Rivers Laurie, the public health nurse most closely associated with the infamous Tuskegee Syphilis Study, was born November 12, 1899, in Early County, Georgia, the oldest of three daughters born to Albert and Henrietta Rivers. As a child, she was sent to a church-run boarding school in Fort Gaines, Georgia, by her father, a farmer and sawmill worker, determined to provide better opportunities for his children. After a bout of typhoid fever, Rivers attended a mission school in Thomasville, Georgia. When Albert Rivers learned that nearly all of her teachers were white, he arranged for his daughter to enter the Tuskegee Institute in Tuskegee, Alabama. Late in her life, Rivers recalled how her father's mistreatment at the hands of the Ku Klux Klan had shaped his determination to see his daughters succeed.

In 1918 Rivers enrolled at the Tuskegee Institute, founded in 1881 to provide educational and vocational training for blacks. After a year studying handcrafts and other practical skills, Rivers, at her father's insistence, transferred to the nursing program. Although initially reluctant about a career caring for sick and dying patients, Rivers quickly excelled in her new endeavor, attracting favorable notice from faculty and hospital staff. After receiving her nursing degree in 1922, she was hired by the state of Alabama as part of a program to bring social services to rural blacks. As a member of Macon County's Movable School, Rivers, together with a home economics agent and a carpenter, spent several years driving around the state in a specially appointed bus, stopping to provide instruction in basic nursing and hygiene to families in their homes. Later Rivers joined the staff of the state health department's Bureau of Vital Statistics. In Alabama most black women gave birth attended by midwives rather than physicians. In order to collect accurate information about births in the black population, Rivers made visits throughout the state, instructing midwives in basic hygiene and teaching them to record births and deaths. In 1931, worsening economic conditions led the state health department to discontinue the program, and she was forced to seek a new position.

In 1932 Rivers was offered the job of night supervisor in a general hospital in New York. She chose to remain in Alabama, taking a post as supervisor of night nursing at the John A. Andrew Memorial Hospital, built on the campus of the Tuskegee Institute to serve the health needs of the students, faculty, and staff. In 1932, after eight months at the hospital, Dr. Eugene Dibble, head of the Andrew Hospital and one of four black physicians on the staff, asked Rivers to become a scientific assistant to the study of untreated syphilis being organized in Macon County under the auspices of the U.S. Public Health Service. Given her lack of experience with research in syphilis, Rivers expressed some reservations about the position but was persuaded by Dr. Dibble to assume the task.

In 1930 the Public Health Service, with support from the Julius Rosenwald Fund, undertook a syphilis control demonstration project among Negroes in six southern counties. Initial plans called for a diagnostic survey, followed by a one-year treatment program. With the onset of the Great Depression, however, funds for treatment were no longer available. The unexpectedly high prevalence of the disease in Macon County, Alabama, where the Tuskegee Institute was located, led Public Health Service investigator Dr. Taliaferro Clark to propose a short-term study of untreated syphilis in the black population. From this developed the longest-running nontherapeutic experiment in American history, the Tuskegee Syphilis Study.

In her capacity as scientific assistant, Rivers performed a number of duties. In addition to transporting the men recruited for the study to and from the hospital for testing, she helped Dr. Raymond Vonderlehr, a venereal disease investigator, perform extensive physical examinations on the men. In order to ensure that the men would return for the lumbar punctures deemed essential for making the diagnosis, Vonderlehr sent each of the participants a form letter about their "last chance for a special free treatment," a letter that did not disclose that the "spinal shots" the men received had no therapeutic value. Rivers recalled that for a number of the men, the shots were enormously painful, leading, in some cases, to debilitating headaches. The experience with the spinal punctures led many of the subjects to distrust the government doctors, a distrust that Rivers had to work to overcome when the decision was made to continue the study indefinitely.

Vonderlehr's appointment as acting director, and later director, of the Venereal Disease Division of the PHS ensured that both the study and Rivers's association with the project would continue. Recognizing the crucial importance of the nurse to the ongoing success of the project, Vonderlehr quickly reappointed Nurse Rivers on a two-thirds-time basis at an annual salary of $1,000. For her initial work with the study, Rivers had received an annual salary of $1,200, plus an additional $600 reimbursement for driving expenses, a good wage for a black nurse in the depression era. Her new assignment was to maintain contact with the men between the annual visits of government doctors and to assist the investigators with their examinations when they visited Tuskegee. Rivers was also entrusted with the sensitive task of obtaining the family's permission for autopsy when one of the study participants died. She found this one of the most difficult aspects of her work, although her job was made considerably easier after 1935 when the PHS, with support from the Milbank Memorial Fund, offered burial stipends of $50 to families who agreed to allow an autopsy. Given the bleak poverty of most inhabitants of Macon County, the burial stipend gave families an opportunity to provide a funeral for their loved ones. Most families took advantage of the offer; Rivers noted in 1953 that only one of the

146 families she approached for permission to conduct an autopsy refused to cooperate with the study's request for a postmortem.

By all accounts, Rivers developed an extraordinary rapport with the men—399 with the disease and some 201 controls—enrolled in the study. She administered government-provided tonics and other "incidental medications," visited the men in their homes, listened to their complaints, sat at their bedsides during illness, and attended their funerals with their families. In addition to her contact with the men, she knew many women in the community through her continuing position as a public health nurse at Andrew Hospital. She participated in programs in the public schools and in the maternity and well-baby clinics at the hospital. In 1952 she married Albert Laurie, an orderly at Andrew Hospital and the son of one of the controls in the study, further cementing her ties to the Tuskegee community.

During her years with the Tuskegee Syphilis Study, Rivers also earned the respect of the white Public Health Service investigators, who continued to make periodic visits to Macon County to examine the physical manifestations of the disease as the men aged. In 1953 she appeared as lead author of an article in *Public Health Reports*. In the article, Rivers and her coauthors emphasized the importance of nurse-physician cooperation in a study in which the scientific personnel changed from year to year. The nurse's knowledge of the individual subjects and their "eccentricities" and her ability to "bridge the language barrier" between doctors and subjects allowed the study to continue. In 1958 Rivers became the third person to receive the newly established Oveta Culp Hobby Award from the federal Department of Health, Education and Welfare. Rivers traveled from Tuskegee to Washington, D.C., to receive $200 and an engraved certificate for "notable service covering twenty-five years during which through selfless devotion and skillful human relations she has sustained the interest and cooperation of the subjects of a venereal disease control program in Macon County, Alabama." Rivers received other awards over her lifetime, but she regarded the Hobby prize as the most meaningful.

In 1965 Rivers resigned her position with the Public Health Service and was eventually replaced by a second black nurse, Elizabeth Kennebrew. Seven years later, in 1972, newspaper reports about a forty-year study of untreated syphilis in four hundred black men made the Tuskegee Syphilis Study a national scandal. Amid harsh public criticism of the study, the Department of Health, Education and Welfare appointed an ad hoc panel, headed by distinguished black educator Broadus N. Butler, to review the study. The panel quickly recommended the discontinuation of the study and directed the federal government to provide medical care to the surviving subjects. In 1973 Defense Secretary Caspar Weinberger instructed the PHS to provide all necessary care for Tuskegee participants; two years later, the government extended a similar offer to subjects' wives who had contracted syphilis and to their children born with congenital syphilis. Angered by the government's role in an experiment to withhold treatment from black men, Senator Edward M. Kennedy of Massachusetts held public hearings in February and March 1973 at which a number of interested parties, including two surviving research subjects, informed a congressional subcommittee about the systematic deception of subjects that marked the government study of untreated syphilis. Rivers did not testify at these hearings. In Tuskegee, where she had continued to live after her retirement, prominent civil rights attorney Fred Gray filed a $1.8 billion lawsuit against the federal government, federal agencies, the state of Alabama, and the Milbank Fund on behalf of the survivors and their families. Not named in the suit were predominantly black institutions like Tuskegee or black professionals, including Eunice Rivers.

In an oral history interview conducted in 1977, Rivers expressed the opinion that much that had been written about the study had been unfair. She accepted that racial considerations had shaped the decision to proceed with the Tuskegee study, noting the interest in seeing whether syphilis affected blacks and whites in different ways. But she emphasized that the investigators had expressly selected men who were in the secondary stages of the disease, when syphilis had already "done its damage." She explained that men who participated in the study received "good medical care," including electrocardiograms and other tests and procedures they would never have received without their participation in the study. Rivers explained that the men had in fact received "better medical care than some of us who could afford it." Rivers continued to live in Tuskegee until her death on August 28, 1986.

In the 1980s and 1990s, Nurse Rivers and her role in the Tuskegee Syphilis Study became the subject of documentaries, drama, and continuing discussion. Playwright David Feldschuh's *Miss Evers' Boys*, first produced in 1989, introduced a fictionalized Nurse Rivers to many more Americans. Although Feldschuh has emphasized that the character of Miss Evers was inspired by Eunice Rivers and is a work of fiction, the similarity of the names and the playwright's use of a number of primary sources from the Tuskegee Syphilis Study make it likely that audiences (the play has been performed around the country and at a number of colleges) identify Miss Evers with the real Nurse Rivers. Historians and other commentators have addressed the question of Nurse Rivers's knowledge of and responsibility for the Tuskegee Syphilis Study. Although some have been critical of her cooperation with the white doctors in the study and her active participation in the deception of the men, including some of the surviving research subjects, a number of historians have emphasized her relative powerlessness as a nurse at a time when nurses were viewed as the physician's subordinate and as a black woman in segregated Alabama. There is no disagreement, however, about Rivers's abilities as a public health nurse and her superb communication skills. Not only her father, who had first steered her into a nursing career, believed that she was a "born nurse."

BIBLIOGRAPHY

There is some biographical material on Rivers in the archives of Tuskegee University, Tuskegee, Alabama. In addition, Rivers participated in two oral histories, both conducted after the Tuskegee Syphilis Study gained public notoriety in 1972: "Interview with Daniel Williams and Helen Dibble," January 29, 1975, Tuskegee, Alabama, Tuskegee University Archives; and Eunice Rivers Laurie, "Oral History Interview," October 10, 1977, Black Women Oral History Project, Schlesinger Library, Radcliffe College, and available in *The Black Women's Oral History Project* (Westport, CT: Meckler Publishing, 1991), 7: 231–242.

Writings by Eunice Rivers

(with Stanley Schuman, Lloyd Simpson, and Sidney Olansky). "Twenty years of Followup Experience in a Long Range Medical Study." *Public Health Reports* 68 (1953): 391–395.

Writings about Eunice Rivers and Related Topics

Brandt, Allan M. "Racism and Research: The Case of the Tuskegee Syphilis Study." *Hastings Center Report* 8 (1978): 21–29.

Feldschuh, David. *Miss Evers' Boys.* New York: Dramatists Play Service, 1995. (See also *American Theatre Magazine* [November 1990].)

Hammonds, Evelynn M. "Your Silence Will Not Protect You: Nurse Eunice Rivers and the Tuskegee Syphilis Study." In Evelyn C. White, ed., *The Black Women's Health Book*, pp. 323–331. Seattle: Seal Press, 1994.

Hine, Darlene Clark. *Black Women in White: Racial Conflict and Cooperation in the Nursing Profession, 1890–1950.* Bloomington: Indiana University Press, 1989.

Jones, James H. *Bad Blood: The Tuskegee Syphilis Experiment.* New ed. New York: Free Press, 1993.

Reverby, Susan M. "Laurie, Eunice Rivers." In Darlene Clark Hine, ed., *Black Women in America: An Historical Encyclopedia*, pp. 699–701. Brooklyn, NY: Carlson Publishing, 1993.

Smith, Susan L. "Neither Victim Nor Villain: Nurse Eunice Rivers, the Tuskegee Syphilis Experiment, and Public Health Work." *Journal of Women's History* 8 (1996): 95–113.

Susan E. Lederer

ALBERT B. SABIN
(1906–1993)

Albert B. Sabin, one of the great figures of twentieth-century virology, was born in Bialystok, Poland. He received part of his early education in that country but emigrated to the United States (New Jersey) while still a boy to escape religious persecution following the end of World War I. After his graduation from Paterson High School, he was supported by a dentist uncle in studies at the dental school of New York University. However, after three years, during which he was exposed to microbiology and the other medical sciences, Sabin quit dental school to pursue a career in medicine. Following a year in the microbiology laboratories at the invitation of Dr. William H. Park, he was admitted to New York University's school of medicine, from which he graduated in 1931, supported in part by a scholarship and in part by working as a laboratory assistant in return for room and board.

After a year's internship at Bellevue Hospital, he spent a year at the Lister Institute in London. He returned to the United States for a four-year stint on the scientific staff at the Rockefeller Institute (now University) in New York City (1935–1939) and then began a long association with the Cincinnati College of Medicine and the Children's Hospital Research Foundation in Ohio. This was interrupted only by service with the U.S. Army as an investigator of epidemic diseases during World War II (1943–1946). In 1970 he became president of the Weizmann Institute in Israel, a position he held until 1972. He continued to be active thereafter, particularly in a number of national and international health care agencies, until his eightieth birthday, when he ceased his full-time activities. Despite his formal retirement, brought on by a series of serious illnesses, he continued to be sought for advice and lectureships until his death at the age of eighty-six in 1993.

Although his pioneering work on understanding the pathophysiology and epidemiology of poliomyelitis (''infantile paralysis'') and his development of an orally administered live attenuated vaccine for its prevention remain his greatest achievements, Sabin's interests and accomplishments in many other aspects of infectious disease were notable. His ability at research was demonstrated when, still a medical student, he developed an improved rapid method for typing pneumococcal infections. This improvement was significant because, at the time, specific antisera represented the only effective treatment of these pneumonias. His mentor at New York University, Dr. Park, turned him toward the study of viral infections, including polio. In 1932 Sabin discovered a new virus, the B(rebner) virus, which had resulted in the death of a laboratory associate working at NYU. This resulted in his first publication in virology.

It was poliomyelitis, however, that remained Sabin's chief interest and, overturning previously entrenched beliefs, he demonstrated that it was not transmitted by the nasal route, but by the fecal-oral human route with multiplication of the virus within the intestinal tract. In much of this work, he was assisted by Dr. Robert Ward, who had joined him in Cincinnati shortly after his arrival. In the development of an effective vaccine against polio, Sabin was influenced by the knowledge that, following an infection, protective antibodies could persist for twenty years or more, as had been demonstrated by a single outbreak among Alaskan Eskimos. Therefore, his approach to prevention was based on the development of an attenuated live vaccine rather than a killed vaccine, whose effects might be much shorter lasting. Furthermore, a live vaccine could be administered by mouth, and perhaps spread from those who had been given the vaccine to others, enhancing the effect of such a program.

While Sabin worked to perfect his oral vaccine, Dr. Jonas Salk, who had had great success with a killed virus against influenza, embarked on a similar approach against polio under the sponsorship of the National Foundation for Infantile Paralysis. While Sabin's work was still substantially incomplete, Salk had achieved notable success with a killed vaccine administered by injection. By 1953 Salk had demonstrated the safety of his vaccine, and in 1954 a nationwide trial demonstrated its efficacy. Between 1954 and 1961 a dramatic decrease in the incidence of paralytic polio occurred as a result of the Salk vaccine program. By 1957 Sabin had completed his initial work on an oral vaccine and had demonstrated its safety. However, the National Foundation for Infantile Paralysis, which had committed itself to the Salk vaccine program, ignored, if not actually discouraged, new approaches to the prevention of this dreaded disease. The World Health Organization, however, endorsed extensive trials of the oral vaccine. These trials were undertaken with Sabin's participation in Czechoslovakia, Mexico, and especially the Soviet Union. By the end of 1959 about 145 million people in the USSR had received the vaccine; the protective effect was considered excellent, and there were no reports of paralytic polio as a result of the vaccine. Later, in the United States, it was shown that there was a very small but real risk of vaccine-induced paralytic polio; between five and ten such cases may occur annually in the United States as a result of the vaccine. In view of this, the future direction of vaccination against polio will probably incorporate an injection of inactivated vaccine for initial protection, followed by the oral live attenuated vaccine for long-term protection.

Although his work on polio remains Sabin's crowning achievement, his interest and accomplishments in a variety of other infectious diseases were broad and intense. Among the other achievements of this tireless investigator must be mentioned his work on arthropod-borne viruses and the human diseases they cause (dengue, sandfly fever, Japanese encephalitis, and others). Other work by Sabin led to his discovery of a unique dye test for the toxoplasma antibody. He also contributed to the understanding of the genetics of natural resistance to certain viruses and experimental arthritis.

Lost amid the universal praise of Sabin's research accomplishments is his unwavering dedication to the eradication of the human misery caused by infectious diseases, especially among the children of the Third World. Even in the face of advancing age and disability, he strove to introduce measures to control diseases that continued to flourish among the less fortunate nations of the world after the developed countries had adopted preventive measures into their public health procedures and routine medical care.

Dr. Sabin received forty-six honorary degrees from the United States and numerous foreign countries. Among these were the U.S. National Medal of Science (1971), the Presidential Medal of Freedom (1986), Order of Friendship among Peoples from the USSR (1986), and, from Brazil, the Ordem Nacional do Cruziero do Sol, Grau Grande Oficial (1986), and Gra Cruz do Ordem do Rio Branco (1991). The one great award that did escape him (and Salk) was the Nobel Prize in Medicine, which many observers believe has been granted to individuals whose accomplishments merited it much less than those of Sabin and Salk. But perhaps the greatest encomium that Sabin might have wished for was that made to him by another distinguished polio researcher, Dr. John R. Paul of Yale, who noted, "No man has ever contributed so much effective information and so continuously over so many years to so many aspects of poliomyelitis as Sabin."

BIBLIOGRAPHY

The most comprehensive review of the poliomyelitis story is contained in John R. Paul's *History of Poliomyelitis*. An updating is included in my chapter on poliomyelitis in *Medical Odysseys*. Additional insights may be obtained from Saul Benison's oral history, *Tom Rivers*. My transcribed interview with Dr. Sabin in 1987 is on record with the Smith Library of the University of Medicine and Dentistry (Historical Section), Newark, New Jersey. A collection of Dr. Sabin's papers may be found at the University of Cincinnati, to which they were donated by his widow.

Writings by Albert B. Sabin

(with A. M. Wright). "Acute Ascending Myelitis Following a Monkey Bite, with the Isolation of a Virus Capable of Reproducing the Disease." *Journal of Experimental Medicine* 59 (1934): 115–136.

(with others). "Live, Orally Given Poliovirus Vaccine: Effects of Rapid Mass Immunization on Population under Conditions of Massive Enteric Infection with Other Viruses." *Journal of the American Medical Association* 173 (1960): 1521–1526. (This report on the success of the oral vaccine is among the most important of Sabin's publications.)

"Oral Polio Vaccine: History of Its Development and Prospects for Eradication of Poliomyelitis." *Journal of the American Medical Association* 194 (1965): 872–876. (The text of the speech given by Sabin at the presentation of the Lasker Award to him in 1965.)

Writings about Albert B. Sabin and Related Topics

Benison, Saul. *Tom Rivers: Reflections of a Life in Medicine and Science.* Cambridge, MA: MIT Press, 1967.

Paul, John R. *History of Poliomyelitis.* New Haven, CT: Yale University Press, 1971.

Weisse, Allen B. "Polio: The Not-So-Twentieth-Century Disease." In A. B. Weisse, *Medical Odysseys: The Different and Sometimes Unexpected Pathways to Twentieth Century Medical Discoveries.* New Brunswick, NJ: Rutgers University Press, 1991.

Allen Weisse

MAHENDRALAL SARKAR
(1833–1904)

Mahendralal Sarkar was a pioneer in spreading science education throughout India and in motivating young men to pursue careers in science. Before Sarkar's birth, teaching modern science was almost unknown in India. In the eighteenth century, large numbers of Christian missionaries came to India to preach and to proselytize. The group also contained some learned men who introduced studies of various subjects that were uncommon in India.

On November 2, 1833, Sarkar was born in Paikpara, a small village near Calcutta. He was the eldest of two sons. After his father, Ramtarak Sarkar, died, Sarkar went to Calcutta with his mother and lived with his maternal uncles, Iswar Chandra and Mahesh Chandra Ghose, who undertook the entire responsibility for Sarkar's education and development.

Sarkar began his education in a local Bengali school at Nebutala. To learn English, he was placed under the tutelage of Thakurdas Dey, one of the most erudite English teachers of the time. In 1841, Sarkar was admitted into the David Hare School and studied there until 1849. Then he joined the Hindu College after obtaining a junior scholarship. He studied there for five years and showed outstanding proficiency in English composition and pronunciation. His excellence attracted the attention of his professor of mathematics, J. Sutcliffe, who made arrangements for him to study geometry, astronomy, and natural sciences. He became bent upon joining the Calcutta Medical College to study medicine and related applied sciences.

In 1854 he was admitted to the medical college, where he studied until 1860 and received the diploma of L.M.S. (licentiateship in medicine and surgery). The Calcutta Medical College then offered the diploma of L.M.S. and the degrees of M.B. and M.D. A student who was a matriculate during his entry received an L.M.S. diploma; a student who had a first arts diploma (F.A.) received a bachelor of medicine degree (M.B.); and, by the British standard, the postgraduate degree was a doctor of medicine (M.D.). The L.M.S. and the M.B. were virtually the same. Sarkar studied under such famous teachers as W. C. B. Eatwell, E. Goodeve, Surya Kumar Chakraborty, and N. Chatterjee. After successfully passing the L.M.S. examination, he started preparing for the M.D. examination. In 1863 he qualified in the M.D. examination with highest honors. He was the second M.D. from Calcutta University; Dr. Chandra Kumar Dey was the first. Sarkar's brilliant career at the medical college impressed his teachers, who gave him opportunities to study more advanced areas in medicine.

During his lifetime, both the indigenous Ayurvedic system of medicine and the *Hekimi*, or *Unani* system, which had been imported from Persia and Arabia during the period of Muslim rule (eleventh to fourteenth centuries) were popular in India. *Unani* medicine combined Arabic or Tibbi medicine with Greek medicine. Some exchanges between Ayurvedic and Greek medicine can be traced back to the time of Hippocrates.

At the beginning of the nineteenth century, homeopathic medicine was developed by Dr. Samuel Hahnemann. A German geologist stationed in Calcutta introduced homeopathy to India. The progress of homeopathy was slow until the 1840s, when Rajendralal Dutta, a learned citizen of Calcutta, became interested in it and made extensive studies that ultimately led him to practice homeopathy. Since he had no basic knowledge of medicine, he asked Sarkar to practice homeopathy. During this period, British doctors stationed in India practiced only allopathic medicine. At first Sarkar was not very keen on homeopathy, but he made some critical clinical tests using homeopathy and some radical changes. After revisions and extensive study, he became convinced that it was an effective and rational system of medicine. In 1867 he spoke on the system to a large gathering of local medical practitioners. Allopathic colleagues immediately opposed him and made him an outcast. His friends, former teachers, and old patients abandoned him. But in 1868 he published a new medical journal and wrote prolifically about homeopathy.

Like other learned Indians, Sarkar was greatly in favor of science education. Raja Ram Mohun (Raja Ram Mohun Roy, 1772–1833), social reformer and landlord, was the forerunner of this movement. Sarkar had great respect for ancient Indian science, but he was eager to introduce European scientific study. In 1869 he called for the formation of a national association of science for the study and practice of science. He suggested that the association should arrange for regular lectures, experiments, and the inclusion of young Indians within its fold. He collected lavish donations from local rich people. On July 29, 1876, the Science Association was founded at the junction of Bow Bazaar and College Street and was renamed the Indian Association for the Cultivation of Science (IACS). From a small beginning, it grew gradually through donations and the support of the local government that helped import expertise from England.

The curriculum was approved by the Calcutta University. Many contemporary experts in the scientific field came forward to teach, including Dr. J. C. Bose, a physicist; Dr. P. C. Roy, a chemist; Dr. C. L. Bose, an organic chemist; P. N. Bose, a geologist; and G. C. Bose, a botanist. Sarkar made a renewed appeal for funds to appoint permanent teachers to the faculty. Even twenty-five years after the association's founding, he was not fully satisfied and continued his endeavors until his death on February 23, 1904. Many prominent Indian scientists such as Sir A. Mukherjee, Sir G. D. Banerjee, Dr. J. C. Bose, and others continued Sarkar's support of science education. C. V. Raman (1888–1970), who was awarded the Nobel Prize in Physics in 1933, performed his research on light scattering at the IACS. In 1950–1951, Dr. M. N. Saha moved the association to its present location at Jadavpur, near Calcutta.

Undeniably, Sarkar's efforts paved the way for modern scientific studies and research in India during the nineteenth and twentieth centuries. He was honored with many titles and awards during his lifetime: for example, Companion of the Indian Empire, member of the Legislative Assembly in Bengal, "first citizen" of Calcutta and an honorary magistrate, a doctor of laws, fellow of the Calcutta University Syndicate, fellow of the Asiatic Society in Calcutta, trustee of the Indian Museum in Calcutta, and life member of the British and French Science Societies. Besides being a doctor and a scientist, he was also a poet; over ten of his songs written in Bengali have been set to Indian classical tunes and are still extant. Today, one is still awed by the determination and single-mindedness of Sarkar in introducing science education to India.

BIBLIOGRAPHY

Although Sarkar was a prolific author, his writings are now quite rare and virtually inaccessible. Sarkar's writings included *The Physiological Basis of Psychology, Treatment of Cholera with Notes on Diarrhoea, Dysentery and on Acute Intestinal Disorders, Therapeutics in Plague, Sketch on the Treatment of Cholera,* and *Moral Influences of Physical Sciences.* He also wrote numerous editorials in the *Calcutta Journal of Medicine.*

Writings about Mahendralal Sarkar and Related Topics

Ghosh, S. C. *Life of Dr. Mahendralal Sarkar, MD, DL, CIE.* 2d ed., Calcutta: Hahnemann Publishing Co., 1935.

Hosten, Fr. H. *Memories of the Asiatic Society of Bengal* 3, no. 9 (1914): 313ff.

Sarkar, Jaladhi. *The Physician of Sri Ramakrishna, Mahendralal Sarkar.* (In Bengali.) Calcutta: Udbodhan Karyalaya, 1990.

Sen, B. C. "Medical College in the Past Sixties." *Calcutta Medical Journal* 4 (1907): 193–204.

Sen, Samarendra Nath. *The Doyen of science Dr. Mahendralal Sarkar.* (In Bengali.) Calcutta: IACS, 1985.

ACKNOWLEDGMENTS

Sipra Mitra, the librarian of the Indian Association for the Cultivation of Science, is gratefully acknowledged for her kind help.

Asoke K. Bagchi

HENRY ALFRED SCHROEDER
(1906–1975)

Henry Alfred Schroeder, M.D., pioneer in aerospace physiology, was a medical scientist known for many contributions to the prevention and treatment of hypertension and the prevention of chronic diseases caused by imbalances of trace elements. A native of Short Hills, New Jersey, Schroeder graduated from Yale College in 1929 with majors in English and biology. He earned his medical degree from the College of Physicians and Surgeons, Columbia University, in 1933. Schroeder's graduate medical education consisted of a two-year internship at Presbyterian Hospital, New York City, a one-year fellowship in pharmacology at the University of Pennsylvania Medical School, and a two-year residency at Rockefeller Institute Hospital. He then served on the staff of the last-named institution as an assistant in medicine from 1939 to 1942. While at Rockefeller, Schroeder collaborated with Professor Isaac Starr in the early development of the ballistocardiogram, an instrument designed to detect abnormalities in cardiac function.

During the next four and one-half years, Schroeder was on active duty in the U.S. Navy, attaining the rank of commander. As a flight surgeon, he studied the high accelerative forces that build up in turns, diving pull-outs, and crashes. He was one of the three developers of the standard aviator's anti-blackout suit, which protects pilots against loss of vision during high G forces. Schroeder established standards for aircraft seats and harnesses to prevent injury from crashes. He wrote and directed a four-reel training film with sound and color, *G and You*, which later received a prize at an international film festival. He recommended standards for astronauts' space suits and participated in the construction of the world's largest human centrifuge. After World War II but long before *Sputnik*, he was one of three medical consultants to the Department of Defense on problems to be encountered during space flight. From 1946 to 1958, Schroeder was a faculty member of the Department of Medicine at Washington University School of Medicine in St. Louis. During the last seventeen years of his life, he was a member of the Physiology Department at Dartmouth Medical School.

Schroeder's first major contribution to the prevention of chronic disease was his development of the low-sodium diet, widely used today, for amelioration of hypertension and cardiomyopathy. Between 1937 and 1958, he published over one hundred papers on hypertension in major medical journals. In 1951, he developed the first successful drug therapy for this disease.

Early in the 1950s, Schroeder became interested in the possible roles of trace elements in hypertension and other chronic diseases. In part, this interest developed from his observation that drugs with efficacy in these diseases often contain metal-binding sites. But as Schroeder told colleagues, when driving through Indiana he saw signs urging Indiana farmers to "feed your hogs zinc." He observed that although a zinc requirement had been established by veterinary scientists at Purdue University to prevent a serious chronic disease of hogs (parakeratosis), knowledge of the roles of trace elements such as zinc in human health and disease was conspicuously lacking. In 1956–1957, he traveled extensively through Asia and the Middle East collecting human autopsy material for trace element analyses. He collaborated with Professor Isabel H. Tipton, University of Tennessee and Oak Ridge National Laboratories. His data were combined with those obtained from autopsy material from other regions of the world. The combined results became an important baseline for all subsequent studies.

In 1958, Schroeder established the Trace Element Laboratory. Two years later, he built a metal-free, environmentally controlled animal laboratory on a remote hill near Brattleboro, Vermont. Rats reared in this pollution-free habitat had excellent health and extended longevity. However, Schroeder discovered that the addition of a small amount of cadmium to drinking water duplicated in the rats the symptoms of human hypertension and that the disease could be cured by administering a zinc-containing preparation. A deficiency of chromium also caused the rats to develop diabetes and atherosclerosis, again duplicating human lesions. Schroeder studied the lifetime exposure of rats and mice to each of twenty-six trace elements to determine their ability to produce cancers. Depending on the route of entry, the dosage, and the chemical form, trace elements such as beryllium, nickel, arsenic, selenium, and chromium could, he reported, be carcinogenic in rodents and humans.

Schroeder emphasized that, in some cases, a small amount of an element such as chromium or selenium is essential for health and a large amount is hazardous. He noted also that essential elements are provided by the mother to the fetus, whereas nonessential elements in polluted environments accumulate in the tissues as the individual ages. Schroeder's work stressed the biologic uniqueness and nonexchangeability of the roles of each trace element. Moreover, his research repeatedly called attention to the danger not only of ingested toxic trace elements but of those inhaled from tobacco smoke, internal combustion engine exhausts, and mining dusts.

By the 1960s, epidemiological studies in Japan, the United States, Canada, Sweden, the Netherlands, and South America had confirmed that persons who drink "soft" or acidic waters have a two-to threefold greater risk of dying from cardiomyopathy and hypertension than those who drink "hard" water. Based on his rat model, Schroeder recognized that cadmium is most likely the hazardous "water factor." This element is eluted from the pipe solder upon corrosion by acidic water. Accordingly, he and other medical scientists have recommended that municipalities add lime and magnesium to make water less corrosive, harder, and more alkaline. Schroeder predicted that by this simple procedure, a reduction of 25 percent in death rates from cardiovascular decay would ensue.

Of the various diseases Schroeder showed to be caused by industrial trace element pollution, the most important is lead poisoning. From the 1920s until the mid-1970s, lead was discharged from the tailpipes of motor vehicles at an annual rate of about 4.4 pounds per car. It was then inhaled by drivers, passengers, and animals and humans living or working near heavy traffic. Lead is much more hazardous when inhaled than ingested, because the intestinal mucosa permits only 5 to 10 percent absorption, whereas the lung allows 30 to 50 percent entry into the circulatory system. In the United States, even the 35 million pounds per year of lead that remained in motor oil was dangerous because discarded oil is re-refined for lubrication. Thus, lead had a second chance to escape into the air when recycled oil was used.

Early in the 1960s, Schroeder had demonstrated and reported that lead poisoning in animals is associated with decreased longevity, greater susceptibility to infection, and accelerated cardiovascular deterioration. In humans, he and others reported, infection is frequent, and central nervous system problems occur, including fatigue, apathy, depression, mental retardation, and paralysis. Schroeder found up to 200 parts per million of lead in grass growing along a secondary highway near Brattleboro, an amount sufficient to abort a pregnant cow. He noted that the quantity of lead at that site had quintupled in a decade, whereas an isolated pasture five miles away had no detectable lead.

In his book *The Poisons Around Us* (1974), Schroeder recounted his ten-year struggle with the well-financed and entrenched lead industry. For decades, scientists employed by the Kettering Institute, the Lead Industries Association, and the Ethyl Corporation had maintained that "lead attributable to emission and dispersion into ambient air has no harmful effects." Incredibly, the National Academy of Sciences selected employees of the lead industry to compile and write the 1970–1971 National Research Council advisory report for the U.S. Environmental Protection Agency (EPA). Not surprisingly, this panel concluded that airborne lead "poses no hazard to the general population."

The National Academy of Sciences report and similar undocumented statements by the lead polluters were protested vigorously by Schroeder and two other independent, knowledgeable scientists, but not by the American Medical Association. During that period, Schroeder was interviewed by the National Broadcasting Company and the British Broadcasting Company. The interviews were broadcast in Australia and England, but, to avoid offending oil company sponsors, not in the United States. Eventually Schroeder persuaded the EPA to consider documented evidence rather than the biased advice of the National Academy of Sciences. EPA administrators promised to reduce the lead in gasoline by half by 1978. By the mid-1990s, only a small quantity of leaded gasoline was sold in the United States. The use of internal combustion engines has increased vastly since the 1970s. Had Schroeder's counsel not been heeded by the EPA in 1973, lead pollution would certainly have had an appalling impact on human health.

The work of the Trace Element Laboratory, plus Schroeder's ability to evaluate laboratory and environmental data objectively, were instrumental in defining the effects of mercury. In the late 1940s, methylated mercury had been discharged into two rivers in Japan by plastic manufacturing plants. Several hundred humans, as well as other mammals and birds, died from ingesting this highly toxic form of mercury. Other chemical compounds of mercury, however, are far less dangerous, and small amounts are found in healthy fish. Unfortunately, some analytical chemists assayed the element in fish by a procedure that caused the mercury to become methylated during the assay. The Food and Drug Administration (FDA) officially condemned various game fish, large batches of tuna, and all swordfish. Schroeder commented that one of the silliest projects of the "mercury fiasco" was the demonstration by the government of the United States that the hair of some healthy human residents of Alaska had ten times as much mercury as the FDA allowed in edible fish. Fortunately, Schroeder convinced the FDA that small background levels of some forms of mercury in fish and consumers of fish are natural and harmless. The bans on marketing such fish were eventually lifted.

On the other hand, fish contaminated with cadmium and nickel are extremely dangerous to eat. In 1971, the Trace Element Laboratory demonstrated that fish in the Hudson River downstream from Foundry Cove were dangerously contaminated with these highly toxic elements. Schroeder's testimony and analytical data persuaded the EPA to order the companies that were making cadmium-nickel-plated equipment to stop discharging the elements into the river and to remove the contaminated mud from Foundry Cove.

Schroeder was the author of three books on hypertension and four on the impact of trace elements on health and disease. His studies of trace elements were reported between 1955 and 1975 in over one hundred publications in distinguished medical journals. He served as a consultant on trace elements to the World Health Organization, the International Commission on Radiological Protection, the International Atomic Energy Agency, the President's Council on Environmental Quality, the Food and Drug Administration, the Federal Water Quality Board, the National Air Pollution Control Administration, the Environmental Protection Agency, the U.S. Department of Agriculture, the Senate Subcommittee on the Environment, the Senate Committee on Nutrition and Human Needs, and the Center for the Study of Responsive Law. Although much of his time and energy was devoted to pioneering research and to making his findings known to the scientific and political establishments, Schroeder also pursued an alternative vocation. He was a licensed lay reader in the Episcopal church and a member of the Vermont Diocesan Commission on the Ministry, and, in the winter months, he served a congregation in St. Thomas, the Virgin Islands. Moreover, his fine voice was considered an asset to his church choir.

BIBLIOGRAPHY

Dr. Schroeder was the sole or coauthor of 214 scientific publications. A complete list of these can be obtained from Eugene D. Weinberg.

Writings by Henry Alfred Schroeder

(with L. A. Peters). *Shirt Tail and Pig Tail.* New York: Minton Balch and Co., 1930.
Hypertensive Diseases: Causes and Control. Philadelphia: Lea and Febiger, 1953.
Mechanism of Hypertension. Springfield, IL: Charles C. Thomas, 1957.
A Matter of Choice. Brattleboro, VT: Stephen Green Press, 1968.
Pollution, Profits and Progress. Brattleboro, VT: Stephen Green Press, 1971.
The Trace Elements and Man. Old Greenwich, CT: Devin-Adair Co., 1973.
The Poisons Around Us. Toxic Metals in Food, Air, and Water. Bloomington: Indiana University Press, 1974.

Eugene D. Weinberg

MICHAEL ABRAHAM SHADID
(1882–1966)

Michael Abraham Shadid was the innovative father of prepaid and cooperative medical care, as well as the founder of Hospital Haramoon, a badly needed facility in South Lebanon. Shadid was born in Judeidat, a small town of a few thousand inhabitants in Marj'yoon County, now in South Lebanon and, before the end of World War I, in the Ottoman Empire's province of Syria. The exact date of his birth is not known; he was the twelfth child and was born a few months after his father died. The first nine of his brothers died in infancy. His family name, *Shadid*, means "strong." His mother's father and brother were Greek Orthodox priests. Shadid later recalled that when his father died, he left only a one-room house, two mules, and twenty thousand piasters (about one thousand dollars). His mother was frugal and hard working and managed to make the money last for ten years. "Among my earliest memories," he wrote some sixty years later, "are many that have to do with poverty. Why was I barefoot . . . ? Why were my clothes shabby and my lunch meager compared with that of other children? Why was my mother menial?" So many questions worked their way into the subconscious of the young boy; they most probably shaped his future ideals in life and resulted in his valiant struggle to establish social justice in his environment.

Shadid studied in his hometown's Greek Orthodox school; later, he went to the preparatory section of the Syrian Protestant College, which was founded in Beirut by American missionaries in 1866. In 1898, at the age of sixteen, he emigrated to America, where the fiery young man literally peddled his way through college by selling jewelry and linens and into Washington University's Medical School in Saint Louis, from which he obtained his M.D. in 1906. After graduation he took postgraduate courses in medicine and in surgery in Chicago (1911, 1912), New York (1912), Philadelphia and Chicago (1922), and Vienna (1928). He went to Vienna because "at that time the opportunities in Vienna for good training were unmatched anywhere."

He started working in Maxville, Missouri, where in 1907 he married Adeeba (Edna) Shadid, the girl to whom he had been betrothed in Syria on the day she was born. Soon after his marriage he moved to Oklahoma, where he practiced medicine, purchased a Ford, and bought an oil and gas lease around Sayre, Oklahoma, for $300. He later sold the lease to Skelly Oil Company for $21,000. With this money he bought four business buildings. During the influenza epidemic of 1918, he used intravenous typhoid vaccine with good results in at least nine cases. He worked in Mangum (1923) and then in Elk City, where his income doubled to $20,000 per year. He opened a small hospital, Elk Sanitarium, where he did surgery. His reputation as an excellent physician became widespread over the area. In 1928, he went, with his daughter Ruth, on a vacation to Lebanon, Damascus, Haifa, Jerusalem, Egypt, and Vienna.

During the Great Depression, his intense beliefs and fierce dedication drove him into the snowdrifts and the dust storms of the so-called short grass country of western Oklahoma. In 1929, in order to give the common people of America better medical care for less money and remove the temptation to perform unnecessary surgery, Shadid devised a prepaid, cooperative medical plan. He called a meeting of a number of his farmer-patients on October 29, 1929, in the basement of the Carnegie Library in Elk City. A few thousand farmers subscribed at $50 a share and built and equipped the Community Hospital in Elk City, Oklahoma, the first cooperative hospital in the United States. A family member would prepay an average of $25 per year, which covered room, board, nursing care, doctors fees, X-rays, and laboratory fees. Dentures could be had for $25, major surgery for $20, minor surgery for $10, daily hospitalization for $3 a day, and a dental filling for $1. The annual hospital expenses, including salaries, medicines, surgical supplies, and so forth, amounted to $110,000.

The opposition of organized medicine to this innovation was strong, vicious, and unbecoming; the battle went on for twenty-three years. Dr. Shadid began to feel the sting of his medical colleagues before 1930. False rumors that the plan was a hoax and that bankruptcy was inevitable were circulated. Many slurs were made about Shadid's ethnic origin, and he even received death threats. The Beckham County Medical Society excluded him from membership by disbanding and reorganizing without him. The Oklahoma Medical Association, in collusion with the Beckman County Medical Society and the American Medical Association, tried to revoke his license to practice medicine. This battle lasted four years and ended in 1940 by a court writ. The hospital was blockaded to prevent him from obtaining physicians, dentists, nurses, and technicians. The Oklahoma State Board of Medical Examiners stopped certifying doctors they suspected were headed for the community hospital. On that account, the hospital's physicians were denied admission to many postgraduate courses and malpractice insurance. Most of the hospital's physicians were drafted into the military, including Shadid's son and nephew. Shadid was called "a peddler of rugs," "a communist," "a Nazi," "an atheist," "a fifth columnist," and "the communist Turk." Firecrackers were shot while he was delivering speeches, or the fire siren was turned on. These lies and tricks seemed to spark and motivate him more. The more tenacious the opposition, the harder he fought. Despite all the opposition, the hospital was enlarged seven times between 1934 and 1949. The number of surgical operations rose from 121 in 1932 to 1,000 in 1936. The membership grew to 1,800 families in 1940 to 2,500 in 1949. The nonmember families grew to 2,500. In the final analysis his ideas were vindicated.

In order to inform members and keep them well aware of health matters and hygiene, Shadid published the monthly *Community Hospital Bulletin*. In a letter to Shadid written in 1945, Dr. J. P. Warbasse, the editor of the *American Journal of Surgery*, the *Annals of Surgery*, and the *New York State Journal of Medicine*, said:

This is the most important periodical published in the United States. This is because it is the first and only journal devoted to the interest of the patients and prospective patients, owning a hospital. It is my belief that these patients and prospective patients are the people most concerned for the advancement and perfection of medicine. It is to them that the world must look for the demands of high standards and efficiency in medical practice. They are the people who have to pay the doctor's bills, suffer the pains, and do the dying. They have the greatest stake in the problems of health. . . . I speak not only from experience but also with sincerity.

The national news media coverage caused a flood of inquiries from doctors and communities asking for advice on how to start their own prepaid health group. Shadid traveled throughout Texas, Kansas, Washington, Idaho, Oregon, Minnesota, and Wisconsin, speaking and offering advice and expertise. It was for this purpose that he wrote two pamphlets, *Principles of Cooperative Medicine* and *Co-op Hospital Catechism*. The purpose of cooperative medicine was to bring to the people, at cost and within their means, the services of scientific medicine through periodic payment, group practice, and cooperative control, in order to avoid the dark and unwholesome medical practices prevalent at the time and to provide a safer and more economical system of medical care and hospitalization. The three main principles of cooperative medicine are reducing medical costs by having the people build, control, and manage their hospital; staffing the hospital with salaried physicians, and prepayment.

Staffing the hospital with salaried physicians would cut down on unnecessary surgery, unnecessary medical tests, and unnecessary medication. The physician is thus prevented from thriving on the misfortunes of the sick. In the current system of organized medicine, the physician puts profits before professional duty and before the interests of patients. In the cooperative system the physician no longer has financial incentives to prolong the treatment and hospitalization of patients. The physician is no longer concerned with bookkeeping, collections, rent, administrative chores, and overhead expenses. Competitors become colleagues. Physicians have more spare time to rest and take vacations. They have no pecuniary reason to lead the patient to think he or she is sick. The hospital and all medical facilities exist for the sole purpose of the welfare of the public and cease to be institutions for the promotion of private gain. The emphasis is laid on prevention of disease. The incentive and the inducement to give dishonest advice are eliminated.

The third principle, prepayment, periodic in nature, would allow the patient to seek medical help early on. The lack of money is no longer an impediment to seek medical help, whereas in the current system, the patient does not avail himself or herself of medical help except in emergencies. In the new system, money is no longer an obstacle to early consultation. Patients no longer self-medicate from fear of the high cost of medication and surgical operations. They are not afraid of costs; the annual prepayment has removed the economic factor, and they know that physicians have no pecuniary motive in recommending treatment or operation. They seek medical help early. In the current system, medicine becomes very expensive because the physician has to involve many other health care providers in the treatment of the patient; this includes the diagnostic arms, the specialists, and the hospital. In the cooperative plan, the people can budget themselves for ill health and unpredictable illness. For example, members of a prepayment plan seldom come to the hospital with a ruptured appendix, whereas 50 percent of the cases of appendicitis that come from patients seeing physicians on a fee-for-service basis are ruptured. These principles became widely known and resulted in the establishment of the Group Health Association in Washington, D.C. (1937), the Kaiser Foundation Medical Care Plan (1942), and the Group Health Cooperative of Puget Sound (1940s).

In 1943, in a concise and elegant article about Shadid, Dr. Paul de Kruif* wrote, "Courageously, resourcefully, Dr. Shadid and these Oklahomans have pioneered a way to beat our shortage of country doctors. They have proved that even a poor community can build its hospital, pay for it, and hire a staff of competent physicians and surgeons . . . made possible by prepaid group practice—the country medicine of tomorrow." In 1944, J. D. Ratcliff wrote in *Collier's*: "A crusading Oklahoma doctor proves that health protection and Grade A medical care are within the reach of every purse. The first American Co-Operative Hospital is a resounding success today and a milestone for tomorrow." In 1954, a play, *Oracle Junction*, written by playwright Sari Scott from Los Angeles, based on Shadid's book, *A Doctor for the People*, was performed on stage at the Margo Jones Theater in Dallas. In 1978, Dr. Shadid was initiated into the Cooperative Hall of Fame. In 1982, Raouf J. Halaby wrote, "The unique role played by Dr. Michael Shadid in the establishment of the Community Hospital and the great impact it had on the lives of thousands of farmers in the Western region of Oklahoma is an unprecedented feat in the annals of medical history. Equal in significance is the tremendous influence which the philosophy and practice of Cooperative Medicine exerted at the national level." T. R. Mayer and G. G. Mayer wrote: "Thus, in 1929, before the origins of traditional health insurance, came the *medical shot heard around the nation* in the small community of Elk City." The story of Dr. Shadid had such an impact that, in 1990, Ralph Nader wrote, "If Hollywood is looking for both drama and historical significance in the life of one immigrant to this country, the saga of Dr. M. Shadid has to be a leading candidate."

Shadid was an honest, straightforward physician. Unlike the rank and file of contemporaneous physicians, who in essence put their own interests before those of their patients, he put the interests of the patient first. It took a vast amount of courage to carry the fight to its logical end, despite the numerous attempts by organized medicine to impede and sabotage his efforts. At great expense to his health and the well-being of his two physician sons who were drafted into the military, and despite the vile egotism of the medical profession, he continued with diligence, persistence, and persuasion his fight for the legal rights of patients and followed up his ideals to their logical and fruitful conclusion by founding the Cooperative Health Federation of America (1946), of which he was elected the first president (1946–1949). This was a significant step in the evolution of medical care.

When Shadid retired in mid-1946 after a heart attack, his son, Dr. Fred V. Shadid, took over the reins and immediately renewed efforts to reverse the ostracism against the Community Hospital, but to no avail. In 1950, on August 28, he finally filed a lawsuit against the Beckham County Medical Society for unlawful conspiracy. On April 22, 1952, just prior to going to court, the opposition folded, and an out-of-court settlement was arranged. All the doctors of the Community Hospital were admitted to full membership privileges in the society. The long, hard struggle came to a victorious end. Unfortunately, the damage had already become critical. Dr. Fred V. Shadid retired in 1953, after a heart attack. The hospital closed its doors in 1955. Dr. Fred Shadid attributed this to "lack of dedication and sincere beliefs in the fundamental concepts of the cooperative ideas by members of the staff and the lack of leadership."

The impediments and the difficulties of the struggle to establish cooperative medicine did not halt the enthusiasm of Dr. Shadid, who in the twilight of his life realized his benevolent and charitable dream by founding Hospital Haramoon (called today "Marjøuyuwn Government Hospital"). From his visit to Lebanon in 1928, he realized how badly his native town needed a hospital. Later, he began to assess how much the immigrants in his area were willing to contribute to such a project. From the beginning, he was opposed by no less a person than the multimillionaire president of the Orthodox church of St. Elijah in Oklahoma City, B. D. Eddie. This opposition stirred him all the more to increase his vigor in soliciting funds for the project. Shadid went on a solicitation trip to Wichita, Canada, and New York. Because of Eddie's opposition, the total amount collected was less than $17,000. In the summer of 1951, Shadid flew to Brazil where, with the help of Faris Dabague (Dabagiy; also spelled DeBakey in the United States), $32,000 was collected. Unfortunately, the local committee (President Dabague and Secretary Rashid Abukessm) put the money in the bank, and in 1955, the exchange rate was such that the value of the fund had dropped to $12,000. Shadid wanted to call the proposed hospital "Marjøuyuwn Hospital," but when Dabague asked whether it could be called "Hospital Haramoon" (Brazilian style), Shadid agreed.

After fourteen months of negotiating with the architects, builders, and others involved in the project, changing the deed of the Zalaf property, which had been so generously donated, tearing down the Zalaf house, and dealing with the lot, Shadid turned over the remaining money to President Camille Chamoun. Dabague sent $15,000 and promised to send another $10,000 later. The construction of Hospital Haramoon was finished in 1959. The hospital was inaugurated in 1960. Since then, it has been enlarged several times under the able supervision of Sister Marguerite Nader and Dr. Khayrallah Mady.

Having completed the two major accomplishments of his life—the founding of the Community Hospital in Elk City and the founding of Hospital Haramoon in Judeidat Marj'yoon—Shadid established in 1958 a $50,000 scholarship fund at the American University of Beirut. Shadid had several other ideas, such as the democratization and equitable admission of physicians to the hospital staff and the nationalization of the medical license. He also pleaded against privilege, monopoly, and intolerance. Throughout his life, Shadid battled against the greed of physicians. In 1922, his fight with diabetes started. He had heart attacks in 1944, 1945, and 1946. In 1963, he lost a limb, and on August 13, 1966, he died while playing cards with friends. "We bow our heads," wrote Freda Ameringer, "a great man lived among us, gone now to a well-earned rest."

The saga of the extraordinary Dr. Shadid reflects the image of his childhood as an underprivileged and poor child. All his life he strove to obtain better medical care for the underprivileged. "He dared break through the barriers of decaying medical tradition," wrote Ralph Nader, "and suffered persecution and ostracism so that the way might be cleared to wide opportunities for . . . service to the public and the profession. The idealism of the past can help nourish the motivation of the future. No better example of service can be recounted than that rendered, amidst a maelstrom, by Dr. Shadid and his sons. They practiced medicine as if only people mattered." The epilogue to this story has not yet been written. A time will come when the people will awaken from under the yoke of the traders in health, to revive Dr. Shadid's concept of a cooperative health system based on prepayment and nonprofit.

BIBLIOGRAPHY

Memorabilia pertaining to Dr. Michael Shadid and to the Community Hospital of Elk City were donated in 1984 by his son, Dr. Fred V. Shadid, to the Western History Collections, University of Oklahoma libraries.

Writings by Michael Abraham Shadid

"Protein Shock Therapy in Influenza and Pneumonia." *Clinical Medicine and Surgery* 36 (1929): 332–333.
Principles of Cooperative Medicine. Chicago: Cooperative League of the USA, 1938.
Doctors of Today and Tomorrow. Superior, WI: Cooperative Publishing Association, 1947.
Crusading Doctor: My Fight for Cooperative Medicine. Foreword by Ralph Nader. Boston: Meador Publishing Company, 1956. Reprint ed. Oklahoma City: University of Oklahoma Press, 1992.

Writings about Michael Abraham Shadid and Related Topics

de Kruif, Paul. "Cooperative Health Harvest." *Reader's Digest* (September 1943): 97–100.

Mayer, T. R. and G. G. Mayer. "HMOs: Origins and Development." *New England Journal of Medicine* 312 (1985): 590–594.

Nader, Ralph. Foreword to Michael Shadid, *Crusading Doctor: My Fight for Cooperative Medicine*. Boston: Meador Publishing Company, 1956.

Ratcliff, J. D. "Co-op Hospital." *Collier's Magazine*, July 31, 1943, pp. 24–26.

Scott, Sari. *Oracle Junction*. Unpublished play. 1954.

Shadid, Fred V. *First Rural HMO—a Co-op Hospital*. Santa Monica, CA: Fred V. Shadid, 1991.

Farid Sami Haddad

HILLA SHERIFF
(1903–1988)

Hilla Sheriff, pediatrician and public health officer, was one of the most influential medical women in the history of the American South. As a member of what historians sometimes call a "lost generation" of feminists—women who came of age immediately after the suffrage victory in 1920—Hilla Sheriff surmounted numerous structural and psychological obstacles in order to practice medicine in South Carolina. Despite her relative isolation, the presence of all of the practical problems still encountered by women who pursued careers as physicians, and the additional disincentives of institutional barriers, hostile colleagues, and public prejudice, Sheriff persevered. She rose to prominence in the 1930s as the state's first female county health officer. Sheriff's ability to tailor programs to diverse communities—women who bore double burdens as textile workers and mothers, isolated farm families, mountaineers dependent on weak agricultural markets and a sagging coal industry, and African Americans denied medical care by the paucity of accessible facilities in the Jim Crow South— serves as a timeless example for those committed to a more egalitarian system of health care delivery.

The programs Sheriff developed in Spartanburg County during the 1930s became models for South Carolina's responses to calls for inclusion across racial and class lines and the integration of services in the decades after World War II. Her presence at the head of the South Carolina Board of Health's Division of Maternal and Child Health during the postwar decades ensured progressive responses to the region's most pressing health care needs despite the conservatism of the state's social and political systems.

Born in the Appalachian foothills of Pickens County, South Carolina, and raised in Orangeburg, an agricultural settlement near the center of the state, Sheriff attended the College of Charleston for two years before transferring to the Medical College of the State of South Carolina (now the Medical University of South Carolina), where she graduated in 1926. Sheriff never finished the bachelor's degree because, believing her disapproving parents might withdraw their support at any time, she sought to expedite her medical training. After an internship at the Hospital of the Women's Medical College of Pennsylvania, Sheriff completed residencies at the Children's Hospital in Washington, D.C., and New York City's Willard Parker Contagious Disease Hospital. She returned to South Carolina in 1929 and opened a pediatrics practice in Spartanburg, a county seat town at the edge of the Appalachian mountains surrounded by some of the region's largest textile mills.

The poverty of most of her patients and an offer in 1931 to direct the first American units of the American Women's Hospitals (AWH) facilitated Sheriff's quick move from private practice to public health. She traveled into the mountain hollows and examined mothers and children in the AWH's healthmobile, a motorized trailer set up to serve as a doctor's office. Although by 1916 the South Carolina and Mississippi studies of Public Health Service epidemiologist Joseph Goldberger* had resulted in abundant evidence linking pellagra to a prolonged dietary deficiency, the disease reappeared with the downturn of the textile industry in the 1920s. In 1929, Spartanburg County claimed 2,438 of South Carolina's 7,763 pellagra cases. In that year, 909 people died of that disease in a county with a population of just over 115,000. As the Depression intensified, 300,000 cases of pellagra were reported throughout the South (Hill 1995: 580, 583). Until the mid-1930s, physicians did not know that insufficient nicotinic acid or niacin caused pellagra, but Sheriff and her contemporaries understood that fatback pork, corn bread, and molasses, all staples of the diet of the southern poor, required augmentation with fresh vegetables, lean meats, and dairy products. Sheriff staffed the healthmobile with nurses and nutritionists to teach mothers to can vegetables and use pressure cookers to cook inexpensive, vitamin-rich dried peas and beans more quickly. She arranged for loans of milk cows to isolated mountain families whose children showed symptoms of pellagra. The "gospel of nutritional health" spread by Sheriff and her female medical team was remarkably well received by mill workers and farm families, who suspected the expertise of "outsiders" and considered both piety and domesticity "womanly" traits. Sheriff adapted the familiar metaphor of a religious crusade, which had been used successfully by the Rockefeller Sanitary Commission in its campaign to eradicate hookworm in the South during the 1910s and 1920s, to her pellagra prevention work (see Ettling 1981). Even without an upturn in textile fortunes or cotton prices, pellagra was reduced by one-half in Spartanburg County between 1931 and 1933 (Sheriff May 1933: 209–212).

As the deputy and later chief health official for Spartanburg County between 1933 and 1940, Sheriff's responses to endemic pellagra, diphtheria, and tuberculosis, innovative maternal and child health campaigns, and contraceptive research for the Milbank Memorial Fund attracted national attention and spawned programs based on her models throughout the South. Sheriff established the first family planning clinic associated with a county health department in the United States. Public opposition was eliminated when Sheriff organized a committee of leading club women and executives to oversee the project. Sheriff used South Carolina's high maternal death rates to "embarrass" policymakers into allowing her to teach birth-spacing techniques as part of postpartum clinics. Clinics based on Sheriff's model were organized in county health departments around the state beginning in 1936, and, three years later, South Carolina followed North Carolina's lead and became the second state to make birth control an official public health service.

In 1936, officials with the U.S. Children's Bureau recommended Sheriff for one of four Rockefeller Foundation fellowships to study public health at Harvard. She became the second woman (the first American woman) to earn an

M.P.H. (master of public health) from Harvard the following year. Sheriff's experience and training attracted the attention of state officials, and in 1940 she moved to Columbia as the assistant director of the Board of Health's Division of Maternal and Child Health. She was promoted to director the following year. Sheriff continued to head state programs for women and children until 1967, when she was promoted to deputy commissioner of the renamed state Department of Health and Environmental Control and simultaneously as chief of the Bureau of Community Health Services. She held these positions until her retirement in 1974.

Sheriff's efforts to train and license the state's lay midwives during the postwar decades reveal interesting tensions between professional goals that stressed the importance of a physician's presence during childbirth and a feminist consciousness that appreciated the control women retained over the process of giving birth at home assisted by other women. As had been the case in Spartanburg County, Sheriff's pragmatism often guided her policy. By the 1940s, most South Carolina midwives were African American women whose patients were denied the option of an attending physician by poverty and segregation. Sheriff argued that outlawing lay midwifery in the Jim Crow South would not end the practice but would simply ensure that most midwives remained beyond the reach of state health officials. She established training and licensing procedures that sanctioned the use of midwives during routine deliveries (thus raising their status and ensuring high levels of participation), linked lay practitioners with local nurse midwives and physicians willing to attend in the case of difficult births, and screened the ranks of South Carolina midwives for carriers of contagious diseases.

Sheriff also organized pre-and postnatal clinics and child health clinics, during which inoculations for smallpox, whooping cough, diphtheria, poliomyelitis, and tetanus were given and literature on infant and child care distributed to mothers. After the use of antibiotics became widespread, the Division of Maternal and Child Health focused on accident prevention, poison control, family planning services, and programs to eliminate child abuse.

Late in life, Sheriff recalled that she used to take care of sick and injured farm animals, always named the father in her family of paper dolls "the doctor," and could not remember a time when she did not want a career in medicine. Her brothers and parents predicted that she would be married before she finished her first year in medical school. Sheriff did marry, but not until she was thirty-seven years old and partially immune to southern society's traditional expectations of wives. Her spouse from 1940 until his death in 1953 was George Henry Zerbst, an ophthalmologist and public health officer who had been one of Sheriff's medical school instructors. Correspondence during an eighteen-year friendship before their wedding indicates that both were keenly aware that marriage would have a negative impact on Sheriff's career, if she was perceived primarily as a wife instead of as a doctor.

Sheriff is remembered for her hands-on style and strong will combined with a graciousness associated with the South. Catherine Greene, a public health nurse who worked with Sheriff, recalled, "She was a very persuasive person and yet a very feminine, sophisticated Southern lady. She managed to maintain all of that and yet it was known she was the person in command." During the mid-1930s, Sheriff took Greene and the rest of her staff to a Thanksgiving lunch at a black schoolhouse. It was the first time most of the white public health nurses had shared a meal with African Americans. According to Greene, "We felt very much in place because Dr. Sheriff made everyone feel we were doing exactly the right thing. . . . It didn't faze her at all to go into any one of the colored schools." Some members of the health department refused to examine black patients or inoculate black children until Sheriff instructed them that health care was a right of all of the state's citizens. She routinely asked those with reservations to accompany her to a clinic at an African American school. Greene added, "She made you feel like no one but you could do the job she was giving you." Dr. James Padgett, who succeeded Sheriff as the state director of maternal and child health, described his mentor as "a very powerful woman and a very smart woman. When you're with her, you're still at her feet because you know what she's going to say is going to be worthwhile. . . . I think Scarlett O'Hara could take a few lessons from her" (Buice 1986).

Sheriff served as vice president of the American Medical Women's Association in 1950 and as president of the National Association of State Maternal and Child Health and Crippled Children's Directors between 1960 and 1962. She was a fellow of the American Public Health Association and a diplomate of the American Board of Preventive Medicine and Public Health. She presided over the South Carolina Public Health Association in 1947, served as secretary and treasurer of the South Carolina Pediatric Society between 1941 and 1946, and was vice president of the Columbia Medical Society during 1962–1963. Sheriff represented South Carolina at White House Conferences for Children and Youth in 1940, 1950, and 1960.

Accolades included the first Ross Award, presented at the 1969 annual meeting of the southern branch of the American Public Health Association, outstanding employee of the South Carolina Department of Health and Environmental Control (1974), outstanding female employee for 1974, the University of South Carolina School of Medicine's William Weston Distinguished Service Award for Excellence in Pediatrics (1983), and the Order of the Palmetto (South Carolina's highest honor). The Medical University of South Carolina continues to award a scholarship bearing Sheriff's name.

BIBLIOGRAPHY

Hilla Sheriff's papers are housed at the University of South Carolina's South Caroliniana Library, Columbia. The collection includes correspondence between 1912 and 1987, twenty-nine topical files, Sheriff's publications, a diary, college and medical school notes, clippings, meeting programs, awards, calendars, photographs, and Henry Zerbst's sketchbook and poetry written for his wife. The Archives and Special Collections on Women in Medicine at the Medical College of Pennsylvania, Philadelphia, hold the records of the American Women's Hospitals. Files on AWH work in the southern Appalachians contain Sheriff's correspondence with AWH leaders during the 1930s, when she directed units in South Carolina's Spartanburg and Greenville counties. AWH minutes and financial records for that decade detail the relative priority accorded and resources allocated to Sheriff's work.

Writings by Hilla Sheriff

"American Women's Hospitals in South Carolina." *Medical Review of Reviews* 39 (May 1933): 209–212.

"The Tuberculin Skin Test." *Journal of the South Carolina Medical Association* 29 (November 1933): 253–257.

"Immunization against Diphtheria." *Journal of the South Carolina Medical Association* 30 (November 1934): 219–221.

"Trends in Maternal and Child Health." *Journal of the American Dietetic Association* 34 (December 1958): 1304–1308.

"The Abused Child." *Journal of the South Carolina Medical Association* 60 (June 1964): 191–193.

"Laboratory Diagnosis in Toxoplasmosis." *Journal of the American Medical Women's Association* 27 (December 1972): 638–640.

(with G. Thomas Moore, Jr.). "Toxoplasmosis, the Laboratory and You." *Journal of the South Carolina Medical Association* 69 (April 1973): 111–114.

Writings about Hilla Sheriff and Related Topics

Beardsley, Edward H. *A History of Neglect: Health Care for Blacks and Mill Workers in the Twentieth-Century South.* Knoxville: University of Tennessee Press, 1987.

Buice, Allison. "Dr. Sheriff: Health Pioneer." *Spartanburg Herald-Journal*, June 22, 1986.

Etheridge, Elizabeth. *The Butterfly Caste: A Social History of Pellagra in the South.* Westport, CT: Greenwood Press, 1972.

Ettling, John. *The Germ of Laziness: Rockefeller Philanthropy and Public Health in the New South.* Cambridge, MA: Harvard University Press, 1981.

Hill, Patricia Evridge. "Go Tell It on the Mountain: Hilla Sheriff and Public Health in the South Carolina Piedmont, 1929 to 1940." *American Journal of Public Health* 85 (April 1995): 578–584.

———. "Invisible Labours: Mill Work and Motherhood in the American South." *Social History of Medicine* 9 (1996): 235–251.

Morantz-Sanchez, Regina M. *Sympathy and Science: Women Physicians in American Medicine.* New York: Oxford University Press, 1985.

More, Ellen S., and Maureen A. Milligan, eds. *The Empathetic Practitioner: Empathy, Gender, and Medicine.* New Brunswick, NJ: Rutgers University Press, 1994.

Terris, Milton, ed. *Goldberger on Pellagra.* Baton Rouge: Louisiana State University Press, 1964.

Patricia Evridge Hill

HENRY ERNEST SIGERIST
(1891–1957)

Henry Ernest Sigerist, the medical historian who established the history of medicine as an academic discipline in the United States and pioneered the social history of medicine, was born in Paris, France, on April 7, 1891. His father, Ernst Heinrich Sigerist, a native of Schaffhausen, Switzerland, was a shoe merchant in Paris, and his mother, Emma Wiskemann Sigerist, was a native of Zurich. Henry was the eldest of their two children. When Sigerist was ten years old, his father became mortally ill, and the family moved to Zurich. In 1916 Sigerist married Emmy M. Escher of Zurich. They had two daughters, Erica Elizabeth (Campanella) and Nora Beate (Beeson).

After beginning his education in Paris at the Cours Delarbre (1897–1901), the move to Zurich introduced Sigerist to the German-speaking world in the Von Beust'sche Privatschule (1901–1904) and the Literargymnasium (1904–1910), a public school that emphasized studies in Greek and Latin. In 1910 he matriculated at the University of Zurich as a student of Oriental philology, studying Arabic, Hebrew, and Sanskrit, and in 1911 he studied Chinese at University College, London. During his lifetime, he learned fourteen languages, half of which he spoke fluently. He was also greatly interested in science, and for a career decided to study medicine, which he felt embraced the broadest scientific range. He obtained his M.D. degree from the University of Zurich in 1917. Between 1912 and 1922 he served periodically in the Medical Corps of the Swiss Army, an experience with ordinary people that strongly influenced his subsequent interest in the social history of medicine.

In the summer of 1914, while visiting Venice as a temporary escape from clinical studies at the University of Munich, he decided to combine all his interests by studying the history of medicine. Seeking advice, he contacted Dr. Karl Sudhoff, an eminent medical historian who was the director of the Institute for the History of Medicine at the University of Leipzig. The institute had the only graduate department in the history of medicine at that time. After the war, in December 1919 Sigerist traveled to Leipzig and spent several months as Sudhoff's student, conducting philological studies of medical manuscripts of the early Middle Ages.

Returning to Zurich, Sigerist began to explore Swiss medico-historical source material and in 1923 published his first book, *Studien und Texte zur frühmittelalterlichen Rezeptliteratur* (Studies and texts for the early medieval prescription literature), which he had written as his *Habilitations-schrift* (qualifying essay) to become a *Privatdozent* (unsalaried lecturer) at the University of Zurich in 1921. In 1924 he became titular professor, but as titulary or nominal professor he had no prescribed duties or responsibilities. In 1910, Sigerist began to publish articles and reviews in *Neue Zürcher Zeitung* (New Zurich Newspaper). In 1923 he published a critical edition of the 549 Latin letters in the Zurich Zentralbibliothek (Zurich Central Library) that Albrecht von Haller had written to his lifelong friend Johannes Gesner, as well as a German translation of Ambroise Paré's treatise on gunshot wounds that was published in Sudhoff's *Klassiker der Medizin* (Classics of Medicine) series. He also initiated *Monumenta Medica* (Medical Monuments), a series of facsimiles of historical medical books. With his friend Charles Singer, he prepared a festschrift for Sudhoff's seventieth birthday in 1923.

In 1925 when Sudhoff retired from his Leipzig chair, Sigerist was appointed to succeed him. Between 1925 and 1932, Sigerist filled the Leipzig Institute with his dynamic energy. A brilliant, friendly lecturer who spoke with graceful gestures, he attracted both medical students and the public to medical history. Among his Leipzig students were Erwin H. Ackerknecht, Owsei Temkin, and Walter Pagel, all of whom became eminent medical historians.

Believing that knowledge of the history of medicine was essential to the education of all physicians and public health personnel, Sigerist began to write general works: *Einführung in die Medizin* (1931), which was translated into six languages (Man and Medicine: An Introduction to Medical Knowledge, 1932), and *Grosse Aerzte*, 1932 (Great Doctors, 1933), which contained sixty medical biographies intended to interpret the evolution of modern medicine. Residing in post–World War I Germany and observing the effects of poverty and the problems of providing medical care led to Sigerist's intense interest in the relationship between medicine and the social environment. His history of American medicine (*Amerika und die Medizin*, 1933; *American Medicine*, 1934) dealt with the social history of medicine, which became one of the main themes of all his projects, including trips to the Soviet Union in the summers of 1935, 1936, and 1938 to study Soviet medicine (*Socialized Medicine in the Soviet Union*, 1937).

In 1931 Sigerist was invited by Dr. William H. Welch, director of the new Johns Hopkins Institute of the History of Medicine in Baltimore, Maryland, to give a series of lectures, which were followed by a lecture tour in the United States. Sigerist was so successful that he was invited to become Welch's successor as professor of the history of medicine at the Johns Hopkins School of Medicine and director of the institute. Inspired by the American medical environment and deeply concerned about the rising popularity of Hitler's Nazi beliefs, Sigerist accepted the Hopkins position and moved to Baltimore in 1932.

Sigerist immediately began what he regarded as his basic tasks: to professionalize the history of medicine in America and to change attitudes concerning the provision of medical care. Although much had been published by American physicians interested in history, Sigerist considered their work amateurish. In a friendly, inoffensive way he tried to raise the professional level of the history of medicine, teaching by example rather than with criticism. In addition to bringing Owsei Temkin, his former Leipzig student and colleague, and Ludwig Edelstein, a Berlin classicist, and Erwin H. Ackerknecht to teach in the Hopkins Institute, he invited numerous European scholars to give lectures and created Graduate Weeks in Medical History, which were attended by physicians, librarians, and others who were interested in medical history. He also created the *Bulletin of the History of Medicine* (1933) and gradually reorganized the American Association for the History of Medicine.

As Sigerist successfully made the Hopkins Institute the mecca for medico-historical activities in the United States, his interest in the social history of medicine shifted his focus from the past to the present. Since he was an advocate of socialized medicine, the rumor that he was a communist began to spread in the medical community. He never succeeded in persuading critics that he was not a member of any political party but a historian studying sociological aspects of medicine. So that others could learn from the Soviet medical experience, in 1943 he helped create the Soviet-American Medical Society and became the first editor of the *American Review of Soviet Medicine*. In the same year he became a U.S. citizen.

His 1938 Terry Lectures at Yale (*Medicine and Human Welfare*, 1941) and his 1940 Messenger Lectures at Cornell (*Civilization and Disease*, 1943) discussed the connections between disease and the social, economic, and cultural aspects of society. At Hopkins he taught courses on medical economics and sociology to students of the School of Medicine and the School of Hygiene and Public Health. He received international recognition for this expertise in 1944, when he was called as medical planning consultant to the Canadian province of Saskatchewan and to India.

During World War II, Sigerist's duties increased enormously as faculty members became engaged in wartime functions. He was named acting director of the Welch Medical Library and went to Washington one day a week as a consultant to the Board of Economic Warfare; in November 1943 he was relieved of this position when the Civil Service Commission declared him unfit for government service because of his activities in so-called communist-front organizations. After the war ended, in poor health and depressed because his plans to write comprehensive works on the history and sociology of medicine were constantly being thwarted by administrative duties, Sigerist decided to resign from Hopkins and return to Switzerland. In the summer of 1947 he settled near Pura, a village overlooking Lake Lugano, and began his projected eight-volume social history of medicine. At the time he held the title of research associate (professorial rank) at Yale University. In 1945 he rejected the leadership of an institute at the University of London, and later he turned down chairs at Jena, Zurich, Berlin, and Leipzig.

Unfortunately his cardiovascular disease progressed, and Sigerist was able to complete only one volume of his *History of Medicine* and part of a second (Vol. 1: *Primitive and Archaic Medicine*, 1951; Vol. 2: *Early Greek, Hindu, and Persian Medicine*, 1961). In 1952 he gave the Heath Clark Lectures at the University of London (*Landmarks in the History of Hygiene*, 1956), and in 1954 he attended the International Congress of the History of Medicine in Rome and Salerno. He died from a cerebral hemorrhage two and a half years later.

Recognized throughout his life for his many talents, Henry Sigerist was elected to membership and received awards from many European, South American, and North American societies, including the American Philosophical Society. He received honorary doctorates from the University of Madrid (1935), University of the Witwatersrand, Johannesburg, South Africa (1939), Queen's University, Kingston, Ontario (1941), and the University of London (1953). Henry Sigerist was the leading medical historian of his generation who introduced graduate studies in medical history to the United States, promoted the social history of medicine, and sought to make medical history an integral part of American medical education.

BIBLIOGRAPHY

The major sources of archival material relating to Henry E. Sigerist are the Historical Library of Yale Medical School, the Alan Mason Chesney Archives of Johns Hopkins Medical Institutions, the Karl Sudhoff Institute of the University of Leipzig, and the University Archives of Zurich. Additional materials are in the possession of his nephew, Dr. Marcel H. Bickel of Bern, Switzerland, and his daughter, Nora Sigerist Beeson of New York. The Henry E. Sigerist Valedictory Number of the *Bulletin of the History of Medicine* (1948, 22: 1–93) contains a complete bibliography of publications of the Johns Hopkins Institute during Sigerist's tenure. After his death, the *Journal of the History of Medicine and Allied Sciences* (1958, 13: 125–250) commemorated him. Intense interest in Henry E. Sigerist's ideas has stimulated a number of publications in recent years in both Europe and America. These include a colloquium at Leipzig in 1991 (see Hahn and Thom 1991) and four doctoral dissertations at Cologne, Zurich, Leipzig, and Stanford universities (Elisabeth Berg-Schorn 1978; Marianne Christine Wäspi 1989; H. Wissel 1968; and Fernando G. Vescia 1975). A group called the Sigerist Circle meets annually with the American Association for the History of Medicine to discuss sociological aspects of medicine. Its biannual *Newsletter* includes a bibliography of current publications. Extremely useful published information includes *Henry E. Sigerist: Autobiographical Writings*, selected and translated by Nora Sigerist Beeson (1966), and *A Bibliography of the Writings of Henry E. Sigerist*, edited by Genevieve Miller (1966).

Writings by Henry Ernest Sigerist

Man and Medicine. An Introduction to Medical Knowledge. Introduction by William H. Welch. New York: W. W. Norton, 1932.

Great Doctors. A Biographical History of Medicine. New York: W. W. Norton, 1933. 2d ed., Garden City, NY: Doubleday, 1958.

American Medicine. New York: W. W. Norton, 1934.

Socialized Medicine in the Soviet Union. New York: W. W. Norton, 1937. Rev. ed., *Medicine and Health in the Soviet Union*. With the cooperation of Julia Older. New York: Citadel Press, 1947.

Medicine and Human Welfare. New Haven, CT: Yale University Press, 1941.

Civilization and Disease. Ithaca, NY: Cornell University Press, 1943.
The University at the Crossroads: Addresses and Essays. New York: Henry Schuman, 1946.
A History of Medicine, vol. 1: *Primitive and Archaic Medicine.* New York: Oxford University Press, 1951.
Landmarks in the History of Hygiene. London: Geoffrey Cumberlege, Oxford University Press, 1956.
On the History of Medicine. Edited by Felix Marti-Ibañez. New York: MD Publications, 1960.
On the Sociology of Medicine. Edited by Milton I. Roemer. New York: MD Publications, 1960.
A History of Medicine, vol. 2: *Early Greek, Hindu, and Persian Medicine.* New York: Oxford University Press, 1961.

Writings about Henry Ernest Sigerist and Related Topics

Beeson, Nora Sigerist, ed. *Henry E. Sigerist: Autobiographical Writings.* Montreal: McGill University Press, 1966.

Berg-Schorn, Elisabeth. *Henry E. Sigerist (1891–1957), Medizinhistoriker in Leipzig und Baltimore, Standpunkt und Wirkung. Arbeiten der Forschungsstelle des Instituts für Geschichte der Medizin der Universität zu Köln,* vol. 9 (Medical historian in Leipzig and Baltimore, point of view and effect: Works of the Research Center of the Institute for the History of Medicine of the University of Cologne). Cologne, 1978.

Fee, Elizabeth, and Theodore M. Brown, eds. *Making Medical History: The Life and Times of Henry E. Sigerist.* Baltimore: Johns Hopkins University Press, 1997.

Hahn, Susanne, and Achim Thom, eds. *Ergebnisse und Perspektiven sozialhistorischer Forschung in der Medizingeschichte* (Results and prospects of social history investigation in the history of medicine). Leipzig: Karl-Sudhoff-Institut, 1991. (The product of a colloquium held at Leipzig in 1991 to celebrate Sigerist's one hundredth birthday. It includes an extremely useful bibliography of books and articles about Sigerist.)

Miller, Genevieve, ed. *A Bibliography of the Writings of Henry E. Sigerist.* Montreal: McGill University Press, 1966. (Contains detailed data concerning Sigerist's society affiliations and so forth.)

Terris, Milton. "The Contributions of Henry E. Sigerist to Health Service Organization." *Milbank Memorial Fund Quarterly* 53 (1975): 489–530. (Milton was a student of Sigerist.)

Vescia, F. G. *Henry E. Sigerist: The Years at Hopkins (1932–1947).* Palo Alto, CA, 1975.

Wissel, H. "Das Werk Henry E. Sigerists—Höhepunkt der bürgerlichen Medizingeschichtsschreibung" (The work of Henry E. Sigerist—The high point of civil medical history writing). Phil. diss., Leipzig University.

Genevieve Miller

JAMES MARION SIMS
(1813–1883)

James Marion Sims was one of a handful of physicians responsible for the definition and establishment of the modern profession of gynecology. His life spanned the nineteenth century and embodied many of the century's central themes in the United States, such as the rise of professionalism, the emergence of modern medicine, the end of slavery and the Civil War, Victorian culture, and newly defined roles for women and men.

J. Marion Sims was born in Hanging Rock, South Carolina (the Lancaster district), on January 25, 1813. He was the oldest of eight children and came from Scotch-Irish ancestry. His parents were of middling income, so Sims grew up in the antebellum South in a family with a few slaves. His mother was able to read and write, but his father was illiterate.

Being the oldest was important because his parents urged him in particular to obtain an education. As a youth, he went to the Franklin Academy near his home, where he first met Theresa Jones, the woman who later became his wife. Searching for a career after graduating from South Carolina College at Columbia in 1832, Sims decided to become a physician. His mother died within two months of his graduation, so he answered to his father alone for his commitment to a career. Sims's recollection of his father's dissatisfaction with his career choice is frequently cited today as an example of the low reputation of physicians in the first half of the nineteenth century. His father was shocked that his son would go to college to become one of those who traveled "from house to house through this country, with a box of pills in one hand and a squirt [syringe] in the other" (Sims 1884: 116). Sims stood his ground and attended Charleston Medical College in Charleston, South Carolina, in late 1833 and early 1834. Instead of completing his degree there, he moved to Philadelphia, where he studied from October 1834 through March 1835 at Jefferson Medical College. Jefferson was a new medical school and quickly gained a reputation for excellence. One of Sims's chief mentors was George McClellan, a surgeon. Although Sims graduated with a general degree in the practice of medicine, he eventually emulated McClellan and became a surgeon. Between and after his studies he returned to the small town of Lancasterville, South Carolina, where his family and friends lived, to study under a preceptor and to gain experience practicing medicine on his own.

After his formal education, Sims's career paralleled that of many other young physicians of his time in that he learned more from his mistakes and mentor relationships with physicians than he had in college, and his patients included a few casualties along the way. Sims moved from one place to another before becoming established in his career. In 1835 he moved from South Carolina to the so-called black belt of rural Alabama to serve as a plantation physician. After a long negotiation between Sims and her mother, Theresa Jones married him in 1836, and they lived together in Mt. Meigs, where they had two children, before moving to the relatively settled town of Montgomery in 1841. Alabama was frontier country, and the Deep South suffered epidemics of various diseases. While living there, Sims contracted malaria and a form of dysentery that threatened his life off and on for several years and took the life of one of his children.

After his move to Montgomery, Sims's practice began to change as his clientele broadened and his surgical expertise increased, eventually becoming a specialization in gynecological surgery. He established at least two clinics and did surgeries on conditions ranging from tumors of the jaw to harelip and trismus nascentium in newborn infants. Sims laid the foundation for his career when he perfected a surgical remedy for vesicovaginal fistula, a condition appearing in women after giving birth. Women who incurred the disability almost always experienced a prolonged labor during which the fetal head pressed against the pelvic floor, robbing it of oxygen for many hours. Within a few days of the delivery, these same women sloughed dead tissue from the vagina and began to suffer incontinence (sometimes rectal tears were also involved). The condition was seldom life threatening, but it did result in discomfort and often isolation for the victim. Although many physicians and surgeons had attempted to find a surgical cure, none had been successful. Today such fistulae are uncommon in developed countries, except as the results of surgery, but in the nineteenth century these tears between the vagina and the bladder were fairly prevalent.

Sims reported in his autobiography that slaveholders begged him to attempt a surgical remedy (Sims 1884: 231). Even though he did not have an expertise in the delivery of infants or female complaints, his surgical skills were remarkable. Sims therefore began to treat what we now describe as gynecological disorders with experimental surgery. He set up a small hospital where he kept several slave women. From 1845 to 1849, Sims repeatedly operated (without anesthesia) on these women, trying different techniques to close their vesicovaginal fistula and render them productive (and reproductive) once again. Three of these women, Anarcha, Betsy, and Lucy, remained with Sims for the duration of his experiments. In 1849 Anarcha's surgery was successful and healed well. What Sims thought pivotal for his success was the use of silver sutures instead of silk or other types of metallic sutures. He also devised a sigmoid catheter to drain the area after surgery. Sims now declared that he had created a cure for vesicovaginal fistula. With this achievement, Sims eventually made his name among elite physicians in the Western world and helped to define gynecology as an area of surgical expertise.

As Sims recalled his life in his autobiography, his health failed drastically just as he perfected the surgery. Seeking a cure, he moved from one place to another, until he came to rest up North. First he lived in Philadelphia for a short while, where he wrote an article describing his surgical technique for correcting vesicovaginal fistula. His article in the *American Journal of the Medical Sciences* informed a national audience of his medical prowess. Sims next went to New York City and decided to establish a practice there because of his belief that the city's Croton water had saved his life.

After several years of struggling to gain recognition and acceptance among the powerful and elite New York physicians, Sims won the support of Sarah Doremus and other philanthropic reform-minded women, who helped establish a hospital where Sims could practice surgery. Several prominent physicians also joined in support of the institution, including Valentine Mott, Fordyce Baker, John W. Francis, and Alexander Stephens. Sims had impressed them with his surgical abilities and the significance of his novel methods. As a result, the Woman's Hospital of the State of New York opened in 1855; it was the first hospital in the United States specifically devoted to the treatment of women. The State of New York granted a charter for the institution in 1855, and the Woman's Hospital Association, with a female board of managers, supervised the hospital until the opening of a new building in 1868 forced reorganization and the addition of an all-male board of governors. The female administrators continued to have some voice, but by the middle of the next decade their authority had greatly lessened.

At the Woman's Hospital, Sims continued to operate for vesicovaginal fistula. His hospital served a wide range of patients, with roughly 45 percent of them Irish immigrant women. The hospital operated on a type of sliding scale with arrangements for patients of means as well as charity patients. Sims appointed Thomas A. Emmet, a younger physician with considerable experience in managing childbirth, as his assistant. Working together from 1855 until 1860, they expanded their range of gynecological surgeries. Emmet became a renowned surgeon in his own right. In fact, the hospital became a kind of workshop for surgical gynecology, with many physicians observing surgeries to learn technique.

The coming of the Civil War provided the backdrop for the early history of the hospital and Sims's New York success. In 1858 Sims delivered a renowned honorary address before the New York Academy of Medicine called "Silver Sutures" in which he described the development of his surgical technique and alluded to this therapy as a possible way to bring the North and South back together. In the late 1850s Sims visited England and France, ostensibly to research architectural alternatives for the new hospital, but also out of a kind of restlessness. After the outbreak of the war in 1861, Sims left the United States again. He felt he could no longer fit into either northern or southern society. Abroad as a southerner with French connections, the State Department took him under surveillance. In 1862 his wife and seven children came to Paris, where they lived until the 1870s.

During Sims's preliminary trips to Europe, he met many famous physicians. He demonstrated his technique before James Y. Simpson, Alfred Velpeau, and Jobert de Lamballe and was courted by royalty for his medical abilities. Thus, Sims left a hospital in New York, where he had developed gynecological surgeries, often practicing on women of little means, to take up a European practice in which he served princesses and women of the upper classes. In fact he moved from treating disorders resulting from childbirth to treating sterility and what is now called frigidity. While in Europe, he wrote a textbook for medical students. This book, *Clinical Notes on Uterine Surgery* (1866), appeared in installments in the British medical journal *Lancet*. Although there was a fair amount of discord in response to Sims's descriptions of his surgeries, particularly cervical incisions, the textbook was a success and ultimately was translated into several languages.

During his stay in Paris, Sims helped to create the Anglo-American Ambulance Corps in which he served as surgeon in chief during the Franco-Prussian War. He was decorated by the governments of France, Italy, Spain, Portugal, and Italy for his medical service. Leopold I, king of Belgium, sought to knight Sims but was thwarted by the U.S. government because of Sims's pro-southern sentiment until 1880, when Sims finally received this honor.

When Sims returned to the United States after the war years, he frequently encountered conflict. In 1869 the Ethics Committee of the New York Medical Society censored him for public statements he made concerning surgery for breast cancer on Charlotte Cushman, a popular actress. Among physicians at the time, speaking publicly about a patient's breast removal was not acceptable behavior, and Sims was not even Cushman's physician. Trouble also brewed at the Woman's Hospital. After the governing board determined that Sims's absence in the 1860s was going to be lengthy, they named Emmet as chief surgeon. In 1872 they created a medical board, which named four surgeons as surgeons in chief. Sims shared the position with Emmet, E. R. Peaslee, and T. Gaillard Thomas, all of whom were or became gynecologists of high repute. The development of the Woman's Hospital as a learning center for the medical specialty continued.

The Board of Lady Supervisors (as the women governors were now called) objected to the large audiences in attendance at surgeries and the public exposure of patients to physician spectators. Furthermore, they watched with concern in the 1870s as the new hospital (now in the Wetmore Pavilion) witnessed more major surgeries. Previously, few of the hospital's patients had died, but now Sims and his colleagues began to practice abdominal surgeries in which the risk of death was quite high. The introduction of anesthesia and antisepsis made abdominal surgery more feasible than before but still uncertain in outcome. Sims was eager to treat many different female conditions, including cancer. The women administrators, the Medical Board, and the board of governors objected to Sims's particularly large audiences and the hospitalization and treatment of cancer patients. There was also controversy between Sims and his colleagues about his use of what was known as "normal ovariotomy" (as devised by Robert Battey): the removal of healthy ovaries in patients diagnosed with various conditions, such as mental imbalance or epilepsy. Sims felt that he alone should determine the parameters of his conduct and practice, and he resigned from the Woman's Hospital in 1874. Although he sought to be reinstated, not until 1881 did he again become a practicing physician at the hospital originally established for him.

Despite Sims's mixed reception at the Woman's Hospital and among some medical practitioners, he won many professional honors. He was president of the American Medical Association in 1875. In 1876, Sims, Emmet, and Thomas were founding members of the American Gynecological Society (AGS). In 1880 he was named president of the AGS. Sims died in New York City in 1884. Memorials stand to his life in Columbia, South Carolina; Montgomery, Alabama; and near the New York Academy of Medicine in Central Park, New York City.

J. Marion Sims built his medical career on the surgical treatment of women. In doing so, he helped many women to recover from damage caused by childbirth. Today we also recognize his treatment of cancer victims as well founded. At the same time, however, he exploited certain groups of women by conducting repeated experimental surgeries on them without the benefits of anesthesia and when they were held in bondage, or sometimes simply in poverty. He also typified Victorian standards by bypassing the authority of the woman patient altogether and deciding for her what was in her best interest. Although he helped some women out of the misery of incontinence and treated several disorders of the female reproductive system successfully, he victimized others with heroic efforts at impregnation and mechanical surgeries to remedy conditions that were later recognized as pathologies of the endocrine system. His long history of radical experimentation leaves a mixed legacy. Certainly he contributed significantly to the creation of gynecology as a medical specialty.

BIBLIOGRAPHY

Archival material and published sources pertinent to the life and career of J. Marion Sims are rich and abundant. Sims published extensively during his lifetime as both a physician and a chronicler of his own life. In addition there are annual reports from the Woman's Hospital. Unlike Sims, Thomas A. Emmet kept meticulous records; his publications include *Vesico-Vaginal Fistula* (1868), which describes cases of vesicovaginal fistula that he and Sims treated at the Woman's Hospital in the 1850s and 1860s. T. Gaillard Thomas and E. R. Peaslee also published extensively. The library and special collections of St. Luke's Hospital in New York City hold many original documents from the Woman's Hospital, including case records from the 1850s, records of the Woman's Hospital Association, and notes from the women governors, photographs, annual reports of the institution, and various pamphlets and materials from earlier historians of the institution, particularly James Pratt Marr. Other records can be found at the New York Academy of Medicine, the New-York Historical Society, the Philadelphia College of Physicians and Surgeons, Jefferson Medical College, and the University of Alabama Reynolds Library Special Collections.

Writings by James Marion Sims

Clinical Notes on Uterine Surgery. New York: Wm. Wood & Co., 1866.

The Story of My Life. New York: D. Appleton & Co., 1884. Reprint ed., New York: DeCapo Press, 1968.

Silver Sutures in Surgery: The Anniversary Discourse before the New York Academy of Medicine. New York: Samuel S. & Wm. Wood, 1858.

"On the Treatment of Vesico-Vaginal Fistula." *American Journal of the Medical Sciences* 45 (January 1852): 59–82. Reprinted in *Medical Classics* 2 (1938): 677–712.

Writings about James Marion Sims and Related Topics

Barker-Benfield, Ben. *The Horrors of the Half-Known Life: Male Attitudes toward Women and Sexuality in Nineteenth Century America.* New York: Harper & Row, 1976.

Emmet, Thomas A. *Vesico-Vaginal Fistula from Parturition and Other Causes.* New York: Wm. Wood & Co., 1868.

Harris, Seale. *Woman's Surgeon: The Life Story of J. Marion Sims.* New York: Macmillan, 1950.

Hartman, Mary S., and Lois Banner, eds. *Clio's Consciousness Raised: New Perspectives on the History of Women.* New York: Octagon Books, 1976.

Kaiser, Irwin H. "Reappraisals of J. Marion Sims." *American Journal of Obstetrics and Gynecology* 132 (December 1978): 307–310.

McGregor, Deborah Kuhn. *Sexual Surgery and the Origins of Gynecology: J. Marion Sims, His Hospital and His Patients.* New York: Garland, 1990.

Marr, James Pratt. *Pioneer Surgeons of the Woman's Hospital.* New York: F. A. Davis Co., 1957.

Russett, Cynthia Eagle. *Sexual Science: The Victorian Construction of Womanhood.* Cambridge, MA: Harvard University Press, 1989.

Deborah Kuhn McGregor

THEOBALD SMITH
(1859–1934)

Theobald Smith, medical doctor and comparative pathologist, helped to introduce the germ theory of disease and practical microbiology into American agriculture, sanitation, and medicine. The germ theory of disease arguably
demarcates the beginning of modern times more than any other idea. Its applications in medicine and sanitation made health a more achievable goal, and
ultimately created the twentieth century's unique achievement: the dramatic rise
in human life expectancy. Certainly it influenced all subsequent aims and
achievements. Louis Pasteur, Robert Koch, and Joseph Lister were the illuminati
of germ theory; no American matched their stature. Yet Theobald Smith, the
son of German immigrants to New York, conducted a fundamental study of
insect-vectored disease, organized one of the first bacteriology departments at
an American medical school, differentiated the human and bovine tubercle bacilli, and ran pioneering pathological laboratories in Washington, Boston, and
New York. In nearly 300 publications, he unraveled mysteries of infectious
agents and host immunity, and applied that knowledge to clinical practice.

Theresa Kexel Schmitt gave birth to her second child and only son in Albany,
New York, on July 31, 1859. She and her husband, Phillip, named the baby
after a friend, Jacob Theobald, and anglicized their surname to Smith. The boy's
schooling began at a German-speaking academy and continued at the Albany
Free Academy, from which he graduated as class valedictorian in 1876. Theobald Smith entered Cornell University on a scholarship the following year, and
after graduating in 1881, completed a two-year M.D. course at the Albany Medical School. He intended to pursue a second degree at Cornell with his undergraduate mentor, microscopist Simon Gage, but instead, with Gage's urging and
help, he took a position with the U.S. Department of Agriculture's newly established Veterinary Division in Washington, under Daniel Salmon (D.V.M.,
Cornell, 1876). In 1884, Congress redesignated Salmon's division the Bureau
of Animal Industry (BAI) and charged it with controlling several epizootics that
had devastated livestock growers since the Civil War. Smith's professional career began in 1884 as he took charge of the BAI's Pathological Laboratory at
the Benning Veterinary Experiment Station in the District of Columbia. For the
next eleven years, his work focused on two major livestock diseases: "swine
plague" and "Texas" cattle fever.

Because the humoral theory of disease, the prevailing medical philosophy at
the time, placed so much emphasis on blood, various maladies of pigs exhibiting
septicemia tended to be lumped together as "swine plague." In 1878, Koch
isolated a bacillus responsible for septicemia in mice during his research on
anthrax, raising the possibility that this also caused plague in pigs. However, a

few years later, Pasteur discovered another organism associated with hemorrhagic septicemia in pigs. Gram's stain, developed in 1884, confirmed that the pathogens were distinct. But Smith's research turned up yet another suspect: a bacillus that was motile and Gram negative like Pasteur's, but with a flagellum that Pasteur had not seen. To determine if this was simply a different strain, Smith ordered vaccine from Pasteur's laboratory and used it to immunize two healthy pigs. He then exposed those animals to others already sick with plague; soon they all died. These results suggested that not only had he discovered a new organism, but that it probably caused the extremely deadly swine disease American farmers called hog cholera. With that in mind, Smith named the pathogen *Bacillus choleraesuis*.

The etiology of swine plague quickly became a trilateral dispute between researchers in Germany, France, and the United States, with several opposing camps in each country. Later it was shown that Pasteur had been correct: the microbe he discovered, eventually named *Pasteurella multocida*, caused swine plague (pneumonic pasteurellosis). Koch's organism, *Erysipelothrix rhusiopathiae*, was responsible for another acute septicemia named swine erysipelas, and Smith's germ, renamed *Salmonella choleraesuis*, often appeared as an opportunistic infection (Salmonellosis) in swine already suffering from hog cholera but was not itself the cause of the deadlier disease. Not until 1905 did BAI researchers demonstrate that hog cholera arose from a filterable virus, which was unknown as a pathogenic class until 1892. If Smith suffered any embarrassment in this controversy, he recovered quickly, and the research taught him useful lessons about producing pure cultures, testing killed bacillus vaccines, sorting out etiologies, and learning the means of transmission, all of which served him well as he turned to an equally enigmatic disease, "Texas" cattle fever.

The name *Texas fever* stirred confusion. Unlike "swine plague," which was several diseases passing as one, "Texas fever" was one disease that had been known variously as Carolina distemper, Georgia murrain, and Spanish fever (implying Florida) for about two hundred years. Farmers had long suspected ticks, as either a cause or a result of the sickness, though that opinion did not stand up well against the observation that tick-infested southern cattle did not suffer from the disease. The trouble appeared among northern cattle only after they had come into contact with animals from the South. Before germ theory, no one could have known that a protozoan was the pathogenic agent that ticks spread from cow to cow, or that southern calves developed passive immunity from their mothers' milk until their own antibodies provided protection. Farmers realized that colder winters in the North killed the ticks, but that seemed largely irrelevant.

In 1889, Smith began examining the spleens of cattle that had died of the fever. He could see that, whatever the cause, the animals' red blood cells appeared severely damaged. To test the possibility that ticks might be involved, he set up a trial using three fenced fields, with a few head of insect-infested southern cattle and some healthy northern animals in the first, and a similar mix in the second, but with all the ticks removed before exposing one group to the other. Shortly, the northern stock in field 1 became covered with ticks and died; those in the second remained healthy. On the third field, where no cattle had grazed, he sowed ticks over the grass and then drove in the northern survivors from field 2. Again, the vulnerable animals got sick and died. He repeated these experiments and others over the next three summers, using cows and calves, feeding some stock minced ticks to see if ingestion was the means of transmission, studying the life cycle of the insect, and examining the red blood cells of the healthy and the diseased cattle. He observed the protozoan culprit, *Babesia bigemina*, in the first summer of these trials, but it took subsequent clues to put together a complete picture. In 1893, he and his collaborator, F. L. Kilbourne, published the results as a BAI report, *Investigations into the Nature, Causation, and Prevention of Texas or Southern Cattle Fever*. It completely explained the etiology and epidemiology, pathogenesis, clinical findings, diagnosis, and treatment, and, as such, it was the first correct assessment of any disease by American researchers. This was not, however, the original observation that an insect might be implicated in the transmission of disease. A decade before Smith's work, English physician Patrick Manson, found that mosquitoes spread the filarial worms that cause human elephantiasis, and it was Manson's investigations that led Ronald Ross to understand the mosquito-borne transmission of malaria in 1897. Still, Smith's accomplishment did more than identify a vector; he demonstrated the complex relationship between a parasite and its host's immune response, a point that he would build upon again and again.

While working for the BAI, Smith also set up a bacteriology division at the National Medical College (now the medical school of George Washington University) and taught there from 1886 until 1895. The first bacteriology course, at Harvard's Medical School, preceded Smith's by only one year. Apparently Koch's discovery of the cholera bacillus and his demonstration of how cholera spread through drinking water prompted Smith's 1887 study of Washington, D.C.'s water supply (the Potomac River) and his later examination (1893) of the Hudson River for the New York Health Department, using a coliform assay to detect pollution. This work, possibly more than his veterinary research, led to the next phase of his career.

Controversy over the hog cholera findings may have weighed in Smith's decision to leave the BAI in 1895, though Salmon's overarching ego could have had something to do with it as well. If Smith felt some dissatisfaction earlier, his happy marriage to Lilian Hillyer Egleston in 1888 and the birth of two daughters in Washington (their third child, a son, was born later) probably postponed any thoughts of moving. With a rising reputation, though, enticements came, and when the Massachusetts Board of Health offered him a position as director of the state Antitoxin and Vaccine Laboratory, with a concurrent professorship of comparative pathology at Harvard Medical School, he jumped at the chance. Though he was an M.D. who never relished practicing medicine, the opportunity to move into the public health field was attractive; Emile Roux had just developed the method for making diphtheria antitoxin, and Koch seemed on the verge of producing a vaccine against tuberculosis. It was at this time too that Smith met William Henry Welch, recently returned from studies with Koch and newly appointed as dean of the Johns Hopkins Medical School— on his way to becoming the most influential medical administrator in the nation. Welch chaired a committee of the American Public Health Association that developed standard methods of water analysis; Smith served as a member, bringing his experience in analyzing coliforms in the Potomac and Hudson rivers. This contact with Welch eventually opened the third phase of Smith's career, but, while in Boston Smith focused on diphtheria and tuberculosis.

Diphtheria, an acute contagious disease, became increasingly troublesome in the later nineteenth century, as more and more children attended consolidated schools, creating susceptible pools for epidemics. Frederich Löffler and Edwin Klebs discovered the responsible pathogen, *Corynebacterium diphtheriae*, in 1883, and a few years later Löffler showed that the bacillus actually produced an exotoxin that caused the clinical symptoms of sore throat, cough, fever, and, often, death within a week. Emil von Behring proved the existence of a serum antitoxin in 1890, which opened the way for producing an effective treatment. In 1894, the New York City Health Department was first in the United States to produce diphtheria antitoxin in the laboratory headed by William H. Park. Smith's laboratory, like Park's, offered physicians diagnostic kits to detect the disease, and antitoxin when they found it. Boston, the first city to have medical inspectors for its schools (1894), soon dramatically cut into diphtheria's mortality.

While the laboratory mostly served as a production and testing facility, Smith studied the nature of diphtheria, observing a type of anaphylaxis and noting, as others had, that a mixture of diphtheria toxin and antitoxin produced active immunity in laboratory animals. Nearly thirty years later, Leon Ramon demonstrated that formaldehyde-treated diphtheria toxin created a "toxoid" that could prevent the disease. Perhaps Smith missed this finding because he devoted more attention to keeping diphtheria bacilli alive so he could study their variations than to figuring out ways to check them. But if so, the same strategy contributed to his most important scientific finding: that two distinct species of tubercle bacilli existed in mammals.

In 1896, Smith tentatively proposed the hypothesis that a more virulent and invasive tubercle organism existed in cattle than the faster-growing type found in human lung lesions. (It was already known that birds contracted a third form.) Yet nearly all bacteriologists who knew about tuberculosis, and most notably Robert Koch, supposed that variation existed because of the parasite's adaptation to different host species. Further, the tuberculin test that Koch developed in 1890 could be used on people or cattle. When Smith visited Koch in Berlin in 1896, he proposed that the bovine and human forms seemed to be two distinct species, but Koch rejected that view. Smith returned home, continued experiments, and published a more definitive statement in 1898, "A Comparative Study of Bovine Tubercle Bacilli and of Human Bacilli from Sputum." The controversy continued for several years. Koch reversed his position in 1903 and later credited Smith for the original finding. In time, researchers showed that the bovine tubercle bacillus, transmitted through raw milk, caused the humpback deformity in humans.

In 1901, William Welch, who had become the chief scientific adviser to John D. Rockefeller, invited Smith to organize and head the pathology laboratories in New York City of the newly created Rockefeller Institute for Medical Research. Smith declined, saying that Harvard still offered exceptional opportunities, but he agreed to serve on the institute's board of scientific directors (which Welch chaired from 1901 to 1933). The position went to Simon Flexner, who, quite admirably, concentrated on viral pathogens. When the Rockefeller Foundation made an additional gift to the institute in 1914, to enlarge its research facilities with pathological laboratories in Princeton, New Jersey, Flexner asked Smith to head this new department. It was an extraordinary opportunity that not even Harvard could match, and Smith accepted, moving his family in 1915.

Designing and building the laboratories took nearly two years, and at that point the United States entered World War I. For several months, the Princeton unit mainly made diphtheria and tetanus antitoxin, though Smith found some time to return to a research project he had started in 1894: an investigation of the protozoal disease of turkeys called infectious enterohepatitis, or blackhead. Apparently, though, this was something of a refresher course, as he soon turned to another unicellular pathogen, *Cystiosospora*, responsible for coccidiosis in calves, and transmissible to people. Among his findings was the observation that colostrum, the first milk secreted after birth, provided passive immunity to newborn calves. This, of course, further explained calf immunity to Texas cattle fever as well. After the war, Smith explored yet another major disease of both cattle and humans, brucellosis, trying unsuccessfully to develop a vaccine from weakened *Brucella abortus*. He continued studies of contagious abortion until the end of his career.

At age seventy, Smith retired from active research, though he held an emeritus position and succeeded Welch as president of the Rockefeller Institute's board of scientific directors in 1933. His last and as it turned out his most lasting publication, *Parasitism and Disease* (1934), delineated the lifelong theme of his work: an exploration of the complex relationship between host and pathogen.

Smith received numerous honors and awards: a dozen honorary degrees from European and American universities and the presidency of the Society of American Bacteriologists, the National Tuberculosis Association, and the Congress of Physicians and Surgeons. He received medals and invitations to deliver most of the distinguished lectures in medicine. A self-effacing and reticent man by all accounts, Smith took more joy in the pleasures of discovery than the accolades for his enormous achievements. He died in New York City of colon cancer on December 10, 1934.

BIBLIOGRAPHY

As Paul Franklin Clark noted in 1959, "No definitive biography [has] appeared of this man who has been acclaimed one of the greatest figures in American medicine and certainly the most distinguished of early American bacteriologists." Hans Zinsser's *Biographical Memoir of Theobald Smith, 1859–1934* (1936) remains the most authoritative sketch and lists most of Smith's publications. Paul de Kruif* devoted a chapter to Smith in the classic *Microbe Hunters* (1926). Claude E. Dolman's 1982 article is the most recent assessment. Smith's papers can be found in the U.S. Bureau of Animal Industry records at the National Archives, at Harvard University and the Rockefeller Archives, and in Kremers Reference Files, Institute for the History of Pharmacy, University of Wisconsin, Madison.

Writings by Theobald Smith

"Preliminary Observations on the Microorganism of Texas Fever." *American Public Health Association Report* 15 (1889): 178–185.
"A New Method for Determining Quantitatively the Pollution of Water by Fecal Bacteria." *New York State Board of Health, Thirteenth Annual Report for the Year 1892* (1893): 712–722.
"A Comparative Study of the Toxin Production of Diphtheria Bacilli." *Report of the Massachusetts State Board of Health* (1896): 649–672.
"A Comparative Study of Bovine Tubercle Bacilli and of Human Bacilli from Sputum." *Journal of Experimental Medicine* 3 (1898): 451–511.
(with R. B. Little). "The Significance of Colostrum to the New Born Calf." *Journal of Experimental Medicine 36* (1922): 181–198.
Parasitism and Disease. Princeton, NJ: Princeton University Press, 1934.

Writings about Theobald Smith and Related Topics

Clark, Paul Franklin. "Theobald Smith, Student of Disease (1859–1934)." *Journal of the History of Medicine* 14 (1959): 490–514.
De Kruif, Paul. *Microbe Hunters.* New York: Harcourt, Brace, 1926.
Dolman, Claude E. "Theobald Smith (1859–1934), Pioneer American Microbiologist." *Perspectives in Biology and Medicine* 25 (1982): 417–427.
Zinsser, Hans. *Biographical Memoir of Theobald Smith, 1859–1934* Washington, D.C.: National Academy of Sciences, 1936.

G. Terry Sharrer

ANDREW TAYLOR STILL
(1828–1917)

Andrew Taylor Still, physician and founder of osteopathy, was born in Jones-ville, Lee County, Virginia, to Abram Still, a Methodist preacher, and Martha Poage (Moore) Still. Andrew's father was assigned to serve the farming community of New Market, Tennessee, where Andrew attended grammar school at Holston College. With the westward movement of Methodist circuit riders, Abram was called to attend the Mission Methodist Conference in Macon County, Missouri, in 1837. Andrew, or Drew as he was known to his family, returned to formal schooling in Schuyler County, Missouri, from 1842 to 1848. While not in school, Andrew found life on the Missouri frontier both practically and personally rewarding. As he later recalled,

Before I ever studied anatomy books, I had almost perfected the knowledge from the great book of nature. The skinning of squirrels brought me in contact with muscles, nerves, and veins. The bones, this great foundation for the wonderful house we live in, was always a study for me long before I learned the hard names given to them by the scientific world.

Indeed, it was while enjoying nature as a ten-year-old that Drew experienced a headache while swinging. He took the swing rope down "to about eight to ten inches off the ground, threw the end of a blanket on it, and . . . lay down [with my neck across the rope] . . . and used the rope for a swinging pillow." This action, which relieved his headache, was later deemed to be his "first lesson in osteopathy" (Still 1897:45).

While learning to hew trees, split rails, and build barns, Still became enamored of the new labor-saving technology such as the sewing machine. He constantly tinkered with machines throughout his life; in the 1870s, for example, he invented and marketed an improved butter churn. His interest in machines was central to the development of osteopathy, which he described as "a system of engineering the whole machinery of life" in a harmonious fashion (Still 1910:47).

Still married Mary Margaret Vaughan in January 1849, and they homesteaded near Bloomington, Missouri. After a devastating hailstorm destroyed the prospects of his first crops, he took a local teaching post to help support his family. In 1853, Still left Missouri with his wife and children, Marusha (b. 1849) and Andrew Price (b. 1852), to join his parents, who were tending to the spiritual and health needs of the Indians at the Wakarusa Shawnee Mission near Eudora, Kansas. Mary taught children enrolled at the Indian mission school while Still began farming and assisted his father in treating the Indians, which provided him somewhat of an apprenticeship to his father's textbook-approach medical practice, as well as exposure to a variety of traditional Indian healing methods.

Still supplemented this training with practical anatomical knowledge he obtained from dissecting the bodies of cholera victims he exhumed from Indian graves.

Ever a family on the move, the Stills left the Indian mission in 1854 and were founding members of the community that would become Lawrence, Kansas. In 1857, A. T. Still, together with his brothers John and Thomas, offered tracts of their land holdings as the site for a university to be established in the Kansas Territory. With additional funds from Ohio Methodist John Baldwin, Baker University was established in 1858. Abram Still had developed a staunch antislavery following in Missouri during the 1840s when the Methodist church divided over the issue of slavery. Still joined the Poker Moonshiners, a men's group that organized protection against the Missouri "Border Ruffians." Still, together with some eighty other emigrant settlers, established a free-state Kansas militia in June 1855. In 1857, his efforts to promote the entrance of Kansas to the Union as a free state won him a seat in the Kansas territorial legislature as representative from Douglas and Johnson counties. As a representative, he frequently engaged in verbal, and later military, confrontations with governmental opponents. One such encounter, later known as the Wakarusa War, sparked Still's thinking about a new type of medicine. While hiding in an effort to escape arrest warrants, Still discussed medicine and other matters with fellow free-stater Major James Burnett Abbott. He credited Abbott for stimulating his thoughts about a type of healing that would replace allopathy, eclecticism, and homeopathy, medical practices that neither man deemed efficacious.

In 1859, Still was left the sole provider for his four children, Marusha, Abram, Susan (born 1856), and an adopted daughter, after his wife died following a difficult childbirth. He married Mary Elvira Turner, a New York school teacher who had recently settled in Kansas in 1860. Mary Elvira, the daughter of physician Charles McLeod Turner, was active in various reform movements. Within a year, Kansas achieved statehood, followed soon after by the outbreak of the war between the states. Still enlisted in the Cass County Home Guards, which was attached to the 9th Kansas Cavalry, Company F. After this group disbanded in April 1862, he helped organize the 18th Kansas Militia and was later transferred to the 21st Kansas Militia to patrol the Santa Fe Trail. He gained surgical experience throughout the war, became an active military hospital steward and surgeon, and obtained a major's commission in the Kansas militia. Mary Elvira assisted him as hospital matron.

The deaths of three of Still's children in 1864 from epidemic spinal meningitis devastated him. With a heart "torn and lacerated with grief" and disillusioned at the promise of standard medical therapy, Still temporarily abandoned medical practice. He considered pursuing formal medical education at the Kansas City School of Physicians and Surgeons but became further disgruntled with contemporary medical teachings. His rejection of established medicine, coupled with his family losses, drove him in search of a new, complete therapeutic system. After much thought, he concluded that "all the remedies necessary to health exist in the human body . . . [and] they can be administered by adjusting the body in such condition that the remedies may naturally associate themselves together . . . and relieve the afflicted'' (Still 1897: 110).

Driven by the strong Methodist belief in the possibility of achieving perfection on earth, he regularly confronted clergymen who, though promoting God's works as perfections of nature, administered addictive drugs, calomel, and alcohol to parishioner patients. He attended many postwar lyceum and revival camp meetings where speakers promoted specific alternatives to allopathic medicine, including homeopathy, hydrotherapy, mesmerism, and magnetic healing. He was particularly impressed by magnetic healing, which was based on the belief that an invisible magnetic fluid flowed through the body and that disease stemmed from imbalances or obstructions of this fluid. Still began an ''extended study'' of human mechanics, concentrating on the ''drive wheels, pinions, cups, arms, and shafts of human life'' together with the ''forces, supplies, framework and attachment by ligaments and muscle, the nerve and blood supply, and the 'how' and 'where' the motor nerves receive their power and motion,'' which in harmonious concert perform the ''duties of life'' (Trowbridge 1991: 115). His continued pursuit of anatomical ''research'' through grave robbing was less tolerated in Baldwin City than it had been on the Indian Mission. After facing repeated denouncements for sacrilege, Still left Kansas in 1874 to meet his brother, Edward, in Macon County, Missouri. It was in these surroundings that A. T. Still announced the discovery of his ''new science'' on June 21, 1874.

Still procured certification to practice in Macon County on August 29, 1874. His method of treatment, derived from his ''new science,'' employed a physical manipulative technique, somewhat like that used by magnetic healers and bone setters, to cure patients' ills without the use of drugs. Still always carried his ''bag of bones'' to demonstrate exactly what he intended to do. Though his manipulative technique was successful, his nonconformist dress, habits, and apparently mystical healing powers prompted many, including the local Methodist minister, to speculate that his powers were derived from the devil. Opposition to his mere presence led him to settle elsewhere. Dr. Grove encouraged Still to establish a practice in Kirksville, Missouri. Although local inhabitants were skeptical at first, Still's ability to restore Kirksville's Presbyterian minister, J. B. Mitchell's daughter's ability to walk secured him wide acclaim. Still advertised himself as a ''Magnetic Healer,'' ''Lightning Bone Setter,'' and ''Human Engineer.''

Throughout his nomadic wanderings before settling in Kirksville in 1887, Still debated with anyone who would listen about the extent to which disease was related to the brain, spinal cord, and peripheral nervous system, as well as the displacement of bones and muscles. He reasoned that removal of the impediments to health through manipulation provided ''unlimited freedom of the circulatory system of nerves, blood and cerebral fluid.'' Most important, this therapy evoked the body's natural healing power. In 1885, following the suggestion of a Baker University professor who had come to Kirksville for treatment, Still named his ''new science'' osteopathy (from *osteon*, ''bone,'' and *pathine*, "suffering") (Trowbridge 1991:140). More elaborately, he described osteopathy as

a knowledge of anatomy applied to healing diseases. It is the surgical adjustment of all parts of the body by the anatomist who knows all bones of the human body, their forms, their places and how they are held together, where each joint is, where the muscles are attached and how they act when in their normal places; how a normal limb looks, how it feels to his hand, and how an abnormal limb, hand, foot, spine or neck feels to his fingers in which the sense of touch is developed to a very high degree (Trowbridge 1991: 164)

With the support of the Kirksville community and the financial contributions of his wife, three of his sons, Charles (born 1865), Herman (born 1867), and Harry (born 1867), and two other followers, Still opened the American School of Osteopathy in 1892. His faculty focused on teaching anatomy, diagnosis, and osteopathic manipulative technique. Members of the original class, which records indicate consisted of approximately twenty-one students, including five women, received the diplomate of osteopathy (D.O.) degree. The school became a tremendous success, receiving official status from the state government in 1897 after adding course work in chemistry and surgery, and it attracted increasing numbers of students and patients. By 1894, Kirksville had become a boomtown due to the influence of osteopathy. M. A. Lane, an early professor in the American School of Osteopathy, claimed that osteopathy students could, "with entire confidence in their own powers and the science under it, treat all kinds of infectious disease with a courage, or rather an entire want of fear, that reminds one of the primitive Christians" (Armstrong and Armstrong 1991: 142).

A. T. Still, or the "Old Doctor" as he became affectionately known, promoted osteopathy on many levels, including textbooks written for students, the *Journal of Osteopathy* for practitioners, and articles in popular periodicals such as *Ladies Home Journal*. His acclaim attracted support from national figures, including President Theodore Roosevelt and Mark Twain. Kirksville osteopaths also began treating an increasing number of players from the National Baseball League and college football teams. Still and his "new science" were honored with the declaration of Osteopathy Day at the 1904 World's Fair in St. Louis, Missouri.

After the turn of the century, Still gave up the daily management of the school. Although he kept active in his private dissection room, he expanded his realm of experiments, looking into such matters as the effect of light on the growth of corn and developing and patenting an "antipollution" smokeless coal-burning furnace. Mary Elvira died in 1910, but Still was comforted by his surviving children, Marusha, Charles, Herman, Harry, and Martha, better known as Blanche (born 1876). For many years, Still faced relentless ridicule from allopathic practitioners. Critics of osteopathy became more fierce once new osteopathic schools opened, effectively spreading this practice beyond Kirksville.

Before his death from a stroke, Still saw his disciples carry his medical philosophy to each of the states, as well as to Great Britain, India, Africa, and Australia. In less than a quarter of a century, the ''new science'' of osteopathy had circled the globe.

BIBLIOGRAPHY

The National Center for Osteopathic History, A. T. Still Memorial Library at the Kirksville College of Osteopathic Medicine and the Still National Osteopathic Museum, both located in Kirksville, Missouri, house the world's largest collection of archival materials related to Andrew Taylor Still and osteopathy. Still's *Autobiography* (1897) provides an indispensable starting point for further information. The 1992 Kirksville College of Osteopathic Medicine centenary celebrations included the production of several new volumes, the most historically useful being the family recollections of Charles E. Still, Jr., published in *Frontier Doctor–Medical Pioneer: The Life and Times of A. T. Still and His Family* (1991), Robert V. Schnucker's profusely illustrated edition of *Early Osteopathy in the Words of A. T. Still* (1991), Carol Trowbridge's *Andrew Taylor Still: 1828–1917* (1991), and Georgia Warner Walter's *The First School of Osteopathic Medicine: A Chronicle* (1992). Additional information about the birth pangs of osteopathy are found in Arthur Grant Hildreth's *The Lengthening Shadow of A. T. Still* (1938, 1988), a chronicle by a member of Still's first osteopathy class who became a key osteopathic leader.

Writings by Andrew Taylor Still

Autobiography of Andrew T. Still with a History of the Discovery and Development of the Science of Osteopathy. Kirksville, MO: By the author, 1897.
Philosophy of Osteopathy. Kirksville, MO: By the author, 1899.
Philosophy and Mechanical Principles of Osteopathy. Kirksville, MO: By the author, 1902.
Osteopathy: Research and Practice. Kirksville, MO: By the author, 1910.

Writings about Andrew Taylor Still and Related Topics

Armstrong, David, and Elizabeth Metzger Armstrong. *The Great American Medicine Show.* Englewood Cliffs, NJ: Prentice Hall, 1991.
Booth, Emmons Rutledge. *History of Osteopathy and Twentieth-Century Medicine.* Memorial ed. Cincinnati, OH: Caxton Press, 1924. (One of the most complete of the early descriptive histories of osteopathy.)
Gevitz, Norman. *The D.O.'s: Osteopathic Medicine in America.* Baltimore: Johns Hopkins University Press, 1982. (An encompassing social historical view of the profession.)
Hildreth, Arthur Grant. *The Lengthening Shadow of A. T. Still.* 3d ed. 1938. Reprint ed., Kirksville, MO: Osteopathic Enterprise, 1988. (This chronicle by a key osteopathic leader who was a member of Still's first osteopathy class provides a valuable chronicle of the birth pangs of osteopathy.)

Schnucker, Robert V., ed. *Early Osteopathy in the Words of A. T. Still*. Kirksville, MO: Thomas Jefferson University Press, 1991.

Still, Charles E., Jr. *Frontier Doctor–Medical Pioneer: The Life and Times of A. T. Still and His Family*. Kirksville, MO: Thomas Jefferson University Press, 1991.

Trowbridge, Carol. *Andrew Taylor Still: 1828–1917*. Kirksville, MO: Thomas Jefferson University Press, 1991.

Walter, Georgia Warner. *The First School of Osteopathic Medicine. A Chronicle*. Kirksville, MO: Thomas Jefferson University Press, 1992.

———. *Osteopathic Medicine: Past and Present*. 3d ed. Kirksville, MO: Kirksville College of Osteopathic Medicine, 1993.

Philip K. Wilson

SAMUEL-AUGUSTE-ANDRÉ-DAVID TISSOT
(1728–1797)

Samuel-Auguste-André-David (occasionally wrongly identified as Simon-André) Tissot was a Swiss physician and medical writer who, with several colleagues, influenced the evolution of medicine in ways that none separately would have achieved. Chief among Tissot's fellows were Daniel Bernoulli (1700–1782) of Basel; Albrecht von Haller (1708–1777) of Bern; Hans Kaspar Hirzel (1725–1803) of Zurich; Théodore Tronchin (1709–1781) of Geneva (then a Swiss ally); Jean-André Venel (1740–1791) of Orbe; and Johann-Georg Zimmermann (1728–1795) of Brugg.

Through a unifying context of close epistolary contacts and a common political (Swiss) and religious (Reformed) background, these doctors were able to reach a consensus on how to apply their medical expertise to the service of their community, private and public health practice, and professional training. The sustenance they gained from each other helped to turn their dreams into concrete proposals and their ideas into published books. This intellectual group was primarily concerned with professionalizing and popularizing medicine. These two goals may appear antithetical, yet it was necessary to define and teach a "new correct" medical art for doctors and patients to adopt, so as to change the mentality of both providers and recipients of health care; only then could physicians dispense and patients accept novel ways of preventing and curing diseases.

Tissot is the most appropriate focal point for a study of this group; he was its most prolific writer and the one most concerned with medical praxis. The others are closely associated with other fields: Bernoulli with mathematics, Haller with physiology, Hirzel with politics, Tronchin with urbanity, Venel with education, and Zimmermann with philosophy. Each man's special interest helped define the goals and broaden the appeal of medical professionalization and popularization.

Tissot was born in Grancy (Pays de Vaud) into a family of local officials and pastors; he died in Lausanne. After receiving his master of arts from the Geneva Academy, Tissot went to the University of Montpellier to study medicine. There he boarded in the household of the nosologist François Boissier de Sauvages (1706–1767) and served as surgeon in the town's hospitals, while following the regular course of lectures that led to his medical degree in 1749. Upon his return to the Pays de Vaud, Tissot began practicing medicine, moving soon to Lausanne. He lived there until his death, except for a stay in Paris (1779–1780) and a two-year tenure as professor of clinical medicine at the University of Pavia (1781–1783).

Bernoulli was born in Basel into a family of mathematicians; he died in Basel. He studied medicine in Basel and in Heidelberg and mathematics with his relatives. After some years spent abroad (Russia, Dutch Republic), Bernoulli returned to Basel to become professor of anatomy. He contributed to the use of probabilistic methods in medicine to measure the validity of procedures such as inoculation.

A member of a patrician family, Haller was born and died in Bern. He studied medicine in Leyden under Hermann Boerhaave (1668–1738). A poet and physiologist, Haller developed the concept of irritability experimentally while he was, from 1736 to 1753, the first professor of anatomy, botany, and physiology at the recently founded University of Göttingen. He sustained a lifelong interest for observing, in vivo, the physiological effects and functional impairment due to tying or sectioning nerves, to poisoning and/or irritating with various substances, or to bloodletting, which he also studied as an attempt at reviving the dead.

Hirzel, scion of a family of notables, was born and died in Zurich. He studied medicine at Basel, then returned to his birthplace to practice. Later he became town physician and a statesman who promoted public health measures.

Born in Geneva, Tronchin came from a family of statesmen and bankers; he died in Paris. He studied medicine at Leyden under Boerhaave, later turning down the offer to succeed his mentor. Tronchin introduced the practice of inoculation in continental Europe. He is best known for his commonsense advice on preventive medicine for his wealthy patients, such as sufficient exercise, enough sleep, and moderate eating, and he is best remembered for dispensing medicine to the poor, free of charge.

Venel, the son of a surgeon, was born and died in the Pays de Vaud. He was trained as a surgeon and male midwife in Geneva, Montpellier, Paris, and Strasbourg. He founded the first Swiss Midwifery School in Yverdon (1778) and established the first (anywhere) Orthopedic Hospital in Orbe (1780). He published works on midwifery, orthopedics, and female education.

Zimmermann was born in Brugg to a family of jurists; he died in Hanover where he was court physician. A graduate from the Bern Academy, he studied medicine at Göttingen with Haller, who closely associated him with his physiological research. Under the name of Ritter von Zimmermann, he is remembered as a philosopher and political pamphleteer.

Contacts between Tissot and the others began in the 1750s. The practice of inoculating smallpox and the controversy it aroused presented the right ingredients for the pursuit of both medical popularizing and professionalizing. Aware that the medicine at his disposal was better at preventing than curing disease, Tissot was eager to learn about a practice that was meant to mitigate the devastations of smallpox.

Having heard of Tronchin's inoculating practice in Amsterdam, Tissot took the opportunity of Tronchin's visiting Geneva to contact him about the best way to inoculate; Tronchin wrote back with the information requested. He and Tissot developed close medical ties, particularly in the advocacy of a proper regimen (diet and exercise) in maintaining health and curing sickness. Tissot also studied the available literature on inoculation, noting that most of these works were for either physicians or theologians. He therefore decided to write his own book to inform the general public about the value of inoculation. He sent a draft to Haller asking for suggestions. Haller answered, praising the enterprise, yet mercilessly pointing out the deficiencies. From Haller, Tissot learned to be precise and concise in order to circumscribe adversaries' attacks. Even so, Tissot was drawn into fierce battles over inoculation by the Leyden-trained and Vienna-based physician Anton de Haen (1704–1776).

In 1754, Tissot published in Lausanne *L'inoculation justifiée* (Inoculation vindicated), which Voltaire praised as ''a service rendered to humanity.'' To spread his views and increase his visibility, Tissot sent copies of *L'Inoculation justifiée* to colleagues in Switzerland and abroad. Zimmermann acknowledged the ''honor'' and informed Tissot that he was preparing for publication in Zurich, a long extract, in German, of *L'Inoculation justifiée*. The drive to popularize medicine bounded the two into a friendship that lasted until Zimmermann's death.

The subject of inoculation gave Tissot the occasion for both popularizing and professionalizing medical practice. With the publication of *L'Inoculation justifiée*, he reached the educated public, and with the professional contacts he acquired from it, he was able, through medical open letters often written in Latin and addressed to Haller, Hirzel, or Zimmermann, to advocate the practice to a readership of physicians.

When Tronchin wrote the article ''Inoculation'' for Diderot's *Encyclopédie* (vol. 8, pp. 755–771), he followed the argument of Tissot's *L'Inoculation justifiée* closely. Bernoulli's mathematical work on the efficacy of inoculation to lessen the morbidity and mortality of smallpox, together with their epistolary contacts, helped Tissot buttress his arguments in favor of the practice.

Tissot's next attempt at popularizing medicine came with *Avis au peuple sur sa santé* (1761) (*Advice to the People on Their Health*, English edition, 1765). Tissot aimed at educating the social and religious elite in the ''correct'' approach to preventing and curing diseases, for their personal use and in their charitable deeds. He wanted to wean his readers from almanacs' and charlatans' advice and to lead them to choose instead a neo-Hippocratic style of observing symptoms and proposing mild interventions. He hoped that the medical interactions between wealthy and poor carried out according to his prescriptions would also teach the indigent the proper attitude toward their health care. *Avis* is the most widely published and translated of Tissot's works; the second is *Onanisme*, which he published in 1760. Today Tissot is more often studied or cited for his treatise on masturbation than for his efforts at raising the level of modern medical understanding of society.

Soon after the publication of *Avis*, Hirzel requested from Tissot the privilege of translating it into German; the two exchanged many letters until Tissot's death. The Lausanne physician of the poor and the Zurich town physician shared a concern for the people's health; they aimed at providing urban and rural populations with the best health care that local circumstances allowed. Both recognized that often the meager quality and quantity of food were the main problems leading to the people's poor health. Tissot advised the authorities about the safety of the food supply, while Hirzel popularized physiocratic means to increase crops in a book entitled *Wirtschafteines philosophischen Bauers* (1761, The economic policy of a farmer-philosopher). Later, Tissot wrote two other popular medical treatises, *De la Santé des gens de lettres* (1768) (*On the Diseases Incident to Literary and Sedentary Persons*, English edition, 1768) and *Essai sur les maladies des gens du monde* (1770) (*Essay on the Disorders of People of Fashion*, English edition, 1770) in which he explained the intricacies of keeping healthy through lifestyle choices. Contrary to *Avis*, which was published in English after a four-year delay, both *Gens de Lettres* and *Gens du monde* appeared in English the same year as the original French edition.

Tissot, Venel, and Zimmermann were especially concerned with the training of medical personnel; they had encountered in their practice cases made worse by the bungling of ignorant physicians. Zimmermann was the first of the three to popularize in order to professionalize. In 1764, he published *Von der Erfahrung in der Arzneykunst* (*A Treatise on Experience in Physic*, English edition, 1782) in which he expounded a diagnosis method based on neo-Hippocratic bedside observations, clarified by past physicians' and personal experiences, and construed by Baconian induction guided by intuition. The professionalize-popularize intent of the German medium chosen by Zimmermann was carried over when *Erfahrung* was translated into Dutch, English, French, and Italian, but not Latin.

Venel, aware as a male midwife of the demand for and the lack of properly trained midwives, called on Tissot and Haller to help persuade the Bernese authorities to sponsor a midwifery school. The school was founded in 1778 in Yverdon with Venel as director and instructor; for the benefit of his students, he wrote *Précis d'instruction pour les sages-femmes* (1778) (Handbook for midwives).

Tissot thought that in order to reach diagnosis and prescribe a proper treatment, physicians needed to comprehend not only the pathological but also the physiological phenomena that lay under the symptoms. He extended his popularizing and professionalizing endeavor to the writing of *Traité des nerfs et de leurs maladies* (1778–1780) (Treatise on the nervous system and its diseases) and *Essai sur les moyens de perfectionner les études de médecine* (1785) (Essay on the means of improving medical education). These two books were never published in English. Tissot rendered accessible most of Haller's experiments (previously available in Latin only) on the nervous system, allowing for better insights into the causes and treatments of nervous disorders. Building on his experience at Pavia, he proposed reforms in medical education that Philippe Pinel* later recommended (Weiner 1980).

Tissot and his friends participated actively in the campaign for the medicalization of society that took place in the second half of the eighteenth century. Their writings were meant to inform lay and medical persons alike. They indeed popularized and professionalized the medical field, changing mentalities and leading people to accept a modern perception of medical possibilities.

BIBLIOGRAPHY

Most of Tissot's personal papers, including his vast correspondence, his reading notes, manuscripts, some lectures on clinical medicine, and notes on the deliberations of the Collège de Médecine of Lausanne from its foundation in 1787 to his death in 1797, are kept at the Bibliothèque cantonale et universitaire in Lausanne. Tissot's letters to Haller are at the Burgerbibliothek in Bern; those to Hirzel at the Zentralbibliothek in Zurich and those to Zimmermann at the Niedersächsischelandesbibliothek in Hanover, Germany. Tissot published twenty-five books, some of which went through many editions and were translated into fifteen different languages.

Most of Bernoulli's personal papers are at the Universitätbibliothek in Basel. Most of Haller's papers are kept at the Burgerbibliothek in Bern; others are located at Göttingen Universitätbibliothek. Haller wrote thousands of scientific papers and published multivolume sets of scientific and medical bibliographies. Recently several volumes of his correspondence with various savants have been published. Hirzel's papers are at the Zentralbibliothek in Zurich. Most of Tronchin's papers are at the Bibliothèque publique et universitaire in Geneva. His letters are scattered with the personal papers of his various correspondents. Some of Venel's papers are at the Bibliothèque cantonale et universitaire in Lausanne; others are in Orbe town archives. Most of Zimmermann's papers are at the Niedersächsischelandesbibliothek in Hanover.

Writings by Samuel-Auguste-André-David Tissot and Colleagues

Onanisme. 1st ed. Lausanne: Chapuis. Facsimile ed., Paris: Le Sycomore, 1980. Reprint ed., Paris: Editions de la Différence, 1991.

Avis au peuple sur sa santé. 1st ed. 1761. (The 1782 edition was reprinted in Paris: Edition Quai Voltaire, 1993.)

De la santé des gens de lettres. 1st ed. 1768. (A facsimile of the 1768 edition was published in Genève: Slatkine, 1981, and reprinted in Paris: Editions de la Différence, 1991.)

Bernoulli, Daniel. *Die Werke.* 10 vols. Basel: Birkhauser Verlag, 1982. (Vol. 1, edited by U. Tröhler, contains Bernoulli's contributions to medicine.)

————. ''Essai d'une nouvelle analyse de la mortalité causée par la petite vérole et des avantages de l'inoculation pour la prévenir (Essay on a new analysis of the mortality due to smallpox and of the advantages of inoculation to prevent it)'' In *Histoire de l'Académie royale des sciences, mémoires de mathématique et de physique. Année MDCCLX* (Proceedings of the Royal Academy of Science, section of mathematics and physics, 1760), pp. 1–45. Paris: Imprimerie Royale, 1766.

Writings about Samuel-Auguste-André-David Tissot and Related Topics

Ackerknecht, Erwin H. *Kurze Geschichte des grossen Schweizer Aertze* (A short history of great Swiss doctors) Bern: Huber, 1975.

Bradley, Leslie. *Smallpox Inoculation: An Eighteenth-Century Mathematical Controversy.* Nottingham, UK: University Publications, 1971.

Emch-Dériaz, A. "A propos de *L'expérience en médecine* de Zimmermann." *Canadian Bulletin of Medical History* 9 (1992): 3–15.

———. "L'Inoculation justifiée, or Was It?" *Eighteenth-Century Life* 7 (1982): 65–72.

———. "Health and Gender Oriented Education: An Eighteenth-Century Case-Study." *Women's Studies* 24 (1995): 521–530. (Venel's ideas about education.)

———. *Tissot: Physician of the Enlightenment.* Bern and New York: Peter Lang, 1992.

Holzhey, Helmut, and Urs Boschung, eds. *Gesundheit und Krankheit im 18. Jahrhundert* (Health and illness in the eighteenth century) Amsterdam: Rodoni, 1995.

Porter, Roy, ed. *The Popularization of Medicine 1650–1850.* London: Routledge, 1992.

Saudan, Guy, ed. *L'éveil médical vaudois.* Lausanne: Publications de l'Université, 1987. (Comprehensive treatment of Venel's life.)

Temkin, Owsei. *The Double Face of Janus.* Baltimore: Johns Hopkins University Press, 1977. (Succinct treatment of Zimmermann's medical philosophy.)

Weiner, Dora. *The Clinical Training of Doctors: An Essay of 1793 by Philippe Pinel.* Baltimore: Johns Hopkins University Press, 1980.

Antoinette Emch-Dériaz

ROBERT BENTLEY TODD
(1809–1860)

Robert Bentley Todd, physician and surgeon, physiologist, pioneer in medical education, and founder of the first training institution for nurses, was born in Dublin, one of fifteen children and the second son of Charles Hawkes Todd. Todd senior was surgeon to the House of Industry Hospitals, professor of anatomy at the Royal College of Surgeons in Ireland, and a president of the college.

Todd received his secondary education at a local day school and from a tutor, the Rev. W. Higgins, afterward bishop of Derry. Medicine, to which he was to devote his life so wholeheartedly, was not his first choice as a career. He entered Dublin University in 1825 planning to study law but was forced to switch to medicine the following year when his father died unexpectedly, leaving his large family poorly provided for. Todd graduated with a B.A. from Dublin University in 1829 but received his surgical diploma in 1831 from the House of Industry Hospitals and the Royal College of Surgeons rather than from the university. One suspects that his father's colleagues may have waived their fees for the brilliant but impecunious second son.

Todd had already gone to London and was living on Charlotte Street, without a sixpence to help himself, as he put it, when he became a licentiate of the Royal College of Surgeons in Ireland. Having no introductions or friends in London, he set out to connect himself with a medical school. In 1831 he obtained the post of lecturer in anatomy and physiology at one of the private schools, the Aldersgate Street Medical School. There he lectured for three sessions, attracting the attention of such eminent surgeons as Sir Astley Cooper and Sir Benjamin Brodie. Todd had decided to pursue the new physiological medicine rather than surgery. This approach to scientific medicine, pioneered by the French, was based on research in morbid anatomy with clinicopathological correlations and physical diagnosis. He immediately began planning to get his medical degrees, attending Oxford briefly and receiving his M.A. in June 1832, his B.M. in May 1833, and his D.M. in 1836 from that university.

Todd's lectures at the Aldersgate School were generally well attended, but the school was not successful financially. In 1834, he joined several other medical men, including the eminent surgeon George James Guthrie, of the Westminster Hospital, in setting up a private medical school, which they hoped would become the Westminster Hospital's School of Medicine. A number of the Westminster medical staff who hoped to establish their own profit-making school in connection with the hospital, however, opposed the plan, and the proposal was defeated. In 1836 Todd made an unsuccessful bid to be elected physician to the Westminster. Later in the same year he was appointed professor of physiology and morbid anatomy at King's College, and in 1840 he became physician to the newly opened King's College Hospital.

Other honors of the profession accrued to him. He was admitted a member of the Royal College of Physicians in London in 1833 and became a fellow in 1837. He gave the Gulstonian lectures in 1839, the Croonian lectures in 1842, and the Lumleian lecture in 1849. In 1838 he was made a fellow of the Royal Society, and in 1844 he was elected a fellow of the Royal College of Surgeons. In 1853 he resigned his chair of anatomy and physiology due to the pressures of his large and successful private practice. In order to keep his services, the King's College Council rescinded the rule that a physician to the hospital must be a college professor. Todd resigned this position in December 1859 because of failing health; the council at once appointed him consulting physician to the hospital.

The following month, he died at the age of fifty. Unlike his father, Todd did leave his family well provided for. Todd told his students that if properly followed, no other profession offered better advantages for making a competency (a modest fortune) than medicine, and indeed, he had clearly done well with his private practice. Described by the *Lancet* as dying in the full blaze of success and prosperity, he left an estate of £14,000.

If Todd had arrived in London with no money and no friends or introductions—all prerequisites for a successful medical career at that time—he had one major advantage over his English colleagues, for he had received his basic medical education in Dublin at a time when the Irish school of medicine and surgery was one of the most outstanding in Europe. Midwifery and medicine had been integral parts of the curriculum at the Royal College of Surgeons in Ireland since the eighteenth century, while the triple qualification did not become a legal requirement in England until 1886. Todd also had the benefit of brilliant teachers. In 1826, precisely when Todd was taking up his study of surgery, Robert Adams and Richard Carmichael established the Richmond School of Medicine and Surgery at the House of Industry Hospitals. As well, Todd worked with Robert James Graves, under whose guidance and direction he developed his love of physiology and his commitment to clinical, bedside teaching.

Todd moved beyond the gross anatomy of the early physiologists. Vast improvements in the microscope were providing scientists in the 1830s with the technology that transformed the foundations of biology and medicine in the middle third of the century. Todd was one of the first men in England to appreciate the importance of histology. "Microscopic anatomy, normal and morbid, aided by the minute analyses of organic chemistry, and accompanied with the careful observation and records of symptoms during life," he wrote in 1842, would form the basis for future medical progress (Todd 1842:308). He described the methodology of the new medicine when he explained, "From being little more than a series of vague and ill-founded hypotheses, scarcely deserving even that name, it [anatomy and physiology] has become a well-arranged science, embracing a vast amount of clearly defined facts, which, at once, form a solid basis for a superstructure of sound theory, and throw light upon the various processes of animal and vegetable life'' (Todd 1835–1859, 1: Preface). It was his willingness to call the physiology of the past vague and ill-founded hypotheses that was to cause difficulties for him with more conservative members of the profession and which earned him the title of a fierce controversialist.

Widely read in the work of continental physiologists, Todd was a major figure in the network of leading physicians and surgeons in England. Looking back in 1859, he thought that there had never been such rapid progress in any other branch of science than that in anatomy and physiology during the preceding twenty-five years. Much of that progress stemmed from his own work and the work that he encouraged and assisted his colleagues and students to do. Todd's own discoveries were significant. He introduced the concept of afferent sensitive nerves and efferent motor nerves. He identified postictal paralysis (Todd's paralysis), previously thought to be caused by apoplexy. But he was proudest of his piece of pure, inductive reasoning on the link between lesions in the posterior columns of the spinal cord and tabes dorsalis, later confirmed by the elaborate experiments of Charles Brown-Séquard.

Todd's commitment to professional and academic medical education was to make King's a leading medical school. He introduced the first scholarships for medical students in London; Sir William Bowman was the first King's scholar in 1837. King's, as a new medical department, did not have a hospital of its own. It was largely due to Todd's untiring energies that King's College Hospital was founded in 1840 and the new state-of-the-art facility built in the 1850s. Concerned by the undisciplined life that medical students of the earlier part of the century led, he introduced a collegiate system of education. A dedicated Anglican, he believed that the religious and moral characters of medical men were equally as important as their practical and scientific attainments. He worked closely with leading clergy at King's to provide more religious instruction and closer academic supervision for the students, establishing the office of a dean and arranging for a number of students to live in rooms in the college. The combination of medical education with the cultivation of religious and general knowledge, Todd believed, gave medical education at King's a unique tone and character. King's was the first to introduce a collegiate system for medical students; others were soon to follow its lead.

By the 1850s the medical students at King's were completely integrated into the university system, a goal of Todd since at least 1834. They received their entire education at King's College and had to pass exams in their courses rather than simply presenting certificates of attendance. They alone were eligible to be clinical clerks, dressers, physicians' assistants, and house surgeons to the hospital; these positions were selected by exam and could not be bought or achieved through apprenticeship, as was still common practice. King's was also one of the first to establish a clinical laboratory for microscopical and chemical research.

Todd believed clinical bedside teaching was the only effective way to teach medicine; students had to learn through hands-on practice as well as through academic work. His interest in a teaching hospital, where every attention was paid to the comfort and care of the patients, made him particularly aware of how essential good nursing was. Together with a group of prominent Anglicans, he introduced a radical reform of nursing, based on the same principles as his reforms of medical education: practical bedside training in the hospital combined with religious education and a residential setting where older, upper-class ladies, who were unpaid, could supervise and instruct the paid working-class nurses. Working-class women had always worked as nurses in the London hospitals, while the sisters, or head nurses, came from the lower middle class. Upper-class ladies could not pursue a career or work for a salary without losing their social status. Both the concept of nursing as a professional career for ladies, and having ladies and working-class women work and train together on the wards were radical innovations in mid-nineteenth century England.

The Training Institution that Todd founded in 1848, later known as St. John's House, took the form of a lay Anglican sisterhood. This model was inspired in part by the training schools for teachers that the Anglicans were building across England at this time, and in part by the orders of Protestant deaconesses on the Continent. Systematic training from both doctors and the sisters was required for both lady nurses and working-class nurses, and was designed not only to furnish superior nursing for the patients but to provide legitimate careers for both lady nurses and ordinary nurses.

In 1856 the sisterhood took over the nursing at King's College Hospital with immense success. Almost immediately other London teaching hospitals began adopting some of the St. John's House practices. Visitors came from all over the world to study the order, discipline, and efficiency of the nursing arrangements, which, together with its state-of-the-art building, made King's College Hospital the most modern hospital in London. This nursing system was to be the main inspiration for Florence Nightingale's proposed reforms at St. Thomas's in 1860, and Sister Mary Jones, lady superintendent of St. John's House from 1853 to 1868, became one of her dearest friends.

Todd was considered with his former master, Graves, and Armand Trousseau, one of the three most eminent clinical teachers of the nineteenth century. He was a brilliant lecturer and was said to have charmed unruly medical students into attention. His steady purpose and labor in promoting scientific medicine, his ability to encourage others in the same quest, his rare devotion to the duties of a hospital teacher, and his great gifts as a physiologist and a physician were widely recognized in the 1850s. Bowman, as did many others, spoke of his kindness and generosity, calling him his loved and honored friend and workfellow. Todd's therapeutics, however, were considered questionable, and perhaps they explain why a man so preeminent in his own generation has become forgotten in our time.

Todd's principles of treatment were first, to study sedulously the clinical history of the disease, making a clear diagnosis, then to search for the best way of assisting the curative physiological processes, and finally, to find the best means of upholding vital power. Scientific medicine was transforming the way leading medical men thought of disease and providing them with greater precision in describing disease processes and making diagnoses, but therapeutics and an understanding of etiology lagged behind. Strongly opposed to bleeding and depletion therapies, because he thought they produced exhaustion and failure of vital power, ultimately leading to death, Todd strongly favored supportive therapy.

Unfortunately, he identified alcohol as a premier treatment to uphold vital force and assist curative physiological processes, sometimes prescribing as much as thirty ounces of brandy a day for acute fevers. The one area of received medical wisdom that he never seems to have evaluated critically was the standard belief that alcohol was a stimulant and provided strength and physical stamina. The use of alcohol to uphold strength was standard, but the enormous dosages he prescribed with steadily increasing enthusiasm during his later years were not common practice, and were heavily criticized. The medical students thought he dosed himself with equally large quantities of brandy to fortify his own nervous system under the strain of his extensive private practice, so much so that he was often in a state of semi-intoxication when he drove about to see his numerous patients. In fact, he died of advanced cirrhosis of the liver.

Todd was a prolific writer. His major published works are *The Cyclopaedia of Anatomy and Physiology, The Physiological Anatomy and Physiology of Man*, written with Bowman, and three sets of clinical lectures. Already in 1832 he was projecting his *Cyclopaedia*, recruiting outstanding British scientists to write articles, and traveling to Paris in 1833 to solicit contributions from leading continental men. Publication of the first volume in 1835 established him as a leading physiologist and won him his chair at King's College. In 1892 the *Cyclopaedia* was still considered the largest and most important work of its kind in England and was still valuable for the number and variety of its original articles.

When the young William Bowman arrived at King's in 1837 he brought with him a fine, compound microscope. The following year he became physiology prosector to Todd, and they began planning *The Physiological Anatomy and Physiology* as a textbook for their medical students. This work constituted an epoch in physiology. Its lucid style and its immense superiority in microscopical detail to other works written at the time immediately made it into a standard authority both in England and abroad.

Todd's physiological works were received with unqualified acclaim, but his clinical lectures aroused more controversy, partly because he was working on the intellectual frontiers of medicine and later because of his therapeutics. Conservative men criticized the lectures for their overly clinical approach, putting too much emphasis on naked facts and not enough on the principles, synthesis, and generalization that were so dear to former generations of medical men. Leaders in the field such as William Gull, however, appreciated their scientific and practical approach. Todd's last set of lectures on acute disease were heavily criticized, largely because of his overly enthusiastic advocacy of alcohol, which many thought produced a higher death rate among his patients.

BIBLIOGRAPHY

There appear to be no personal papers extant. The archives of King's College and King's College Hospital hold a number of case notes of Todd's patients, and their minute books document much of his administrative activity. His role in nursing reform is described in the records of St. John's House, a subset of the archives of St. Thomas's Hospital. Todd was a major figure in contemporary medical journals. His letters and lectures were frequently printed, and his books and work discussed and reviewed in such journals as the *Lancet*, the *British and Foreign Medical and Chirurgical Review*, the *London Medical Gazette*, the *Medical Times and Gazette*, and the *Dublin Journal of Medical Science*. The *Dictionary of National Biography* devotes three pages to him, and there is a fine tribute to him in the obituary in the *Lancet*. His death is also described by William Makepeace Thackeray in the *Roundabout Papers*. Historians of medicine have paid little attention to Todd. There is no major work on this outstanding churchman, physiologist, clinical teacher, practitioner, and reformer who played a major role in establishing the new scientific medicine in England and originated the concept of nursing as a professional career for women.

Writings by William Bentley Todd

The Cyclopaedia of Anatomy and Physiology. Edited by R. B. Todd. 5 vols. London: Longman, Brown, Green, Longmans & Roberts, 1835–1859.

"The Physiology of the Stomach." Gulstonian Lectures for 1839. *London Medical Gazette* 25 (1839–1840): 265–270, 314–319, 426–432.

"Lectures on the Anatomy and Physiology of the Intestinal Canal." Croonian Lectures for 1842. *London Medical Gazette* 30 (1842): 305–310, 378–386, 449–456.

(with W. Bowman). *The Physiological Anatomy and Physiology of Man.* 2 vols. London: Parker, 1845–1856.

"On the Pathology and Treatment of Convulsive Diseases." Lumleian Lecture for 1849. *London Medical Gazette* 63 (1849): 661–671, 724–729, 766–772, 815–822, 837–846.

Clinical Lectures on Paralysis, Disease of the Brain and Other Affections of the Nervous System. London: J. Churchill, 1854.

Clinical Lectures on Certain Diseases of the Urinary Organs; and on Dropsies. Philadelphia: Churchill, 1857.

Clinical Lectures on Certain Acute Diseases. London: J. Churchill, 1860.

Writings about Robert Bentley Todd and Related Topics

Coakley, Davis. "Robert Bentley Todd 1809–1860, a Great Clinical Neurologist." In *Irish Masters of Medicine*, pp. 157–162. Dublin: Town House, 1992.

Dictionary of National Biography, 19:910–912. Edited by Sir Leslie Stephen. 1885–1890. London: Oxford University Press.

Helmstadter, Carol. "Robert Bentley Todd, Saint John's House, and the Origins of the Modern Trained Nurse." *Bulletin of the History of Medicine* 67 (1993): 282–319.

Lyons, J. B. "The Neurology of Robert Bentley Todd." In F. Clifford Rose and W. F. Bynum, eds., *Historical Aspects of the Neurosciences*, pp. 137–150. New York: Raven Press, 1982.

Lyle, H. Willoughby. "Robert Bentley Todd, M.D. (1809–1860), Clinical Neurologist and Clinical Teacher." In Sir D'Arcy Power, ed., *British Masters of Medicine*, pp. 110–123. Freeport, NY: Books for Libraries Press, 1936.

Thackeray, William Makepeace. *The Memoirs of Barry Lyndon, Esq.; Roundabout Papers*. London: Nelson, 1899.

Carol Helmstadter

LOUIS-RENÉ VILLERMÉ
(1782–1863)

Louis-René Villermé was a social physician who was an activist against workers' suffering. He was born on May 10, 1782, in the town of Lardy, near Paris. His childhood and his ideals were marked by the troubles brought to his town and his parents by the momentous events of the French Revolution.

After attending a day school in Lardy, Villermé went to a college in Paris, a city still full of the bloody remembrance of the Terror. He wanted to study medicine after the Convention created the new Schools of Health, which took the place of the old Faculties that the French Revolution had suppressed. In the renowned new School of Health of Paris, he learned from many prominent professors, such as Jean-Nicolas Desmarets Corvisart, the creator of the modern anatomical-clinic method; Jean-Noel Hallé, a pioneer in social hygiene; and Guillaume Dupuytren, a surgeon. His classmates included René Theophile Laennec and François Broussais. Villermé became the prosector (assistant) for Dupuytren's anatomical investigations. Throughout his life Villermé remained a faithful disciple of Dupuytren and a friend of Laennec.

In May 1803, the war between France and Great Britain forced many students in medicine and surgery into the army. Villermé was appointed a surgeon of the third class to the 75th Infantry Regiment; by 1806, he rose to the rank of surgeon-lieutenant and was reassigned to the 17th Dragoons Regiment. For twelve years, Villermé was present on the battlefields in Germany, Poland, and Spain. The surgeon general Pierre-François Percy called Villermé one of the greatest surgeons in the army.

At the end of the war, Villermé returned to the obstacle of preparing the doctoral thesis he had been unable to complete during his military service. While working as a town doctor in Paris, he began to write papers for medical and scientific societies. He soon learned that one of his fellow colleagues, the well-known surgeon Jacques Lisfranc de Saint-Martin, had fraudulently claimed to have invented an operation for the amputation of the foot that Villermé had actually invented. Although the Academy of Sciences subsequently validated Villermé's claim and acknowledged his rival's underhandedness, Villermé was so exasperated by the meanness of some of his colleagues that he decided to forsake the private practice of medicine and devote himself to social and scientific research. He was encouraged by his fiancée, Mademoiselle Morel d'Arleux, the daughter of the chief conservator of stamps in the Louvre Museum. Having a small military pension and a little fortune, Villermé and his wife could dedicate their lives to noble causes.

Villermé wrote a book, *Des Prisons telles qu'elles sont et telles qu'elles devraient être* (The prisons, what they are and what they have to be), in which he recalled his dreadful memories of the war and of the prisoners' harsh treatment in Spain. This book became well known in the French scientific community. He also became concerned with the suffering of workers—those who were essentially held captive by the hard world of industry. Some of the workers employed by the factories were only five years old, enduring at times thirteen or fourteen hours of work.

It is sometimes said that Villermé's first studies on the workers' world began around 1840, the year in which he published his well-known investigative report *Tableau de l'état physique et moral des ouvries employés dans les manufactures de coton, de laine et de soie* (Statistical studies of the physical and moral state of workers in the production of cotton, wool, and silk). Actually, the impetus for this study can be traced back to the remarkable statistical analyses of census data for Paris first published as *Recherches statistiques sur la ville de Paris* in 1821 by Gilbert de Chabrol de Volvic, Frederic Villot, and Baron Joseph Fourier. Villermé probably began to explore the major themes of the *Tableau*—the relationships among diseases, occupations, working conditions, and mortality—in the 1820s. These ideas appear in the introduction to Doctor Philibert Patissier's 1822 abridged translation (*Traité des maladies des Artisans d'après Ramazzini*) of Bernardino Ramazzini's (1633–1714) great work, *De Morbis Artificum* (On the diseases of trades, 1700). In his introduction, Patissier describes research carried out by Villermé in the hospitals of Paris, prior to 1822, on the relationship between diseases and particular occupations.

These studies denote a new stage in the knowledge of industrial health, which was previously merely descriptive. Tables of mortality and divisions by sex with regard to hospital patients and by occupations demonstrate that "mortality decreases as the wages of workers increase." The evidence provided by the new statistical approach to industrial health is reflected in the title of William Coleman's excellent book about France and Villermé, *Death Is A Social Disease.* For example, 100 of the 2,159 hospitalized municipal guards died (4.63 percent) while 130 of the 857 hospitalized laborers died (15.17 percent). Felt workers, who worked with mercury salts, had a mortality rate of 29 percent, and mother-of-pearl workers, who inhaled grindstone dust, had a rate of 26 percent. Carriage painters, who worked in confined workshops, had a mortality rate of 25 percent, but building trade painters, who worked outdoors, had a mortality rate of 10 percent. This research was an important forerunner of modern epidemiology and occupational medicine. Throughout his life Villermé applied both the anatomical-clinical and the analytical method to social statistics, demography, and economics.

On June 3, 1823, Villermé was elected to the prestigious Royal Academy of Medicine, founded by Antoine Portal and Louis XVIII. He published extensively in many of the foremost scientific and medical journals, such as the *Archives générales de médecine,* and his fame was acknowledged by many elite societies, including the Royal Academies of Science and Medicine and the free university Athenée Royal. His papers about mortality and health in rich and poor classes, birth distributions in urban and rural areas, and the influence of income or occupation on living conditions were valued not only in France but also abroad.

In 1829, Villermé founded the famous *Annales d'hygiene publique et de médecine légale*, with the physicians Alexis Parent-Duchatelet, Jean Esquirol, and Charles Marc and the chemist Joseph d'Arcet. His research examined the mortality rates of prisoners, the sizes of French men, reapers' health, vaccination, mutual assistance, moral hygiene, the signs of death, and almshouses. With Henri Milne-Edwards, he studied the influence of temperature on the mortality rate of children. He took an interest in hospital architecture and the medical assistance available in Paris. In 1831, he completed another study on birth distribution and conception dates according to climates and seasons. In 1832, as he was preparing a book about statistics and political economy, Europe was shaken by cholera epidemics, which Villermé dedicated himself to fighting.

On December 29, 1832, Villermé was elected to the Royal Academy of Moral and Political Sciences, an original component of the Institut de France, which had been suppressed by Napoleon but reestablished by Louis-Philippe. At first Villermé was a member of the political economy section; he moved the section of moral science in 1851. He continued publishing, chiefly in the *Annales*, about epidemics, cholera, hospitals for the elderly, anthropological research of the pathologist Jacques R. Tenon, and the fatal influence of marshes on children's health. In 1835, he also wrote some chapters on those subjects in the new *Dictionary of Medicine*. The year before, two papers that Villermé wrote about the British population brought him back to the issue of workers' problems, and he shared his ideas on the causes of civilized nations' wealth and poverty with the Academy of Moral Sciences. The academy realized better than the public authorities the heavy weight of adversities that were crushing the life and work of the poor classes, and it wanted to study them thoroughly. On November 8, 1834, the academy decided to spend Prime Minister Guizot's grant of four thousand francs for an inquiry concerning the condition of the working classes. The academy entrusted the inquiry to Villermé and Benoiston de Chateauneuf, a fellow statistician and former army surgeon.

The two began a pilgrimage searching for truth and testimonies. Benoiston explored the western areas near the ocean and the most fertile regions of the country, while Villermé went to the northern, eastern, and southern provinces before going to Zurich, where he could compare the conditions of French and Swiss workers. He traveled for two years. "Everywhere," he wrote, "I ought to have seen the effects of the industry on the workers, and to inquire about poverty without humiliating it. . . . Everywhere judges, doctors, manufacturers, or simple workers tried to help me. . . . I followed the worker from his workshop to his home, I came in there with him." He noted all with accuracy, making thorough studies of the workers, including their physical aptitudes and surroundings. He stated precisely the harmful situations, temperatures, surfaces, hygrometer values, and lighting facing the workers. He denounced vibrations, dust, dangerous postures, repetitive work, and "motions which are rehearsed with an oppressive uniformity in the tight enclosure of one hall." He showed the difference between industrial and service workers. His description of the textile factories, which were then the greatest French industry and were taken by Villermé as the base of his inquiry, was completed with precise accounts of daily life, giving the most faithful picture of the working class and its environment. In many Alsatian factories, Villermé was disturbed by the harsh work of women, who had to labor even at night, and the abominable employment of very young children who worked up to sixteen hours a day. Such workers had to travel more than five miles to work, wore poor clothing, and lived in dirty houses furnished with beds without sheets.

These stories are a contrast to the efforts of Villermé's friends at the Industrial Society of Mulhouse: the Koechlins, Schlumbergers, and Dollfuses, who—in spite of blind laws of competition—created cities, gardens, schools, cooperative societies, and banks for the workers. At Tarare, the weavers seem to be favored by their half-rustic life. But in the north, Villermé found the appalling "Cellars of Lille," mentioned in Victor Hugo's poem, "Les Châtiments." In Reims, as in many other workers' towns and regions, alcoholism devastated families, and many young girls were driven to prostitution, going to filthy houses after they left the factory "to make the fifth quarter of the day." But in Sedan, older workers were provided for, and in Lodève, the working day was no longer than twelve hours and workers carried umbrellas, a sign of wealth during the time of Louis-Philippe. In Lyon, the workshops were small and narrow, allowing only nine cubic meters per worker. The weavers of the Rhodanian city were said to be practicing Malthus's famous "moral restraint." In Zurich, where the lifestyle was frugal, the communal school and social aid brought peerless assistance to workers' families.

For each district, region, and sometimes factory, Villermé recorded many notes and numbers that he placed in detailed tables, which give by example a summary of the wages for all sorts of employments (e.g., 0.6 francs a day for children, 1.25 francs for women, and 2–4 francs for the men in Reims or Lille). These tables also provide the prices of the essential elements of the daily life in accurate and lively documents. In 1840, all these reports were published first in the *Annales d'hygiene* and in the academy's reviews and then in two volumes entitled *Tableau de l'état physique et moral des ouvriers employés dans les manufactures de coton, de laine et de soie* (Statistical studies of the physical and moral state of workers in the production of cotton, wool, and silk). The predominant topic of these pages was the poignant drama of child labor, which Villermé had already exposed during a solemn meeting of the Five Academies on May 2, 1837. Like Marie-Joseph Jacquard who invented a technique that abolished the job of wire-drawing under the looms, Villermé was tormented by the lives of the thousands of children who were working long hours at weaving machines or in mines. Using the English Bill of 1833 as an example, he beseeched the government to impose "a law of humanity" and convinced his friends to send a petition from the Industrial Society of Mulhouse and a Protestant association to the Deputies' Chamber. The cardinal archbishop of Rouen supported Villermé's action by proposing a law that would prevent "killing child workers." After much debate, a law restricting child labor in factories was passed by the two legislative chambers and signed by King Louis-Philippe on March 22, 1841. This law was actually very limited: children could be employed at eight years old in enterprises of more than twenty workers. In 1850, the legal age was pushed up to ten; in 1874, it was raised to twelve, and work inspectors were established to enforce the law.

In the meantime, Villermé undertook studies of other issues related to the welfare of children, such as schools, pensions, and mutual aid societies. After the revolution in 1849, he became suspicious regarding rules for workers' associations. He wrote *Des Associations ouvrières* (On workers' associations), showing a sort of paradoxical independence as to republican public opinion. He also made a study of housing for workers, using the accomplishments of the Industrial Society of Mulhouse as an example.

In 1850, he published a paper, "Accidents Produced in Industrial Work-shops by Mechanical Engines," in the *Journal of Economists*, calling for the construction of "clean machines" that would not produce dust and for preventive plans and the neutralization of risks. These demands reveal Villermé as an excellent safety engineer and mechanic. He wrote about all kinds of modern protective fittings, grates, railings, cages, straps, and ward-lattices for moving machines. He prescribed instructions that forbid greasing or making repairs on working machines. He also recommended inquiries into accidents, the use of close-fitting clothes, the construction of large and well-lit workshops and passages, the prohibition of children working on dangerous machines, and the creation of work inspectors. Villermé ended his paper by reminding industrial leaders of Article 1383 of the Civil Code: "Every man is responsible for damages induced by his actions, by his negligence or by his imprudence."

In the following years, he continued his sociomedical investigations and discussed Malthus and his doctrine with his friends. Even in 1861, he was pushing for reforms: he wrote a paper about lunatic asylums and settlements. As the emperor's doctor, Maxime Vernois, noted, Villermé amazed others with his wisdom and his humor during "long and very affectionate conversations."

After the death of his wife, Villermé lived near his daughter. He died on November 16, 1863. As Flora Tristan wrote, he was "one of the men who have been the most intelligent and devoted to the Holy Workmen's Cause." Villermé said of himself: "My sole purpose has been the truth."

BIBLIOGRAPHY

The main manuscript sources are found in the Army Historical Service of Vincennes, the private archives of the descendants of Villermé, the Archives of the Royal Academy of Belgium, and the Archives of Lardy. These sources are discussed in *Louis-René Villermé* (Valentin 1993), which also lists more than 200 books and articles Villermé wrote.

Works by Louis-René Villermé

Des Prisons telles qu'elles sont et telles qu'elles devraient être: Ouvrage dans lequel on les considère par rapport à l'hygiène, à la morale et à l'économie politique (Prisons: What they are and what they should be). Paris: Méquignon-Marvis, 1820.

Tableau de l'état physique et moral des ouvries employés dans les manufactures de coton, de laine et de soie (Statistical studies of the physical and moral state of workers in the production of cotton, wool and silk). 2 vols. Paris: Jules Renouard, 1840. Reprint ed., Paris: Editions d'histoire sociale, 1979.

"Des Accidents produits dans les ateliers industriels par les appareils mécaniques." *Journal des économistes* 27 (1850): 215–222.

Books about Louis-René Villermé and Related Topics

Ackerknecht, E. H. *Medicine at the Paris Hospital, 1794–1848.* Baltimore: Johns Hopkins University Press, 1967.

Chevalier, Louis. *Laboring Classes and Dangerous Classes in Paris during the First Half of the Nineteenth Century.* Translated by Frank Jellinek. New York: Howard Fertig, 1973.

Coleman, William. *Death Is a Social Disease: Public Health and Political Economy in Early Industrial France.* Madison: University of Wisconsin Press, 1982.

Lécuyer, Bernard, and A. P. Oberschall. "The Early History of Social Research." In D. L. Sills, ed., *International Encyclopedia of the Social Sciences*, 15: 36–53: New York: Macmillan, 1968–1979.

Shapiro, Ann-Louise. *Housing the Poor of Paris, 1850–1902.* Madison: University of Wisconsin Press, 1985.

Valentin, Michel. *Travail des hommes et savants oubliés: Histoire de la médecine du travail, de la securité et de l'ergonomie* (Work of men and forgotten scholars: History of ergonomics and industrial health). Paris: Docis, 1978.

———. *Louis-René Villermé (1782–1863).* Paris: Editions DOCIS, 1993.

Michel Valentin

WILLIAM WITHERING
(1741–1799)

William Withering is best remembered as the physician who first demonstrated the usefulness of digitalis, an extract of the leaves of the purple foxglove plant. The report of his study of its clinical value, *An Account of the Foxglove and Some of Its Medical Uses: With Practical Remarks on Dropsy, and Other Diseases* (1785), is a medical classic. Digitalis is used widely even today to treat a variety of cardiac diseases, principally congestive heart failure. Its name comes from the Latin name for the plant, *Digitalis purpurea*.

Withering was born on March 17, 1741, in the town of Wellington, north of London. William was the only son, and one of three children, of Edward Witherings (sic), a successful apothecary, and Sarah (née Hector). Little is known about his boyhood, aside from the fact that he was educated by a neighboring minister before entering an apprenticeship with a physician at about age seventeen. After four years as an apprentice, he matriculated at the University of Edinburgh to study medicine. The ancient universities of Oxford and Cambridge were then suffering from the effects of the Test Acts, which essentially permitted only Anglicans to attend or to teach. Consequently, Dissenters, and those interested in a more secular education, were forced to attend schools in the provinces and in Scotland. The medical school at Edinburgh was, at the time, the foremost medical school in Great Britain, and among Withering's teachers were Alexander Monroe Secundus, in anatomy, and William Cullen, in medical chemistry. Graduating in 1766, Withering published his dissertation on scarlet fever, *De Angina Gangraenosa*, in Latin, as was the custom.

Following several months of travel abroad, Withering set up a general practice in Stafford, in the Midlands, a region of England about to enter the early phases of the Industrial Revolution. This was also just before the beginnings of modern medicine, if this can be dated from the development of smallpox vaccination by Edward Jenner and Withering's study of digitalis. Both of these medical milestones were the result of clinical trials and were closely followed in time by the work of French physician-scientists like Marie F. X. Bichat, Jean N. Corvisart, and René Laënnec, who were demonstrating that diseases had their origins in organs and tissues and that changes in organ function produced clinical symptoms and signs of disease in the patient.

Withering embarked on his practice at a time when there were relatively few physicians, and most of them came from, and practiced among, the upper classes. During the next nine years, his practice was light enough to allow him ample time to pursue his interest in botany and to collect flora throughout Great Britain. Withering's two-volume *A Botanical Arrangement of All the Vegetables Naturally Growing in Great Britain* (1776) was the first classification of British plants using Linnaean binomial nomenclature, and in subsequent editions was widely used throughout the first half of the nineteenth century.

In 1775, Withering moved to Birmingham where his practice became quite successful, with many demands for his consultative skills coming from the Midlands and western counties. He soon became a member of the Lunar Society of Birmingham, the best known of the provincial associations, which were then fulfilling the role that the ancient universities had abdicated and serving as sources of much ferment, leading to scientific, mathematical, and mechanical advances. At the monthly meetings of the Lunar Society, Withering and fellow members such as James Watt, Joseph Priestley, Josiah Wedgwood, and Erasmus Darwin discussed not only science but also literature and art.

Withering's interest in the foxglove plant as a therapeutic agent was explained in the now-famous introductory paragraph of *An Account of the Foxglove*, which was published after ten years of clinical experience with the drug:

In the year 1775, my opinion was asked concerning a family receipt for the cure of dropsy. I was told that it had long been kept a secret by an old woman in Shropshire, who had sometimes made cures after the more regular practitioners had failed. I was informed also, that the effects produced were violent vomiting and purging; for the diuretic effects seem to have been overlooked. This medicine was composed of twenty or more different herbs; but it was not very difficult for one conversant in these subjects, to perceive, that the active herb could be no other than the Foxglove. (Withering 1785: 2)

How Withering was able to spot the single active drug in such a complex mixture is not known; however, it is presumably related to his vast knowledge of British botanicals. He probably knew the effects of all the other ingredients and concluded that foxglove must be the active agent, as he knew that squill, a plant with mild diuretic activity, also caused nausea and vomiting. Foxglove grew like a weed throughout the English Midlands, so he must have been quite familiar with it.

Withering ground dried leaves of the plant into a powder and initially administered it as either an infusion or a decoction (i.e. soaked, or boiled in water). He later settled on giving the powdered leaf directly in measured doses. In *An Account of the Foxglove*, he described 163 patients from his personal practice who had dropsy. This clinical condition, now known as anasarca or diffuse edema, can be caused by both congestive heart failure and renal failure and was in itself considered an illness in the eighteenth century. Withering reported that 65 to 80 percent of his patients responded favorably to the drug. Most of the cases in which it failed had a clinical history suggesting a cause of edema other than heart failure, such as a large ovarian cyst or ascites from liver failure. Although Withering recognized that the drug had some effect on the heart, he thought of it as a diuretic, particularly effective in dropsy. According to his admiring biographers, "*An Account of the Foxglove* was the first scientific treatise on the treatment of disease written in English, and it remains today as one of the really great English contributions to treatment'' (Peck and Wilkinson 1950: 68). Not only was the drug effective, but Withering's method of studying its effect was a forerunner of today's clinical trials in that all of the patients who received the drug were reported, not just the successful ones, as had been the custom.

Despite Withering's busy medical practice, he performed experiments in chemistry and mineralogy, which resulted in several papers in the *Philosophical Transactions* of the Royal Society. Among them was his discovery of the chemical structure of barium carbonate, subsequently named Witherite in his honor. His mineralogical studies included analyzing the water of several spas. His botanical studies gained him significant attention in Europe, and a plant genus was named *Witheringia* by a French botanist. In 1784 the Royal Society elected him a fellow. Withering began to show symptoms of pulmonary tuberculosis by 1780, and in 1790, after repeated attacks of pleurisy, he gave up his practice. He died on October 6, 1799, age fifty-eight, surrounded by his family, his last words being, ''I am ready.'' He is buried in the old church near his home in Birmingham, and his monument is inscribed with his name and encircled with depictions of the purple foxglove and *Witheringia* plants.

BIBLIOGRAPHY

Some of Withering's unpublished letters are kept at the Birmingham Reference Library. An English translation of Withering's medical school dissertation, his first scientific publication, *Dissertatio Medica Inauguralis, De Angina Gangraenosa* (1766), has been published (O'Malley 1953). The most recent full-length biography of Withering's life (Peck and Wilkinson 1950) describes a decent man with few failings, and, as the authors are also from Birmingham, a good deal of local history. Much of what we know about Withering is derived from the two-volume memoir and collection of his writings published by his son (Withering 1822).

Writings by William Withering

A Botanical Arrangement of All the Vegetables Naturally Growing in Great Britain. 2 vols. Birmingham: For T. Cadell, P. Elmsley and G. Robinson, 1776. (This book appeared in two more editions during Withering's life [1787, 1796]. His son William Withering [1775–1832] brought out four more editions, and subsequent editions were edited by William Macgillivray. Fourteen editions were published by 1877.)

An Account of the Foxglove, and Some of Its Medical Uses: With Practical Remarks on Dropsy, and Other Diseases. London: G. G. J. & J. Robinson, 1785. (Valuable new reprints of this book appeared in the 1980s.)

Works about William Withering and Related Topics

Aronson, J. K. *An Account of the Foxglove and Its Medical Uses 1785–1985.* London: Oxford University Press, 1985. (Aronson's edition includes a facsimile of the original book, along with useful marginal notes explaining the historical allusions, references to eighteenth-century drugs and botanicals, and personal references. It also contains a review of the use of digitalis in medicine into the 1980s, a biography of Withering, and a scientific analysis of the series of patients treated with foxglove and recorded in *An Account of the Foxglove*.)

Estes, J. Worth, and Paul Dudley White. "William Withering and the Purple Foxglove." *Scientific American* 21 (6) (1965): 110–119.

Fulton, John F. "The Place of William Withering in Scientific Medicine." *Journal of the History of Medicine and Allied Sciences* 8 (1985): 1–15.

Mann, Ronald D. *William Withering and the Foxglove*. Hingham, MA: MTP Press Ltd., 1985. (Includes a selection of Withering's letters from William Osler's bequest to the Royal Society of Medicine and facsimiles of some of the letters.)

O'Malley, Charles D. "A Translation of William Withering's *De Angina Gangraenosa*." *Journal of the History of Medicine and Allied Sciences* 8 (1953): 15–45. (Withering did not clearly distinguish between scarlet fever and diphtheria, the other bacterial cause of severe tonsillitis in his medical school dissertation.)

Peck, T., and Douglas Wilkinson. *William Withering of Birmingham M.D., F.R.S., F.L.S.* Bristol: John Wright & Sons, 1950.

Schofield, Robert E. *The Lunar Society of Birmingham*. Oxford: Clarendon Press, 1963.

Withering, William. *A Memoir of the Life, Character, and Writings, of William Withering, M.D., F.R.S., etc., etc. Being a Biography of 248 Pages Prefixed to the Miscellaneous Tracts of the Late William Withering [1741–1799]*. 2 vols. London: Longmans et al., 1822.

Paul G. Dyment

WU LIEN-TEH
(1879–1960)

Wu Lien-teh, plague expert and Chinese public health pioneer, was born in Penang in the Straits Settlements (present-day Malaysia) on March 10, 1879. He was the fourth of five sons in a family of eleven siblings who survived infancy. His father, Ng Khee-hok was a successful goldsmith and jewelry merchant, originally from Guangdong province in China, and his mother, Lam Choy-fan, was born in Penang to parents originally from Guangdong as well. Young Wu received his first schooling at the Penang Free School, a school run along English lines. The family name in Cantonese is romanized as Ng, and his personal name was Leen-tuck, meaning "united virtues." Later in life, Wu adopted the Mandarin pronunciation of his name: Wu Lien-teh. Upon entering the Penang Free School, Wu encountered the first of several mutations in his name; the school clerk romanized the Cantonese, Ng Leen-tuck, into his own Hokien dialect as Gnoh Lean-teik. In an act of compromise, Gnoh Lean-tuck was agreed upon.

While in school in Penang, Wu decided that he would become a physician; as an Asian, he could not enter the civil service but would be accepted into a profession such as law, medicine, or engineering. Being an outstanding student, Wu was awarded one of two queen's scholarships for students from the Straits Settlements for university study in Great Britain. Upon the suggestion of his teachers and advisers in Penang, he applied and was admitted to Emmanuel College in Cambridge. He matriculated there in 1896, and his name underwent a further mutation when the registrar did not realize that Asian names are usually written with the surname first and personal name last; thus Gnoh Lean-tuck became Mr. G. L. Tuck, the name Wu used all during his medical and postgraduate education. He entered the natural science course along with the medical course, and in addition to having lectures in physiology from Michael Foster, in his final year Wu met F. Gowland Hopkins. Hopkins was the supervisor of science studies at Emmanuel College and taught Wu some biochemistry (even though Hopkins was a tutor in anatomy, a subject in which he had become a bit rusty). After his three-year course, Wu received a first-class honors B.A. degree in natural science in 1899 and spent his summer in work on bacteriology and pathology with German Sims Woodhead.

For the final three years of the medical degree, Wu enrolled at St. Mary's Hospital in London where he won a three-year scholarship, which covered all fees and hospital tuitions. He was able to pass the Cambridge medical examinations after two and one-half years and thus completed the M.B and B.Chir. degrees, the basic requirements for medical practice. Intent on learning more about a major infectious disease important in the Straits Settlements, tuberculosis, he secured one of the three positions as house physician at the Brompton Hospital for Consumption and Diseases of the Chest in London, a position he held for six months. His college rewarded his hard work and scholarship with a two year research fellowship, which enabled Wu to pursue his interest in infectious diseases more extensively. For the first year of this fellowship, he went on a grand tour of the major laboratories of Europe: three months with Ronald Ross (Nobel Prize 1902) at the brand new Liverpool School of Tropical Medicine (founded 1899), eight months with Karl Fraenkel (former assistant to Robert Koch) in Halle, and three months at the Pasteur Institute in Paris in the laboratory of Elie Metchnikoff (Nobel Prize 1908).

In Halle, Wu picked a research problem suggested by Fraenkel: the investigation of tetanus in patients receiving gelatin infusions as therapy for aneurysms. The idea was that the thick suspensions of gelatin would induce clot formation in the aneurysmal sac and lead to fibrosis and strengthening of the vessel wall. Wu identified tetanus spores in the gelatin preparations and showed that the usual sterilization methods were inadequate. He continued this research in Paris on French samples of gelatin with similar findings and was able to submit this research for his Cambridge M.D. thesis, "The Occurrence of Tetanus Spores in Gelatine." It was accepted in August 1903, but since the M.D. could not be granted sooner than three years after the M.B., he left England for home with his M.D. to be granted in absentia two years later.

With support from a second-year research fellowship from Emmanuel College, Wu joined the newly established Institute for Medical Research in Kuala Lumpur, capital city of the Federated Malay States. Wu was the one native of the region on the senior scientific staff of five scientists. In collaboration with Hamilton Wright and C. W. Daniels, he undertook a search for an infectious agent as the cause of beriberi. This illness, along with dysentery and malaria, was a major cause of death and sickness in the hospital associated with the institute. Wu also pursued investigations of asymptomatic roundworm infestations in cattle and published a brief report on this work in the annual report of the institute for 1903–1904. This year in Kuala Lumpur was important for the future direction of Wu's career in that he helped organize, and was elected president of, the Selangor Literary and Debating Society, a group of Western and Eastern men living in the State of Selangor. They were dedicated to several liberal causes and advocated reforms, such as cutting off the queue (the long braid of hair worn by Chinese men, originally as a sign of subservience to the Manchu conquerors of China in the seventeenth century), schooling for girls, and curbing official corruption. Wu became a lifelong active advocate for these and other liberal reforms.

With no prospect for a research career in the Straits Settlements, Wu entered the private practice of medicine in Penang. Soon he had developed a thriving practice and a forum for his ideas on social and medical reform. He was especially concerned with the problem of opium addiction, and he openly sought legal and social means to control its use. He founded and was president of the

Penang Anti-Opium Association, and in 1906 he organized the Anti-Opium Conference of the Straits Settlements and Federated Malay States, which drew about 3,000 participants. This anti-opium activity was opposed by local government and business interests, and in a targeted raid, Wu was found to have a small quantity of tincture of opium for medical use in his office. Because he did not have the pro-forma licenses, he was arrested, tried, and fined one hundred dollars. Yet at this same time he received an invitation from the British government to participate in an anti-opium conference in London in 1907. That year too, he received and accepted an offer from Yuan Shih-kai, grand councillor of China, to become vice director of the Imperial Medical College in Tientsin, one of the schools recently established to educate Chinese students in Western medicine. He continued his anti-opium campaigns in China and was sent as a Chinese delegate to the first International Opium Conference in the Hague in 1911.

The opportunity to investigate an epidemic of fatal illness in Manchuria gave Wu a new challenge and a new direction in his work. Manchuria in 1910 was in political turmoil. Officially under Chinese government control, with a viceroy in charge, in reality, both Japan and Russia had troops and other official agents stationed in Manchuria. This situation was one result of the war involving Japan and Russia and the establishment of three major railway routes in northeast China. One railway was controlled by the Japanese, one by the Russians, and one by the Chinese. Russia and Japan had agreed in secret to carve Manchuria into spheres of influence, and Japan had just annexed Korea in the summer of 1910.

The index case of what turned out to be plague, as best as could be determined by contemporary investigation, was a migrant trapper who died in Manchouli in mid-October 1910. At that time, aided by the expanding railroads, Chinese from the south would travel to Manchuria to trap the Siberian marmot for its fur. At the end of the trapping season, these migrants would return to their homes in the south. Plague spread rapidly among the poor and crowded camps of these migrant trappers and was carried south along the railway, in this case, the Russian-controlled one, and it reached Harbin on October 27, 1910, Changchun in mid-December, and Beijing a month later, in January 1911. When people could not get on the trains, they fled south by road and spread the disease into the countryside.

The local Russian and Japanese authorities were implementing local measures, but only the central Chinese government could officially act on a broad scale. In a move to respond to both Chinese and foreign pressure, the Manchu Court through the Ministry of Foreign Affairs sent Wu Lien-teh to Harbin to investigate the plague on its behalf. In late December 1910, Wu and a senior medical student named Lin arrived in Harbin. Lin was particularly valuable because Wu, as an "overseas Chinese," was not fluent in Chinese, especially the local dialects.

On his third day in Harbin, Wu managed to do a limited postmortem examination on a woman who had just died, and he observed massive infection of lung, heart, spleen, and liver with bacteria with the morphology and staining characteristics of Alexandre Yersin's plague bacillus.

As an astute clinician with the most up-to-date education, Wu made the clinical diagnosis of the pneumonic form of plague, while the local Russian doctors in Harbin suspected bubonic plague, and continued to examine patients without respiratory precautions. A senior French physician, Dr. Mesny, sent to Harbin a little later, refused to accept Wu's evaluation and failed to take precautions. He died six days later. This may have been a turning point, because in January 1911 the Chinese government sent troops and police to Manchuria in an attempt to control population movements and enforce quarantines. A new plague hospital was hastily set up and the old one burned down. With the ground frozen, it was impossible to bury the dead. At one point Wu reported seeing two thousand coffins in rows with more dead on the ground because of a shortage of coffins. Worried that rats might become infected by eating the dead bodies, Wu was able to enlist the support of some local officials, and then following the traditional Chinese approach, he wrote a memorial to the throne. Three days later he received an imperial edict allowing mass cremation of the dead bodies.

From the time Wu arrived in Harbin, he carried out investigations on the nature of plague, the bacillus, and its mode of spread. His modern training in Europe provided him with approaches that were admired and accepted by European, American, and Japanese medical authorities. Probably for the first time, Western medicine was learning from Chinese physicians about modern theories of disease.

The International Plague Conference, which was held in Mukden during April 1911, the first international scientific meeting held in China, evolved out of China's political attempts to outmaneuver the Russians and Japanese. During the epidemic, both nations proposed sending "observers" and "investigators." China, reasonably enough, saw these moves as pretexts for further incursions of military units into Manchuria. This fear seemed to prompt the Chinese invitation to the United States and other governments to send experts too. China skillfully played the American researchers against the Russian and Japanese, and soon these foreign advisers were converted to "delegates" to an international plague conference. This, of course, made it harder to include military and police personnel in a purely scientific endeavor. Worried that the conference might pass resolutions, in the name of the international community, that would limit their expansionist control of the South Manchurian Railway, the Japanese at first did not respond to the Chinese invitation, hoping that the absence of Shibasaburo Kitasato, the discoverer of plague germs, would kill the meeting. When it was clear that this tactic had failed, Kitasato was induced to make several disparaging remarks about the ability and even the rights of the Chinese to contribute to the conference. At the conference, however, he was accorded sufficient recognition as chairman of the sections on pathology and bacteriology, "the most important ones," that he put his politics aside and participated in the scientific sessions.

In the first few months of 1911, the Chinese and Americans collected new data on pneumonic plague and thus were in the dominant scientific position when the conference was held in April 1911.

Wu was the president of the conference, and the Japanese were especially upset that a young Chinese should get the international prestige of such a position. By the end of the meeting, however, he had won the respect and acceptance of most of the delegates. The conference lasted three weeks and included demonstrations and ongoing experiments. A tarbagan was even brought to the conference and treated as a mascot and became quite tame. The conference passed forty-five resolutions as recommendations to the Chinese government. These recommendations appeared to be especially sensitive to Chinese positions and were not very politically motivated. Remarkably, the delegates, even though their governments sent them for obvious political reasons, were able to focus on medical and scientific matters rather well. Many of the delegates were personally acquainted or had studied with the same teachers in Europe, thus providing additional extranational loyalties. The success of this conference owed much to Wu's diplomatic skills and his credibility as a medical scientist.

The conference proceedings were published in Manila under Richard P. Strong's editorship, and this document became the major scientific source on pneumonic plague. Wu Lien-teh did not return to the Tientsin Medical School but continued to study plague in Harbin. In the summer of 1912 the North Manchurian Plague Prevention Service was established under Dr. Wu's direction by the imperial Chinese government. In perhaps one of its final acts before the Republican Revolution in October 1911, the imperial regime established Western medicine as official state policy. Wu trained Chinese physicians in research on epidemic diseases, and this service continued until 1931 to be China's premier medical organization against plague as well as cholera. Wu was recognized internationally as the authority on pneumonic plague, and his monograph of 1926 is still a standard reference on that disease.

In addition to his work on plague, cholera, and public health, especially anti-opium work, Wu was an effective organizer and administrator. He was a founding member of the China Medical Association in 1925 and its successor, the Chinese Medical Association in 1932, an advocate for uniform standards in Chinese medical education, and organizer of many special groups to promote health, such as the National Anti-Tuberculosis Association. Wu had an active interest in the medical culture of China and with Wong Chi-min wrote *History of Chinese Medicine* (1932, 1936), a two–part compendium including traditional Chinese medicine and an institutional history of Western medicine in China.

Wu Lien-teh was recruited to China from his home in Penang by the last imperial government of China; he worked efficiently for the Republican government as well as under that of the Kuomintang (Nationalist). Working in Harbin with both Russian and Japanese forces on Chinese territory, Wu was able to avoid political entanglements that might have compromised his public health and medical work. In 1931, however, the North Manchurian Plague Prevention Service was finally disrupted by the increasing factional fighting in China and by the militaristic actions of the Japanese. With the establishment of a new Nationalist government in Nanjing in 1929 and upon the recommendation of an international board of consultants, China established the National Quarantine Service with overall public health responsibility for China. Dr. Wu was appointed to head this new national health organization in 1930. Upon the Japanese invasion of 1937, the seizure of the Quarantine Service, and the shelling of his home in Shanghai, Wu decided to seek refuge in Penang rather than to continue under Japanese authority.

As events led up to World War II, Wu decided to resume general medical practice in Penang after a hiatus of some thirty years. This he continued during and after the Japanese occupation of Malaya. After the war, Wu effectively used his international contacts and his professional stature to advocate improved public health measures in Malaya. To the end of his life he continued his efforts to end one of Asia's major health problems, opium use and addiction.

BIBLIOGRAPHY

The three most extensive and available sources of information about Wu Lien-teh are his autobiography, *Plague Fighter: The Autobiography of a Modern Chinese Physician* (1959), his magnum opus on plague, *A Treatise on Pneumonic Plague* (1926), and the (seven) *Reports of the North Manchurian Plague Prevention Service* (1914–1930). A bibliography of the publications of the Plague Prevention Service is given in an appendix to his autobiography. Wu distributed his papers and collections to several Asian institutions, and these are described in *Plague Fighter*. Over two thousand volumes from his personal library were donated to the Nanyang University of Singapore in 1957 and form the Wu Lien-teh Collection (now in the Central and Medical Libraries of the National University of Singapore) along with about four hundred photographs donated by Wu's family. Material on plague from Harbin, including some biological material, was given to Hong Kong University. Recent publication of a pictorial reminiscence, *Memories of Dr. Wu Lien-Teh, Plague Fighter* (1995), by Wu's daughter, Wu Yu-lin, is a useful supplement to his autobiography. Two sources that give the political and medical context for Wu's work on the Manchurian plague epidemic of 1910–1911 are the monograph by Carl F. Nathan, *Plague Prevention and Politics in Manchuria, 1910–1931* (1967), and the article by Eli Chernin, *Richard Pearson Strong and the Manchurian Epidemic of Pneumonic Plague, 1910–1911* (1989). Two obituaries can be found in the *British Medical Journal* (1960).

Writings by Wu Lien-teh

Reports of the North Manchurian Plague Prevention Service. Tientsin: Tientsin Press. 1914–1930.
A Treatise on Pneumonic Plague. Geneva: League of Nations, 1926.
(with K. Chimin Wong). *History of Chinese Medicine.* 1st ed. Tientsin: Tientsin Press, 1932; 2nd ed. Shanghai: National Quarantine Service, 1936. Reprint ed., New York: AMS Press, 1973.

Plague Fighter: The Autobiography of a Modern Chinese Physician. Cambridge: W. Heffer & Sons, 1959.

Writings about Wu Lien-teh and Related Topics

Chernin, Eli. "Richard Pearson Strong and the Manchurian Epidemic of Pneumonic Plague, 1910–1911." *Journal of the History of Medicine Allied Sciences* 44 (1989): 296–319.

Goh, L. G. "Wisdom and Western Science: The Work of Dr. Wu Lien-Teh." *Asia-Pacific Journal of Public Health* 1 (1987): 99–109.

Ho, T. M. "The Plague Fighter, A Remembrance." *Family Practitioner* 6 (1983): 75–84.

Manson-Bahr, Philip. "Obituary. Wu Lien-teh." *British Medical Journal* 1 (1960): 429–430.

Nathan, Carl F. *Plague Prevention and Politics in Manchuria, 1910–1931*. Cambridge, MA: East Asian Research Center, Harvard University, 1967.

Nixon, W. C. W. "Obituary. Wu Lien-teh." *British Medical Journal* 1 (1960): 655.

Strong, Richard Pearson, ed. *Report of the International Plague Conference*. Manila: Bureau of Printing, 1912.

Wu, Xi-ke. "Dr. Wu Lian-teh, Renowned Epidemiologist and Pioneer of Modern Health Work in China." *Chinese Medical Journal* 100 (1987): 509–512.

Wu, Yu-lin. *Memories of Dr. Wu Lien-Teh, Plague Fighter*. Singapore: World Scientific, 1995.

William C. Summers

HILLEL YAFFE
(1864–1936)

Hillel Yaffe, physician, malaria fighter, and one of the founders of Israel's public health system, was born in the Ukraine to a Jewish merchant's family that granted its children a broad and liberal education. During his childhood, a call for social revolutions and nationalistic movements, accompanied by increased anti-Semitism, swept through Europe. While still a high school student, Yaffe met the Jewish writer Ben-Ami, an active member of the Russian Zionist movement, who urged emigration to Israel (then Palestine) and action to promote the rebirth of the Jewish people. As a result, Yaffe became a Zionist and decided to study medicine and emigrate to Israel.

For Jews, the study of medicine was possible only in Western and Central Europe, because the faculties of medicine in Eastern Europe maintained a "numerous clausus"—a limit on Jewish students of approximately 1 percent. Yaffe selected the Faculté de Médecine Université de Genève in Geneva, Switzerland, one of the best medical schools at the time and preferred by many Jewish students from all over Europe. After graduating with honors in 1889, Yaffe took specialized training in ophthalmology in Paris, having heard that ophthalmology was one of the most severe medical problems in Israel. In 1891, he emigrated to Israel.

At the end of the nineteenth century, the Jewish community in Israel had only about thirty doctors, located mainly in the central cities of Jerusalem, Tiberias, Safed, and Jaffa; only a few were on farms and in villages. After working for the small Jewish community in Haifa, Yaffe went to Tiberias (1891–1893). In 1893 Baron Rothschild of Paris invited Yaffe to serve as principal physician and director of the Jacob Memorial Hospital in Zichron Jacob, one of the Israeli villages founded by the Baron. This hospital was the only medical center for the numerous malaria patients in the area.

Malaria was one of the most severe problems of the first agricultural settlers in Israel, because many Jewish settlement districts were in marshes, the breeding places of the anopheles mosquito that transmits malaria. Many farms and villages were abandoned because of malaria. The death rate from malaria among settlers who refused to leave was generally 60 percent; in Hadera it reached 90 percent. Petah Tikva, the first Jewish village founded in Israel, was abandoned three times because of malaria. Controlling malaria was therefore the key to the continued existence of Jewish settlements in Israel. Baron Rothschild, under whose auspices the settlements functioned, was aware of the malaria problem, and he agreed to finance the fight against it. Thus, Yaffe's appointment was not only part of the fight against malaria but also part of the struggle for the future settlement of Israel.

In the 1890s the battle against malaria generally involved draining swamps by planting eucalyptus trees imported from Australia, spraying swamps with kerosene to prevent the breeding of the anopheles mosquitoes, and administering the antimalarial drug quinine. After consultations with malaria research colleagues in Italy and at the Pasteur Institute in Paris, Yaffe decided to use a systematic combination of these approaches. Because most of the malaria-affected areas in Israel were close to the Mediterranean Sea or to Kinneret Lake (Sea of Galilee), Yaffe decided that besides draining the swamps by planting eucalyptus trees, ditches should be dug in order to drain stagnant waters into the sea. Settlement worker groups were organized to carry out the project as their first priority. Until the swamp-draining projects could be completed, Yaffe organized the systematic spraying of the swamps with kerosene; at the same time, all of the settlers and workers who participated in the project received a registered supply of quinine, along with a warning that they would be dismissed if they did not observe the doctor's orders. Yaffe's system of fighting malaria was eventually adopted by all agricultural settlements in Israel. As a result, malaria was successfully controlled in Israel, and Yaffe's methods have been widely applied in developing countries.

In 1895, Yaffe was elected head of the Israel Zionist Organization to enhance Zionist settlement and organizational activities. Therefore, he left the Zichron Jacob Hospital and moved to Jaffa, where most Zionist institutions were situated. Nonetheless, Yaffe did not relinquish his public health work, especially those related to raising the education level of the settlers' children in order to improve the health status of the Jewish community and boost awareness of preventive medicine.

In 1896, Yaffe founded a girls' school, based on a secular curriculum, which was directed by his wife. Given the traditional social framework of the Orthodox Jewish community in Israel, the education of girls was especially important for improving the prospects of the next generation.

In 1901, Yaffe became director of Shaar Zion Community Hospital (Zion's Gate) in Jaffa, which had been founded six years earlier by the B'nai B'rith Organization. Because of his knowledge of the health needs of the agricultural settlements, Yaffe extended the activities of the hospital to serve areas outside the city. Yaffe created contacts between settlement workers and the hospital by allocating two rooms for sick workers and an additional room for convalescing workers, especially malaria patients, who needed special rest and nutrition before returning to work.

At the time, agricultural workers who were employed in the settlements on a daily basis were not entitled to medical aid services through their work, and they were responsible for the full costs of each visit to a doctor. A sick worker who absented himself from work for more than ten days was registered on a "black list," and his chances of being reemployed were scant. The opening of the Jaffa hospital to sick agricultural workers at lower fees, based on the worker's ability to pay, was vital. Yaffe and other hospital doctors organized a weekly tour of the settlements to learn about the health needs of the workers, assess the incidence of disease, and assist those who were unable to reach the Jaffa hospital. Aware of the daily difficulties encountered by agricultural workers and the health problems associated with their work, Yaffe issued a manual, *Health Care in Israel*, which included explanations and instructions on hygiene, nutrition, and the preservation of health.

In April 1904, as a consequence of disputes with the Jaffa communal council, Yaffe left his position as director of the Shaar Zion Community Hospital and in the Zionist Direction (the Israeli Zionist Organization, which was a branch of the World Zionist Organization), and he returned to the Baron Rothschild Hospital in Zichron Jacob. Yaffe made the hospital the medical center for all the agricultural settlements in Shomron and Galilee and continued to supervise the struggle against malaria.

At the beginning of 1904, the second wave of immigration from Eastern Europe began to arrive in Israel. This wave, which included many well-educated young pioneers with a broad Zionist and socialistic outlook, lasted until 1914. Most of the 2,500 newcomers went into agricultural work in the settlements, organizing themselves in contracting work groups and leading a communal life based on mutual aid. The new workers requested help from Yaffe, as a Zionist leader and pioneer of public health, in dealing with the new medical problems they encountered.

Well informed about the difficulties involved in agricultural work, the dangers of malaria, and the problem of acclimatization facing immigrants in new surroundings, Yaffe organized welfare and aid services for all the worker groups, especially those in the Zichron Jacob area. Because financial resources were scarce and were supervised by both Baron Rothschild and the World Zionist Organization, Yaffe began a series of local actions: extending the hospital kitchen in Zichron Jacob to serve as a workers' kitchen and clinic; extending hospital services and allowing the workers to use them; building washing and bathing facilities attached to the hospital, and arranging for living quarters in various buildings in the settlement; supplying workers with materials for beds and for screening windows to keep out mosquitoes, as well as a steady supply of quinine for workers involved in draining the swamps; and helping newcomers in finding work and organizing a communal kitchen. Yaffe believed that cooperative institutions would facilitate acclimatization, pave the way for supplying food and improved health services at reduced costs, and improve the health of the workers.

Yaffe also suggested training workers in various crafts and home industries. In 1911, Yaffe helped establish a workers' cooperative settlement in Gan Shemuel, Shomron, and convinced Yitshar, the central soap and oil production company, to transfer responsibility for the cultivation of its plantations and orchards, from which it produced oil and soap, to the workers. Thus, Yaffe hoped to ensure continuous employment throughout the year to compensate for the seasonal nature of agricultural work. Yaffe, who totally identified himself with the outlook of the agricultural workers, published articles in the periodical *Hapoel Hatsair* (The young worker) about the foundation of workers' settlements and their vital role in the future of the Jewish community.

Because of the lack of trained medical personnel, such as paramedics, among the workers' groups, Yaffe initiated professional training programs. Some female workers were brought to Zichron Jacob for instruction in first aid and medical treatments, and they were taught the fundamentals of hygiene, nutrition, and preventive medicine so that they could organize and supervise medical services in new settlements. Yaffe's close ties with the workers led to the formation of a public framework that would supply health services to agricultural workers in Israel at an affordable price. In 1909, Yaffe offered the workers of Hadera, a village close to Zichron Jacob, the opportunity to obtain fixed health services for a set annual payment. This arrangement ensured that medical services would be provided by right—and not by charity—and that all Hadera workers, including the unemployed, would have access to necessary services. At the same time, Yaffe initiated the establishment of a Mutual Insurance Fund against Epidemics. By paying a monthly fee, all settlement workers would be able to insure emergency medical aid for the treatment of malaria, typhus, or other epidemic diseases. The Mutual Insurance Fund was one of the first enterprises that led to the foundation of the General Sick Fund in 1911, which still constitutes the central factor in the provision of health services in Israel. By 1995 more than half of the citizens of Israel were insured by the General Sick Fund.

Because Yaffe was dealing with all the workers from the regions of Shomron and Galilee, he needed a way to monitor changes in the health status of agricultural workers. The introduction of personal medical cards was a vital component of his program, because workers frequently changed their residence according to changing work needs. The success of this system induced other doctors to adopt it, and it became the standard system. In 1912, Yaffe lectured on this system at the First Medical Convention in Israel. His main goals were to create a uniform follow-up system among all doctors treating workers and to organize health services so that vital information could be transferred among doctors in a uniform manner in order to promote effective cooperation. Yaffe also published ten scientific papers on the war against malaria, trachoma, and blackwater fever. He was invited by the Pasteur Institute in Paris and various other European scientific organizations to lecture on his research.

Yaffe's extensive efforts to improve the health of agricultural workers in Israel, and his contributions to the foundation of mutual workers' health organizations, were not always accepted by the major landowners who employed settlement workers. The farmers feared that strengthening worker organizations could cause a revolt against the employers on the issues of working conditions and health insurance. As a result, many farmers opposed Yaffe and boycotted his Zichron Jacob hospital, which they referred to as the ''Poorhouse.''

At the outbreak of World War I, the Jewish community in Israel was cut off from its sources of financial support. In order to cope with hunger, epidemics, and rising death rates, Yaffe contacted the Palestine Office, the Jewish Agency functioning in Israel at that time, to obtain food and medicines. Through Henry Morgenthau, the U.S. ambassador in Constantinople, the Palestine Office contacted the American Jewish community and obtained emergency aid. From 1915 to 1917, the U.S. Navy transferred food and medicine to Israel. Simultaneously, Yaffe initiated an orderly distribution of food on a national basis and made special efforts to aid the Yemenite community and pupils of all high schools.

After the British conquest of Palestine in 1918, Yaffe dedicated himself to the reorganization of public health services in Israel. His experience in dealing with malaria control, eye maladies, and public health constituted a valuable asset for the new medical authorities who came to the country. British doctors attempting to learn about the incidence of disease and the war against malaria consulted Yaffe. From 1918 to 1919, Yaffe accompanied the American Zionist Medical Unit, which was sent to Israel to help rehabilitate the public health system, and he established strong ties with Jewish American leaders, including Justice Louis Brandeis. Yaffe hoped that these organizations would take an active part in the reorganization of public health services in Israel, but professional disputes and a lack of mutual understanding between Yaffe and the Hadassah doctors' group led to his withdrawal from the program.

At the end of 1919, Yaffe resigned from his position as director of the Zichron Jacob hospital and went to live in Haifa, where he continued his malaria research and served as physician for the Reali High School. During this period, he published twenty-five scientific papers, eleven of them in the field of malaria and its treatment. Yaffe died in Haifa in 1936. In his testament he asked to be buried in Zichron Jacob, close to the hospital in which he had worked most of his life.

BIBLIOGRAPHY

Yaffe signed his name in an English document as "Yaffe," but German and French reports have given his name as "Yoffe." During his life in Israel, Yaffe kept a daily diary. Recording his strong criticism of the Turkish government was very dangerous, and had the diary been found in the course of a house search, Yaffe would have been put on trial for political activity against the government. Miraculously, the diary, later published as *Brave Generation*, was preserved, and it constitutes one of the central sources for research on the development of the health system in Israel at the beginning of the twentieth century. Archival sources include the Lavon Institute, Labor Archive, Tel Aviv, and the Central Zionist Archive, Jerusalem.

Writings by Hillel Yaffe

Beware of Malaria. Tel Aviv, Israel: Kontress, 1910.

Guarding Health in Israel. Tel Aviv, Israel: Laam, 1911.

Guarding the Health of the Workers in Israel (Palestine). Tel Aviv, Israel: Zionist Direction, 1911.

Brave Generation (A Personal Diary). Tel Aviv, Israel: Dvir, 1939. (in Hebrew.)

Writings about Hillel Yaffe and Related Topics

Kolat, Israel. *Fathers and Founders.* Jerusalem: Hakibutz Hameuchad, 1976. (in Hebrew.)

Margalith, David. *The Way of Israel in Medicine.* Jerusalem: Academy of Medicine, 1970. (in English and Hebrew.)

Shvarts, Shifra. "Kupat Holim: The Worker's Sick Fund in Early XXTH Century Israel." *Sigerist Circle Newsletter* 7 (1994): 5–8.

———. "Who Will Take Care of the Workers? The Establishment of 'Kupat Holim,' the Workers' Sick Fund in Israel 1911–1921." *Journal of the History of Medicine and Allied Sciences* 50 (1995): 525–556.

———. "Health Care System in Israel—An Historical Perspective." In Shyamal K. Majumdar, Leonard M. Rosenfeld, David B. Nash, and Ann Marie Audeth, eds., *Medicine and Health Care into the Twenty-First Century,* pp. 545–562. Philadelphia: Pennsylvania Academy of Science.

Shifra Shvarts

YOSHIOKA YAYOI
(1871–1959)

Yoshioka Yayoi, a physician who founded the first Japanese medical school for women, is important not only as a pioneer educator but also as an activist who spoke out with the authority of an expert on social and political issues and thus helped to legitimate a public role for Japanese women. Tokyo Women's Medical College, the educational institution Yayoi founded, began as Tokyo Women's Medical School in 1900. Thanks to her strenuous efforts, the school won state recognition as a medical school in 1920, thus ensuring that medical education that met licensing requirements was available to women. An officer of numerous women's organizations, Yoshioka was among the handful of women whom the government appointed to committees and commissions in the 1930s and 1940s. Already seventy-five when the war ended and barred from public office by the American occupation forces, she nevertheless played a significant role in the new Japan in which women could vote and run for office.

Born in Hijikata Village in Shizuoka Prefecture in 1871, she was the daughter of Washiyama Yōsai, a physician expert in both Chinese and Western medicine, and his second wife, Mise. She was one of only two girls at her elementary school. Although Yayoi was the daughter of a physician, neither her family background nor her excellent performance in elementary school set her automatically on a path toward her father's profession. Her education after her graduation from elementary school in 1884 conformed to the pattern for any young woman of good family preparing to be a bride: she took sewing lessons from a married woman. In the next few years, however, she decided that she wanted to study in Tokyo to prepare herself to rescue the poor who were so conspicuous in the depressed economic conditions of the 1880s.

She chose a medical career because it was the best option open to her as a woman. In 1887, the highest state-supported educational institution that women could attend was the Tokyo Higher Normal School. She anticipated that because she had no education beyond elementary school, she would not pass the difficult entrance examination. From her older half-brothers who were studying at Saisei Medical School in Tokyo, she knew that there was no such obstacle to winning admission to Saisei, that the school admitted women, and that a few Japanese women, notably Ogino Ginko (1851–1913) and Takahashi Mizuko (1852–1927), had already become licensed physicians. Her father did not immediately agree to her plan, and it was not until 1889 that, with the help of her brother Yatarō, a student at Saisei, she was able to enroll there.

Saisei Medical School presented Yayoi with formidable challenges. A private institution founded in 1876 by Hasegawa Tai (1842–1912), its main purpose was to prepare students for the medical licensing examination from which graduates of university and public medical schools were exempt. Hasegawa, a physician who worked with Nagayo Sensai* in the Home Ministry's Bureau of Public Health, ran his medical school for private profit. He took in as many students as possible and crowded them into inadequate classrooms. Women students, who could not go scrambling across the tops of the desks to secure vacant seats, were at a disadvantage. Moreover, with only an elementary school education, Yayoi had to struggle even to understand the lectures. In these difficult conditions, she made common cause with other women in the medical profession. She founded the Women Medical Students' Friendship Association and secured support for the organization from two women who were already practicing physicians.

By fall 1892, Yayoi had passed both parts of the medical licensing examination, thus becoming the twenty-seventh Japanese woman to qualify as a physician. For a time, she returned home to Shizuoka and helped her father, but in mid-1895, she returned, with her father's permission, to Tokyo. She ran a medical clinic in the evenings and filled her days with lessons, Japanese literature at a private academy, and flower arranging and tea ceremony at the famed Atomi Girls' School. Perhaps with dreams of studying medicine in Berlin, as many aspiring Japanese physicians had done, including her mentor, Takahashi Mizuko, she signed up for German classes at a small private academy, Tokyo Shisei Gakuin.

A new chapter of Yayoi's life began in October 1895 when she married her German teacher, Yoshioka Arata. A native of Saga Prefecture three years her senior, he was the descendant of generations of physicians. He had begun his own medical education at one of the government higher middle schools but had to leave because of illness. Having continued to study on his own, he passed the first medical licensing examination. He founded the Shisei Gakuin to earn living expenses while he studied for the second part of the examination. His own medical studies had been further delayed by his support for his younger brother, who was studying at Saisei Medical School.

Once married, Yayoi dropped her studies at the Atomi school and her clinic work in order to help run her husband's school and to keep house for him, his two younger brothers, and a student. In 1897, to supplement the family income, she opened a small hospital, bestowing on it the same name as her husband's school. When they discovered in 1902 that Arata had diabetes, they closed the school, and the burden of supporting the family fell upon Yayoi and her work at the Shisei Hospital.

The Yoshioka household undertook a new endeavor in 1900 when Yayoi's alma mater, Saisei Medical School, expelled its women students, thus closing off any opportunity for Japanese women to study medicine. Arata and Yayoi responded to this crisis by opening their own women's medical school. Teaching all the classes themselves, they started out with four students in a small room in December 1900. The number of students increased, and they were able to move to better quarters in 1901 and add new buildings in 1903. In 1912, the school was recognized as a medical college, and from 1920 graduates of the school were allowed to become physicians without examination.

The years when Yayoi was bringing her educational institution to maturation were the same ones when she had the responsibilities of motherhood. In September 1901, she gave birth to a son, Hakujin. In April 1922, just months before Arata's death in July left Yayoi a widow, Hakujin entered the prestigious First Higher School, thus ensuring his future professional success.

Even after her husband's death, Yoshioka Yayoi's institutional life remained intertwined with her family life. Early in 1921, her youngest brother-in-law, Yoshioka Masaaki, resigned from his faculty position at the Osaka Prefectural University of Medicine to join the faculty of Tokyo Medical College for Women. The college immediately sent him to Germany to study. He returned to Tokyo in 1923, not long after Arata's death, and thereafter he participated in the administration of the school. A few years later, he married Yamazaki Fusako, a graduate of the Women's Medical College, who was Yayoi's second in command. The couple, who had five children, lived with Yayoi until after the children were grown. When Yayoi retired in 1939, she handed over her work to Masaaki and Fusako.

The considerable support in her work that Yayoi received from her family explains how she was able to find time amid her responsibilities as physician and mother to participate in civic organizations. Her earliest public activities related to women's education, but by the 1920s her civic role had expanded to include organizing women physicians, speaking out on health issues, fighting for the abolition of prostitution, advocating women's suffrage, and forming organizations to prevent delinquency among youth. Her activities took place in an international as well as a national context. She attended the first Pan-Pacific Women's Conference in Honolulu in 1928, and in 1930 she helped to organize the women's section of the League of Nations Society of Japan.

Yoshioka Yayoi's advocacy for women's suffrage and her opposition to prostitution brought her face to face with high government officials as she took part in delegations to the prime minister and other officials. As the government sought to mobilize women on behalf of the state in the 1930s, it recruited Yoshioka into prominent positions in campaigns to fight tuberculosis, purify elections, and form a national women's organization.

Within months after World War II ended, Japanese women received the right to vote and run for office. The newly reconstituted political parties were eager to have some women in their ranks, and several major parties courted Yoshioka. She affiliated herself with one of the parties, but the directors and faculty of her medical school opposed her desire to run for office, and because of her prominence as a leader during the war, the American occupation authorities barred her from public life, including leadership of her medical school. This ban was not lifted until the occupation ended in 1952.

Yoshioka's most important contribution to the practice of medicine in Japan was her medical school. At a time when the state refused to invest in women's medical education, she educated some four thousand women physicians by 1947, most of them Japanese but some of them Korean, Taiwanese, and Chinese. Yoshioka's achievements as a physician and those of her students made modern health care more accessible to women. Some of Yoshioka's early patients were Chinese, Taiwanese, and Korean women residing in Japan who would not have availed themselves of modern medical expertise had it required that their bodies be examined by male physicians. Most of Yoshioka's students worked for either public institutions or private clinics that they shared with their husbands or inherited from their fathers.

Yoshioka's contribution to society at large was the example she set of an educated, professional woman serving as a community leader. As a wife and mother carrying on the traditional work of both her father and her father-in-law, Yoshioka provided a model of modern female leadership that was compatible with Japanese modernity, Japanese national pride, and the Japanese family system. Whereas most of the older women educators with whom she cooperated in civic endeavors were experts on the Chinese classics or Japanese poetry, Yoshioka and her students possessed modern, scientific expertise. In contrast to some of Yoshioka's younger colleagues, who were Christian women educated in Europe and the United States, Yoshioka and her students had expertise transmitted within a traditional Japanese hierarchy. Yoshioka took pride in the fact that the graduates of her school became leaders of their own communities. Branches of her alumnae organization sprang up in various prefectures of Japan, and her students were prominent as heads of women's organizations, suffragists, newspaper columnists, and eventually as politicians. Although Yoshioka herself never held elected political office, she was a major contributor to the civic organizations that prepared some fifty women to take seats in the national legislature in the immediate postwar years.

BIBLIOGRAPHY

Yoshioka Yayoi was so prominent during her lifetime that several English-language biographical dictionaries provide short accounts of her life: *Japan Biographical Encyclopedia and Who's Who* (1958), *Biographical Dictionary of Japanese History* (1978), and *Kodansha Encyclopedia of Japan* (1983). The best source for the details of her life up to 1940 is the biography, written by Kanzaki Kiyoshi, which a committee of her friends commissioned: *Yoshioka Yayoi den* (1967). Yayoi herself supplemented this work with *Kono jūnen* (1952), her memoirs of the decade following the completion of the biography. One other important source is the memoir published by her student, Takeuchi Shigeyo, *Yoshioka Yayoi sensei to watakushi* (1966).

Writings by Yoshioka Yayoi

Kono jūnen (These twenty years). Tokyo: Gakufū shoin, 1952.

Writings about Yoshioka Yayoi and Related Topics

Biographical Dictionary of Japanese History. Tokyo: International Society for Educational Information, 1978.

Garon, Sheldon. "Women's Groups and the Japanese State: Contending Approaches to Political Integration, 1890–1945." *Journal of Japanese Studies* 19, no. 1 (winter 1993): 5–41.

Japan Biographical Encyclopedia and Who's Who. Tokyo: Rengo Press, 1958.

Kanzaki Kiyoshi. *Yoshioka Yayoi den* (Biography of Yoshioka Yayoi). Tokyo: Chūō kōronsha, 1967.

Kodansha Encyclopedia of Japan. 9 vols. Tokyo: Kodansha, 1983.

Takeuchi Shigeyo. *Yoshioka Yayoi sensei to watakushi* (Yoshioka Yayoi and I). Tokyo: Kaneoka, 1966.

Sally Ann Hastings

MARIE ELIZABETH ZAKRZEWSKA
(1829–1902)

Marie Elizabeth Zakrzewska, nineteenth-century pioneer woman physician, was the first resident physician at the New York Infirmary for Women and Children, New York, and founder and first attending physician of the New England Hospital for Women and Children. Dr. Zakrzewska (pronounced Zak-shef'ska) was indefatigable in her commitment to equal access for women to medical training. She was born in Berlin, Prussia, on September 6, 1829. Her mother was of gypsy ancestry, and her father was a Prussian civil officer. Marie was the eldest of their six daughters and one son.

When Zakrzewska was quite young, her father lost his civil career, for reasons of political dissidence, and the family had to rely on his small soldier's pension. To augment the family income, Zakrzewska's mother attended the School for Midwives in Berlin. In 1840, during her mother's absence, Marie suffered an eye infection that temporarily blinded her. She asked to stay with her mother and was allowed to move into the hospital. Marie's physician took her with him on his rounds, coaching her to learn and observe by touch since she could not see. With the encouragement of Dr. Müller, Zakrzewska began to study medicine.

When Zakrzewska regained her health, she resumed her regular schooling. Her memories of these early experiences are mixed. Other students ridiculed her for her plainness and her messy appearance. Sometimes school administrators and teachers also took a dislike to her because of her outspokenness and lack of submissiveness. In her autobiography, however, she tells of the encouragement and mentoring she received from a teacher of history, geography, and mathematics. From him she discovered the high level of her theoretical comprehension and aptitude for the study of mathematics.

After Zakrzewska quit her schooling, she began to assist her mother in her midwifery practice. By 1845, Zakrzewska decided she too would become a midwife. Her father welcomed this decision, but her mother was less certain about her career choice. Zakrzewska and her mother were very close, and perhaps her mother foresaw the many obstacles that lay in the path. In Prussian society at this time, there was much resistance to the female practice of medicine; even in midwifery women were greatly restricted. Zakrzewska's father used his influence to get her into the Berlin School for Midwives, although at eighteen she was too young for the school's formal admission standards. With the advocacy of Professor Joseph Hermann Schmidt, Zakrzewska was admitted in 1849. Dr. Schmidt served as her tutor and mentor at Berlin's Charité, the largest hospital in Prussia at the time. Schmidt considered her a student of exceptional promise, and he immediately devised a plan to make her the head midwife at the Berlin School and professor in charge of the education of more than two hundred students.

In many ways Schmidt's mentorship was a great opportunity for Zakrzewska, and it encouraged her to augment her studies of medicine. Still, many at the school and hospital resented her early success, and they opposed Zakrzewska's appointment for several reasons: she was a single woman, she was too young, and she did not practice religion. Because Zakrzewska's parents were Rationalists, they were not members of any church. Brought up outside conventional religious practices, Zakrzewska was skeptical of religious dogma throughout her life. After she graduated in 1851, Schmidt moved to validate Zakrzewska's appointment as chief midwife at the Royal Hospital of Berlin. Unfortunately, Schmidt's sudden death in 1852, just hours after the arrangements were completed, left Zakrzewska as a vulnerable new administrator. Her enemies were able to join forces, and she left the Berlin School for Midwives six months later. Despite her abrupt departure and the hostility of some of her colleagues, the city of Berlin granted her a substantial monetary award for what she had already done.

While working with Dr. Schmidt, Zakrzewska read about the Female Medical College in Philadelphia. When she lost her position at the School for Midwives, her dream to go to Philadelphia became a possibility. In March 1853, with the help of their father, she and her sister Anna set off on a forty-seven-day voyage to America. Soon after they arrived in New York City, they realized that attending medical school was virtually impossible and that women physicians were not treated with respect. The sisters set up a knitting business and barely supported themselves. After the first year, business began to fail, and Marie and Anna became desperate to better their situation. In 1854 Zakrzewska met Dr. Elizabeth Blackwell and New York City reformer Catherine Sedgewick at the Home for the Friendless. Making a connection with Blackwell was a watershed for Zakrzewska, but she still could not speak much English, and she hid her strong interest in establishing a hospital for women from Blackwell. However, Blackwell had just opened the New York Infirmary for Indigent Women and Children, and she quickly recognized Zakrzewska's potential and their common interests. When she met Zakrewska, Blackwell wrote in a letter she published decades later: "There is true stuff in her, and I shall do my best to bring it out. She must obtain a medical degree" (Blackwell 1895: 201). Zakrzewska and Blackwell agreed on the goal of establishing an institution for women patients and women medical students. Helping Zakrzewska get a medical degree benefited Blackwell's plans for an infirmary. Zakrzewska and Blackwell, along with several others, directed their lives to reforming medical education and providing medical care for women.

Zakrzewska did not always hold to a position of fighting for women's rights. Working with prostitutes in the hospital in Berlin, however, she did come to understand the problems women experienced because of the double standard and the role of class in shaping their lives. In her own career, she met with strong resistance from the Prussian male-dominated medical establishment to her attainment of high professional standing. In the United States she encountered more of the same ideas. In her autobiography she wrote, ''When fathers are unwilling that their daughters shall enter life as physicians, lawyers, merchants, or in any other public capacity, it is simply because they belong to the class that so contaminates the air, that none can breathe it but themselves'' (Zakrzewska 1860: 135–136). Throughout her career, Zakrzewska held to a perspective that cut across class lines and recognized both the vulnerability of women and their potential.

Her involvement in reform activities changed with time. After tutoring her in English, Blackwell made arrangements to send Zakrzewska to Cleveland to study at the Cleveland Medical College (later Case Western Reserve) in October 1854. Emily Blackwell* had recently graduated from this college. Zakrzewska had little money and could still barely speak English. Caroline Severance, a reformer, woman's rights activist, and head of the Physiological Society in Cleveland, supported Zakrzewska financially, initially also providing room and board. Severance introduced her to Dr. Harriet Hunt, a pioneer woman physician. Zakrzewska became involved in abolitionism, spiritualism, and other causes while in Cleveland. During the first year of study, Zakrzewska worked in isolation and spoke very little because of the language barrier and her financial situation. Moreover, her father wrote her an angry letter, condemning her decision to sacrifice so much, as he saw it, to pursue medicine as a career. With the support of friends, she continued her studies and gained some fluency in English.

While Zakrzewska was struggling through her first year in Cleveland, her mother and two other sisters set out to visit Marie and Anna. Tragically, her mother died during the voyage, and Marie was almost unable to continue her work. However, she persevered and completed her M.D. degree in 1856, one of four women in a class of more than two hundred. In honor of her excellence and achievements, the Medical College faculty voted her a monetary award upon her graduation.

Returning to New York with her medical degree, Zakrzewska attempted to establish a practice and encountered what must have become predictable resistance. After a few months, she found herself living in Elizabeth Blackwell's back parlor. Working with the Blackwells, she became the general manager and resident physician at the New York Infirmary and College for Women. At the infirmary on Bleaker Street, she and Emily Blackwell* cared for about twenty-four patients. Living on the funds from her private practice, Zakrzewska donated her time to the infirmary.

In June 1859, Samuel Gregory invited Zakrzewska to come to Boston to take charge of the New England Female Medical College. Gregory was an advocate of the education of women as midwives, but he held a very conservative view of women. Women ought to serve as midwives, he argued, because for men to do so was immoral and a violation of female modesty. Zakrzewska's experiences as a midwife and the creation of Gregory's hospital are both testimonies to the historical context of the early and mid-nineteenth century in which the centuries-old practice of female midwifery met with conflict and criticism from medical practitioners who were almost entirely male and were increasingly involved in the practice of midwifery. This made short-term allies of Gregory and Zakrzewska. Conflict arose within a few years—a conflict of authority between Gregory and Zakrzewska. An advocate of irregular medicine, Gregory was a lecturer in physiology with an honorary medical degree in eclectic medicine. Part of Zakrzewska's framework for the admission of women to medical colleges was that only regular medicine, or allopathic medicine, was suitable in the training of women doctors. During this period, practitioners often drew from many different types of medical therapies. Zakrzewska, however, rejected homeopathy and eclectic medicine and was determined to teach women doctors only orthodox, or scientific medicine, which was the forerunner of today's modern medicine. She envisioned clinical experience as the key to women's medical education.

After Gregory and Zakrzewska locked horns over his refusal to buy a microscope and other equipment, he dismissed her and several members of the governing board. Soon after, in July 1862, Zakrzewska rented a building to establish the New England Hospital for Women and Children. Many of Gregory's former allies supported her efforts. Zakrzewska conceived of this hospital as a training institution for women interns (later doctors), a school for nurses, and a locus for the treatment of women patients. The setting was a hospital where students might gain clinical experience, something medical education generally neglected at this time. This hospital represented Zakrzewska's lasting achievement: "Dr. Zakrzewska brought to the New England Hospital her energy, drive, and persistence; the wisdom of her personal experience; her strong belief in women doctors; her commitment to the highest standards in regular medicine; and her deep sympathy for poor women" (Drachman 1984: 41).

Boston became Zakrzewska's home until her death. From the beginning of her stay in the United States, she maintained a connection with the city through her friend, German radical and now German-American journalist Karl Heinzen, who lived there with his family. Zakrzewska never married, but after 1860 she shared a home in Roxbury with two of her sisters, plus Julia Sprague, an invalid who was a "faithful friend and home companion," and Karl Heinzen, his wife, and his son (Zakrzewska 1924: 297).

In Boston, Zakrzewska continued her connection with many reformers, including the abolitionists and women's rights activists she had met previously while living with Elizabeth Blackwell, as well as William Lloyd Garrison, Caroline Severance, and Caroline Dall. Edna Cheney, another woman's rights advocate, was a strong supporter of the hospital and served as president of the institution for fifteen years and on the board of directors for forty-eight years. Demonstrating the link between women's rights activities and the New England

Hospital, Cheney also served on the executive committee of the New England Woman's Suffrage Association. In addition several medical men, including Dr. Henry I. Bowditch, Dr. Samuel Cabot, and Dr. Edward H. Clarke, stood behind Zakrzewska to support the hospital and her attempts to be admitted to the Massachusetts Medical Society and enroll women students in the Harvard Medical School.

In the next ten years, as the hospital grew in size and reputation, many outstanding women physicians passed through its doors. Because of its clinical basis, Zakrzewska had no trouble attracting women interns (Drachman 1984: 64.) Ironically, in the first few years of its existence, Horatio R. Scorer served as consulting staff gynecologist. In 1866, he resigned in anger when restrictions were put on his surgical practice. The hospital's renowned alumnae included Mary Putnam Jacobi and Susan Dimock. Jacobi went on to specialize by studying therapeutics in Paris, and Dimock went to Zurich, with Zakrzewska's encouragement, to become a surgeon. After completing her studies, Dimock returned to the New England Hospital, where she served as surgeon and professor until her sudden death in 1875. At the same time Dimock was a student, Sophia Jex-Blake was also a student at the New England Hospital. Together they attempted to gain admission to Harvard Medical School but failed. Sophia Jex-Blake went on to become an outspoken proponent of the right of women in Great Britain to have medical education equal to that of men. She played a key role in founding the London School of Medicine for Women.

Other highly reputed women physicians connected to the hospital included Dr. Lucy Sewall who was the hospital's first resident physician and served without salary or vacation. Dr. Eliza Mosher entered the program at New England Hospital and interned there, assisting Lucy Sewall. From there she went on to the University of Michigan in 1875 to get her medical degree. After teaching hygiene at Vassar College, Mosher continued to teach and became dean of women at the University of Michigan in the late 1890s. In 1875 the governing board of the hospital instituted a policy that accepted only women who had already obtained their medical degrees.

"Until it began to lose its appeal in the late 1890's, the New England Hospital . . . was a showplace for quality medical care in the latter third of the nineteenth century" (Morantz-Sanchez 1985: 225). By its twenty-fifth anniversary in 1887, the New England Hospital for Women and Children had attained the goals set by Zakrzewska when she first began to envision a center for the medical education of women. Above all, she had helped to effect a separate curriculum for women who sought medical degrees, and she had established excellence in that course of study, particularly in clinical medicine. The generation of students in the late 1890s began to complain about the internships at the hospital. Students such as Alice Hamilton criticized the absolute separation of women from men and objected to the lack of specialization in the clinical experience. Some of the shortcomings this generation saw resulted from Zakrzewska's inflexibility, but difficulties for the place of women in medicine also arose from the shifting context of medical education.

In 1899, Zakrzewska retired from practice; she died three years later. Her productive life was dedicated to goals for medical education that were ahead of her time. Although her contributions escaped notice for several generations, the historical record now recognizes her as a key figure in the fight for the admission of women to the study of medicine.

BIBLIOGRAPHY

The Countway Library at Harvard Medical School holds the New England Hospital for Women and Children Patient Records and other relevant papers. The Schlesinger Library at Radcliffe College holds papers from the New England Hospital for Women and Children and papers from several students. The Massachusetts Historical Society in Boston holds the Caroline Dall Papers. The Sophia Smith Collection in Northampton, Massachusetts, holds papers from the hospital. In New York City, the Columbia University Rare Book and Manuscript Library holds papers of the Blackwell sisters.

Writings by Marie Elizabeth Zakrzewska

A Practical Illustration of "Woman's Right to Labor"; or A Letter from Marie E. Zakrzewska, M.D., Late of Berlin, Prussia. Edited by Caroline H. Dall. Boston: Walker, Wise, and Co., 1860.
A Woman's Quest: The Life of Marie E. Zakrzewska, M.D. Edited by Agnes C. Vietor. New York: D. Appleton and Company, 1924. (Reprint ed., New York: Arno Press, 1972).

Writings about Marie Elizabeth Zakrzewska and Related Topics

Blackwell, Elizabeth. *Pioneer Work in Opening the Medical Profession to Women: Autobiographical Sketches.* London: Longmans, Green, 1895; reprinted, with an introduction by Mary Roth Walsh, New York: Schocken Books, 1977.
Bonner, Thomas Nevell. *To the Ends of the Earth: Women's Search for Education in Medicine.* Cambridge, MA: Harvard University Press, 1992.
Donegan, Jane B. *Women and Men Midwives: Medicine, Morality, and Misogyny in Early America.* Westport, CT: Greenwood Press, 1978.
Drachman, Virginia G. *Hospital with a Heart: Women Doctors and the Paradox of Separatism at the New England Hospital, 1862–1969.* Ithaca, NY: Cornell University Press, 1984.
Morantz-Sanchez, Regina. *Sympathy and Science: Women Physicians in American Medicine.* New York: Oxford University Press, 1985.
Walsh, Mary Roth. *"Doctors Wanted: No Women Need Apply:" Sexual Barriers in the Medical Profession.* New Haven, CT: Yale University Press, 1977.

Deborah Kuhn McGregor

APPENDIX A
LISTING BY OCCUPATIONS AND SPECIAL INTERESTS

Administration (Academic and Medical)

    Fulton, John Farquhar

    Nagayo Sensai

    Parran, Jr., Thomas J.

    Pisacano, Nicholas J.

Aerospace Physiology or Medicine

    Schroeder, Henry Alfred

African Medicine

    Lambo, Thomas Adeoye

    See also Alternative Medicine

Air Pollution

    Greenburg, Leonard

Alternative Medicine

    Fuller, Solomon Carter

    Greene, Cordelia Agnes

    Gupta, Madhusudan

    Lambo, Thomas Adeoye

    Sarkar, Mahendralal

    Still, Andrew Taylor

Anatomy

    Hunter, John

Ayurvedic Medicine

> Gupta, Madhusudan
>
> *See also* Alternative Medicine

Bacteriology

> *See* Microbiology

Bibliography (Medical)

> Billings, John Shaw
>
> *See also* Literature

Cancer Research

> *See* Oncology

Cardiology

> Boas, Ernst P.

Child Welfare

> Campbell, Kate
>
> Sheriff, Hilla
>
> Villermé, Louis-René

Clinical Investigation and Clinical Medicine

> Finlay, Carlos Juan
>
> Heberden, William
>
> Mitchell, Silas Weir
>
> Pinel, Philippe
>
> Withering, William

Contraception

> *See* Family Planning

Cooperative Medical Services

> *See* Health Care Organization, Financing, and Reform

Education (Medical)

> Blackwell, Emily
>
> Boyd, William
>
> Calderone, Mary Steichen
>
> Gupta, Madhusudan
>
> Haddad, Sami Ibrahim
>
> Heberden, William
>
> Nagayo Sensai
>
> Pinel, Philippe
>
> Pisacano, Nicholas J.

Sarkar, Mahendralal

Todd, Robert Bentley

Yoshioka Yayoi

Yaffe, Hillel

Zakrzewska, Marie Elizabeth

Education (Nursing)

Dock, Lavinia Lloyd

Todd, Robert Bentley

Engineer, Environmental

Greenburg, Leonard

Epidemiology

Francis, Thomas, Jr.

Goldberger, Joseph

Martínez Báez, Manuel

Wu Lien-teh

Family Planning

Calderone, Mary Steichen

Family Practice Medicine

Pisacano, Nicholas J.

Geriatric Medicine

Pinel, Philippe

Gynecology

See Obstetrics and Gynecology

Health Care Organization, Financing, and Reform

Boas, Ernst P.

Butler, Allan Macy

Lambo, Thomas Adeoye

Martínez Báez, Manuel

Parran, Thomas J., Jr.

Sabin, Albert B.

Shadid, Michael Abraham

Sigerist, Henry Ernest

Tissot, Samuel-Auguste-André-David

Yaffe, Hillel

Health Spas

 Greene, Cordelia Agnes

 See also Alternative Medicine

Heavy Metal Poisoning

 Schroeder, Henry Alfred

History (Medical)

 Fulton, John Farquhar

 Haddad, Sami Ibrahim

 Martínez Báez, Manuel

 Sigerist, Henry Ernest

Homeopathy

 Fuller, Solomon Carter

 Sarkar, Mahendralal

 See also Alternative Medicine

Hospital Planning and Administration

 See Health Care Organization, Financing, and Reform

Human Sexuality

 Calderone, Mary Steichen

 Dickinson, Robert Latou

Hydropathic Medicine

 Greene, Cordelia Agnes

 See also Alternative Medicine

Hypertension

 Schroeder, Henry Alfred

Industrial Hygiene

 Greenburg, Leonard

 Villermé, Louis-René

International Medicine and Health Care Policy

 See Health Care Organization, Financing, and Reform

Japanese Medicine

 Nagayo Sensai

 Yoshioka Yayoi

Lead Poisoning

 See Heavy Metal Poisoning

Library Administration

See Literature

Literature (Bibliophiles, Bibliographers, Collectors, Editors, Librarians, Medical Writers, Novelists, Popular Writers, Poets, Publishers, Translators)

Billings, John Shaw

Boyd, William

De Kruif, Paul Henry

Dock, Lavinia Lloyd

Erikson, Erik Homburger

Fenger, Carl Emil

Gupta, Madhusudan

Heberden, William

Mitchell, Silas Weir

Montezuma, Carlos

Sarkar, Mahendralal

Tissot, Samuel-Auguste-André-David

Todd, Robert Bentley

Malaria Control Programs

Yaffe, Hillel

Maternal and Child Health Care Policy

Sheriff, Hilla

Medical Administration

See Administration

Medical Bibliography

Billings, John Shaw

See also Literature

Medical Economics

See Health Care Organization, Financing, and Reform

Medical Education

See Education (Medical)

Medical History

See History (Medical)

Medical Policy and Medical Politics

See Health Care Organization, Financing, and Reform

Medical Reform

See Health Care Organization, Financing, and Reform

Medical Statistics

Billings, John Shaw

Fenger, Carl Emil

See also Literature

Mental Illness

Lambo, Thomas Adeoye

Pinel, Philippe

See also Psychiatry

Microbiology

De Kruif, Paul Henry

Evans, Alice Catherine

Smith, Theobald

Midwifery

Callen, Maude E.

Zakrzewska, Marie Elizabeth

Military Medicine

Beaumont, William

Billings, John Shaw

Gorgas, William Crawford

Native American Rights Movement

Montezuma, Carlos

Neonatology

Campbell, Kate

Neurology

Fulton, John Farquhar

Mitchell, Silas Weir

Nosology

Pinel, Philippe

Nurses

Callen, Maude E.

Dock, Lavinia Lloyd

Rivers, Eunice

Nurse-Midwife

    Callen, Maude E.

Nursing Educator

    See Education (Nursing)

Nursing Professionalization

    See Professionalization (Nursing)

Obstetrics and Gynecology

    Dickinson, Robert Latou

    Sims, James Marion

Occupational Medicine

    Greenburg, Leonard

    Villermé, Louis-René

Oncology

    Park, Roswell

Osteopathy

    Still, Andrew Taylor

    See also Alternative Medicine

Parasitology

    Martínez Báez, Manuel

Pathology

    Boyd, William

    Fuller, Solomon Carter

    Hunter, John

    Smith, Theobald

Pediatrics

    Butler, Allan Macy

    Campbell, Kate

    Sheriff, Hilla

Pharmacology

    Withering, William

Physicians

    Beaumont, William

    Billings, John Shaw

    Blackwell, Emily

    Boas, Ernst P.

Boyd, William

Bustamante, Miguel Enrique

Butler, Allan Macy

Calderone, Mary Steichen

Campbell, Kate

Defries, Robert Davies

Dickinson, Robert Latou

Erikson, Erik Homburger

Fenger, Carl Emil

Finlay, Carlos Juan

Francis, Thomas, Jr.

Fuller, Solomon Carter

Fulton, John Farquhar

Goldberger, Joseph

Gorgas, William Crawford

Greene, Cordelia Agnes

Gupta, Madhusudan

Haddad, Sami Ibrahim

Heberden, William

Lambo, Thomas Adeoye

Martínez Báez, Manuel

Mitchell, Silas Weir

Montezuma, Carlos

Park, Roswell

Parran, Thomas J., Jr.

Pinel, Philippe

Pisacano, Nicholas J.

Sabin, Albert B.

Sarkar, Mahendralal

Shadid, Michael Abraham

Sheriff, Hilla

Sigerist, Henry Ernest

Sims, James Marion

Smith, Theobald

Still, Andrew Taylor

Tissot, Samuel-Auguste-André-David

Todd, Robert Bentley

Villermé, Louis-René

Withering, William

Wu Lien-teh

Yoshioka Yayoi

Yaffe, Hillel

Zakrzewska, Marie Elizabeth

Physiology

Beaumont, William

Fenger, Carl Emil

Poliomyelitis and Polio Vaccines

Defries, Robert Davies

Francis, Thomas, Jr.

Sabin, Albert B.

Pollution

Schroeder, Henry Alfred

Professionalization (Medical)

Fenger, Carl Emil

Pisacano, Nicholas J.

Tissot, Samuel-Auguste-André-David

Professionalization (Nursing)

Dock, Lavinia Lloyd

Todd, Robert Bentley

Psychiatry

Fuller, Solomon Carter

Lambo, Thomas Adeoye

Pinel, Philippe

See also Mental Illness

Psychoanalysis

Erikson, Erik Homburger

Public Health

Bustamante, Miguel Enrique

Callen, Maude E.

Defries, Robert Davies

Dock, Lavinia Lloyd

Evans, Alice Catherine

Finlay, Carlos Juan

Goldberger, Joseph

Gorgas, William Crawford

Greenburg, Leonard

Lambo, Thomas Adeoye

Martínez Báez, Manuel

Nagayo Sensai

Parran, Thomas J., Jr.

Sheriff, Hilla

Wu Lien-teh

Yaffe, Hillel

Public Health Nurses

Dock, Lavinia Lloyd

Rivers, Eunice

Sanitary Engineering

Gorgas, William Crawford

Science Education

Sarkar, Mahendralal

Sex Education

Calderone, Mary Steichen

Dickinson, Robert Latou

Sexually Transmitted Diseases

Parran, Thomas J., Jr.

Surgery

Haddad, Sami Ibrahim

Hunter, John

Park, Roswell

Sims, James Marion

Todd, Robert Bentley

Syphilis Control Programs

Parran, Thomas J., Jr.

Rivers, Eunice

Tropical Medicine

See Parasitology

Unorthodox Medicine

See Alternative Medicine

Urology

    Haddad, Sami Ibrahim

Virology

    Francis, Thomas, Jr.

    Sabin, Albert B.

Vitamin Deficiency Diseases

    Goldberger, Joseph

Workers' Health

    Villermé, Louis-René

    Yaffe, Hillel

APPENDIX B
LISTING BY DATE OF BIRTH

1710

Heberden, William

1728

Tissot, Samuel-Auguste-André-David

Hunter, John

1741

Withering, William

1745

Pinel, Philippe

1782

Villermé, Louis-René

1785

Beaumont, William

1800

Gupta, Madhusudan*

1809

Todd, Robert Bentley

1813

Sims, James Marion

*Year of birth uncertain.

1814

Fenger, Carl Emil

1826

Blackwell, Emily

1828

Still, Andrew Taylor

1829

Zakrzewska, Marie Elizabeth

Mitchell, Silas Weir

1831

Greene, Cordelia Agnes

1833

Sarkar, Mahendralal

Finlay, Carlos Juan

1838

Billings, John Shaw

Nagayo Sensai

1852

Park, Roswell

1854

Gorgas, William Crawford

1858

Dock, Lavinia Lloyd

1859

Smith, Theobald

1861

Dickinson, Robert Latou

1864

Yaffe, Hillel

1865

Montezuma, Carlos*

1871

Yoshioka Yayoi

1872

Fuller, Solomon Carter

1874

Goldberger, Joseph

1879

Wu Lien-teh

1881

Evans, Alice Catherine

1882

Shadid, Michael Abraham

1885

Boyd, William

1889

Defries, Robert Davies

1890

Haddad, Sami Ibrahim

De Kruif, Paul Henry

1891

Sigerist, Henry Ernest

Boas, Ernst P.

1892

Parran, Thomas J. Jr.

1893

Greenburg, Leonard

1894

Butler, Allan Macy

Martínez Báez, Manuel

1898

Bustamante, Miguel Enrique

1899

Fulton, John Farquhar

Campbell, Kate

Rivers, Eunice

1900

Francis, Thomas, Jr.

Callen, Maude E.

1902

Erikson, Erik Homburger

1903

Sheriff, Hilla

1904

Calderone, Mary Steichen

1906

Schroeder, Henry Alfred

Sabin, Albert B.

1923

Lambo, Thomas Adeoye

1924

Pisacano, Nicholas J.

APPENDIX C
LISTING BY PLACE OF BIRTH

Alabama

    Gorgas, William Crawford (1854–1920)

Arizona

    Montezuma, Carlos (1865?–1923)

Australia

    Campbell, Kate (1899–1986)

Canada

    Defries, Robert Davies (1889–1975)

Connecticut

    Beaumont, William (1785–1853)

    Park, Roswell (1852–1914)

Cuba

    Finlay, Carlos Juan (1833–1915)

Denmark

    Fenger, Carl Emil (1814–1884)

England

    Blackwell, Emily (1826–1910)

    Heberden, William (1710–1801)

    Withering, William (1741–1799)

Florida

    Callen, Maude E. (1900–1990)

France

    Pinel, Philippe (1745–1826)

    Sigerist, Henry Ernest (1891–1957)

    Villermé, Louis-René (1782–1863)

Georgia

    Rivers, Eunice (1899–1986)

Germany

    Erikson, Erik Homburger (1902–1994)

    Zakrzewska, Marie Elizabeth (1829–1902)

Hungary

    Goldberger, Joseph (1874–1929)

India

    Gupta, Madhusudan (1800?–1856)

    Sarkar, Mahendralal (1833–1904)

Indiana

    Billings, John Shaw (1838–1913)

    Francis, Thomas, Jr. (1900–1969)

Ireland

    Todd, Robert Bentley (1809–1860)

Japan

    Nagayo Sensai (1838–1902)

    Yoshioka Yayoi (1871–1959)

Lebanon

    Shadid, Michael Abraham (1882–1966)

Liberia

    Fuller, Solomon Carter (1872–1953)

Malaysia

    Wu Lien-teh (1879–1960)

Maryland

    Parran, Thomas J., Jr. (1892–1968)

Massachusetts

    Boas, Ernst P. (1891–1955)

Mexico

Bustamante, Miguel Enrique (1898–1986)

Martínez Báez, Manuel (1894–1987)

Michigan

De Kruif, Paul Henry (1890–1971)

Minnesota

Fulton, John Farquhar (1899–1960)

New Jersey

Dickinson, Robert Latou (1861–1950)

Schroeder, Henry Alfred (1906–1975)

New York

Butler, Allan Macy (1894–1986)

Calderone, Mary Steichen (1904–)

Greenburg, Leonard (1893–1991)

Greene, Cordelia Agnes (1831–1905)

Smith, Theobald (1859–1934)

Nigeria

Lambo, Thomas Adeoye (1923–)

Palestine

Haddad, Sami Ibrahim (1890–1957)

Pennsylvania

Dock, Lavinia Lloyd (1858–1956)

Evans, Alice Catherine (1881–1975)

Mitchell, Silas Weir (1829–1914)

Pisacano, Nicholas J. (1924–1990)

Poland

Sabin, Albert B. (1906–1993)

Scotland

Boyd, William (1885–1979)

Hunter, John (1728–1793)

South Carolina

Sheriff, Hilla (1903–1988)

Sims, James Marion (1813–1883)

Switzerland

Tissot, Samuel-Auguste-André-David (1728–1797)

Ukraine

Yaffe, Hillel (1864–1936)

Virginia

Still, Andrew Taylor (1828–1917)

APPENDIX D
LISTING OF WOMEN PRACTITIONERS

Blackwell, Emily (1826–1912)

Calderone, Mary Steichen (1904–)

Callen, Maude E. (1900–1990)

Campbell, Kate (1899–1986)

Dock, Lavinia Lloyd (1858–1956)

Evans, Alice Catherine (1881–1975)

Greene, Cordelia Agnes (1831–1905)

Rivers, Eunice (1899–1986)

Sheriff, Hilla (1903–1988)

Yoshioka Yayoi (1871–1959)

Zakrzewska, Marie Elizabeth (1829–1902)

REFERENCES AND FURTHER READINGS

Because of space limitations, only a brief list of suggested readings is included here.

Bailey, Hamilton, and Bishop, William J. *Notable Names in Medicine and Surgery*. London: H. K. Lewis, 1944.

Bibliography of the History of Medicine. Bethesda, MD: National Institutes of Health, National Library of Medicine, 1965–.

Bullough, Vern L., Church, O. M., and Stein, A. P., eds. *American Nursing: A Biographical Dictionary*. New York: Garland, 1988.

Chaff, Sandra L. *Women in Medicine: A Bibliography of the Literature on Women Physicians*. Metuchen, NJ: Scarecrow Press, 1977.

Corsi, Pietro, and Weindling, Paul, eds. *Information Sources in the History of Science and Medicine*. London: Butterworth Scientific, 1983.

Erlen, Jonathan. *The History of the Health Care Sciences and Health Care, 1700–1980: A Selective Annotated Bibliography*. New York: Garland, 1984.

Eyler, John M., Gevitz, Norman, and Tuchman, Arleen M. *History of Medicine in the Undergraduate Curriculum: Report of a Survey of Colleges and Universities in the United Sates and Canada during 1990*. American Association for the History of Medicine, 1991.

Fox, Daniel M., Meldrum, Marcia, and Rezak, Ira, eds. *Nobel Laureates in Medicine or Physiology: A Biographical Dictionary*. New York: Garland, 1990.

Garrison, F. H. "Available Sources and Future Prospects of Medical Biography." *Bulletin of the New York Academy of Medicine* 4, no. 5 (May 1928): 586–608.

Gillispie, Charles Coulson, ed. *Dictionary of Scientific Biography*. 16 vols. New York: Charles Scribner's Sons, 1970–1980.

Index Catalog of the Surgeon General's Office. 58 vols. 1880–1955. (Continues as *Bibliography of the History of Medicine*.)

Kaufman, Martin, Galishoff, Stuart, and Savitt, Todd L., eds. *Dictionary of American Medical Biography*. Westport, CT: Greenwood Press, 1984.

Kaufman, Martin, Higgins, L. P., and Friedman, A. H., eds. *Dictionary of American Nursing Biography*. Westport, CT: Greenwood Press, 1988.

Kelly, Howard A., and Burrage, Walter L. *Dictionary of American Medical Biography: Lives of Eminent Physicians of the United States and Canada, from the Earliest Times*. New York: D. Appleton & Co., 1928. Reprint ed., New York: Milford House, 1971.

Marmelszadt, Willard. *Musical Sons of Aesculapius*. New York: Froeben Press, 1946.

Morton, Leslie T., and Norman, Jeremy M. *Morton's Medical Bibliography: An Annotated Checklist of Texts Illustrating the History of Medicine (Garrison and Morton)*. 5th ed. Brookfield, VT: Gower Publishing Company Ltd., 1991.

Pettigrew, Thomas Joseph. *Medical Portrait Gallery: Biographical Memoirs of the Most Celebrated Physicians, Surgeons, etc. etc. Who Have Contributed to the Advancement of Medical Science*. 4 vols. London: Fisher, Son & Co., Whittaker & Co., 1838–1940.

Richardson, Sir Benjamin Ward. *Disciples of Aesculapius*. 2 vols. London: Hutchinson & Co., 1900.

Robinson, Victor. *Pathfinders in Medicine*. New York: Medical Life Press, 1929.

Siegel, Patricia Joan, and Finley, Kay Thomas. *Women in the Scientific Search: An American Bio-bibliography, 1724–1979*. Metuchen, NJ: Scarecrow Press, 1985.

Sigerist, Henry E. *The Great Doctors: A Biographical History of Medicine*. New York: W. W. Norton, 1933.

Talbott, John Harold. *A Biographical History of Medicine: Excerpts and Essays on the Men and Their Work*. New York: Grune & Stratton, 1970.

Thornton, John Leonard. *A Select Bibliography of Medical Biography*. 2d ed. London: Library Association, 1970.

Walker, M. E. M. *Pioneers of Public Health: The Story of Some Benefactors of the Human Race*. London: Oliver and Boyd, 1930.

INDEX

ABOUT THE
CONTRIBUTORS

DAVID P. ADAMS, Ph.D., M.P.H., is research director at the Cabarrus Family Medicine Residency Program, Concord, North Carolina, and consulting associate in the Department of Family and Community Medicine and visiting assistant professor in the medical humanities at Duke University School of Medicine. He has written extensively on the history and sociology of general and family practice in twentieth-century America. Dr. Adams is writing two books: a sociohistorical study of the American Board of Family Practice from 1969 to 1994 and a social history of general and family practice in the United States since 1940.

ASOKE K. BAGCHI, a consultant neurosurgeon residing in Calcutta, has written two books in Bengali on the history of medicine, an encyclopedia on Nobel laureates, a study of great women in science, and a study of medicine in medieval India. He is working on a chronological history of medicine.

TODD BENSON is a lecturer in the History Department at Stanford University. He is the author of *Bitter Medicine: The Federal Government and American Indian Health, 1900–1955* (Michigan State University Press, in press).

ANNE-EMANUELLE BIRN, assistant professor of health policy, New School for Social Research, received a B.A. in the history of science from Harvard University in 1986, an M.A. in history from the University of Canterbury (New Zealand) in 1988, and a doctorate in health policy from Johns Hopkins University in 1993. Her publications include "Public Health or Public Menace? The Rockefeller Foundation and Public Health in Mexico, 1920–1950," *Voluntas* (1996); "The Hook of Hookworm: Public Health and the Politics of Eradication in Mexico,'' (with Armando Solórzano) in *Contested Knowledge: Reactions to Western Medicine in the Modern Period* (edited by Andrew Cunningham and Bridie Andrews, forthcoming); ''Unidades Sanitarias: La Fundación Rockefeller vs. el Modelo Cárdenas en México'' (in *Salud, Cultura y Sociedad en América Latina: Nuevas Perspectivas Históricas*, edited by Marcos Cueto, 1996); and ''Pediatric AIDS in the United States: Epidemiological Reality Versus Government Policy'' (*International Journal of Health Services*, 1990). She is completing a book manuscript on local health and foreign wealth in Mexico, 1924–1951. She previously worked at the Pan American Health Organization, the Catalonia Health Department, and the Baltimore City Health Department.

JANE PACHT BRICKMAN, is professor of history and head of the Department of Humanities at the United States Merchant Marine Academy, Kings Point, New York. She received her undergraduate and master's degrees from Queens College and the Ph.D. degree in history from the City University Graduate Center. Her publications include several articles on the activities of medical reformers and physicians in the 1930s and 1940s. She is at work on an oral history of progressive American physicians who came of age medically in the 1930s and 1940s. Professor Brickman, who served for a decade as the adviser to women students at the Merchant Marine Academy (which has admitted women for two decades), has also written about issues that arise with the integration of women into formerly all-male institutions and women's roles in traditionally male-dominated industries.

VERN L. BULLOUGH is the author, coauthor, or editor of more than 50 books, 150 refereed articles, and many hundreds of nonrefereed ones. He is a former dean at the State University of New York College, Buffalo, and is now SUNY Distinguished Professor, Emeritus. He is a visiting professor at the University of Southern California in the Department of Nursing.

IAN CARR, M.D., Ph.D., FRC Pathology, FRCPC, taught pathology in the Universities of Glasgow, New South Wales, Sheffield, and Saskatchewan. He is now professor of pathology and medical history at the University of Manitoba and editor of *Prairie Medical Journal*. He has published papers and books about the human lymphoid system and the spread of tumors within it.

RANES C. CHAKRAVORTY graduated in medicine from Calcutta University. He has a master's degree in education from Virginia Polytechnic and State University. He trained as a surgeon in India, the United States, England, Belgium, and France. He is a professor of surgery at the University of Virginia Medical School, where he also teaches history of medicine, and was chief of surgery at the Veterans Affairs Medical Center, Salem, Virginia, from 1974 to 1994. His numerous publications in medicine include ''Diseases of Antiquity in

South Asia'' in *The Cambridge World History of Human Disease* (ed. K. Kipple, 1993).

JACQUELINE KARNELL CORN is an associate professor at Johns Hopkins University, School of Public Health, in the Department of Environmental Health Sciences. She has published on lead in the environment, byssinosis, silicosis, vinyl chloride, asbestos, coal mine health, and safety in nineteenth-century America, the social response to epidemic disease in Pittsburgh, Pennsylvania, and municipal organization for public health in Pittsburgh in the nineteenth century. Her books include *Protecting the Health of Workers* (1989), *Environment and Health in 19th Century America* (1988), and *Response to Occupational Health Hazards* (1992). She is working on a book about nonoccupational exposure to asbestos.

PAUL G. DYMENT is professor of pediatrics and vice chancellor for academic affairs at Tulane University, New Orleans, Louisiana. He earned the M.D. at McGill University, Montreal. He has served as president of the Ohio Academy of Medical History and the Handerson Medical History Society in Cleveland, and he founded the Osler Society for students at Case Western Reserve. He has published and lectured extensively in medicine and the history of medicine, and teaches a course on the history and philosophy of medicine at Tulane University School of Medicine.

NANCY ECKERMAN is the special collections librarian of the Ruth Lilly Medical Library, Indiana University School of Medicine. Her A.B. is from Albion College (1970), her M.L.S. from Indiana University (1971), and her M.A.R.S. from Butler University–Christian Theological Seminary (1983). She frequently addresses Indiana historical societies on the medical history of Indiana. She is engaged in original research on Indiana's Civil War surgeons and is building a database on nineteenth-century Indiana physicians. She is active in state and national library groups and has written entries for the *Encyclopedia of Indianapolis* and the forthcoming *Encyclopedia of History and Historians*.

ANTOINETTE EMCH-DÉRIAZ teaches at the University of Florida. She earned a Ph.D. in intellectual history at the University of Rochester. She has written several articles on diverse eighteenth-century medical topics, contributed chapters to books on the history of medicine, and published a monograph on Tissot. She is now editing the forty years of correspondence between Tissot and Zimmermann.

BARRY G. FIRKIN graduated in medicine M.B., B.S., 1954, the University of Sydney, and undertook postgraduate studies in hematology at Royal Prince Alfred Hospital, Sydney, and at Washington University St. Louis, Missouri. He has served as director of the Clinical Research Unit at Royal Prince Alfred

Hospital, chairperson of the Ethics subcommittee of the Australian Red Cross Society, president of the Australian Society of Medical Research, and professor of medicine at the Alfred Hospital, Monash University, Melbourne. In 1992 he transferred to the newly established Department of Medicine at Box Hill Hospital. He has published numerous articles and books, including *A Dictionary of Medical Eponyms* (with Judith Whitworth, 1987).

ANDREW A. GAGE graduated from the University of Buffalo School of Medicine in 1944. He held a faculty position in the School of Medicine in Buffalo and was promoted to professor of surgery in 1972. In 1960 Dr. Gage, in association with William Chardack, M.D., and Wilson Greatbatch, P.E., achieved the first successful implantation of a cardiac pacemaker. Dr. Gage has been deeply involved in cryosurgery since 1964 and has published extensively on the subject. From 1986 to 1994, Dr. Gage was deputy director of the Roswell Park Cancer Institute in Buffalo, a position that provided considerable insight into the history of the institute and its founder, Dr. Roswell Park.

THOMAS P. GARIEPY is associate professor in the program in the history and philosophy of science, Stonehill College, Easton, Massachusetts. Between 1989 and 1996 he was book review editor of the *Journal of the History of Medicine and Allied Sciences*. His publications include "The Introduction and Acceptance of Listerian Antisepsis in the United States" (*Journal of the History of Medicine and Allied Sciences*, 1994). He earned his B.A. from Stonehill College in 1970, his M.Th. and M.A. from the University of Notre Dame in 1973 and in 1976, respectively, and the Ph.D. from Yale University in 1990.

LINDA LEHMANN GOLDSTEIN holds a B.A. in English from the International College in Los Angeles, an M.A. in English, and a Ph.D. in American studies from Case Western Reserve University in Cleveland. Her dissertation, "Roses Bloomed in Winter," explored the role of small midwestern medical schools in facilitating the entry of the first women into the profession of medicine, including Dr. Emily Blackwell and Dr. Cordelia A. Greene. Currently residing in Maine, Dr. Goldstein is the director of corporate and foundation relations and a research associate with the American Studies Program at Colby College, where she also teaches a course on the history of women in medicine.

FARID SAMI HADDAD, M.D., retired urologist, surgeon, and historian, has worked at the Orient Hospital in Beirut, Lebanon, as resident in surgery and as director. He has served as resident physician with the United Nations Relief and Works Agency (UNRWA) for Palestinian refugees in Aleppo, Syria and resident physician with the Arab American Company (ARAMCO) in Saudi Arabia (1951). His career has also taken him to hospitals in Chicago, New York, Saudi Arabia, and Phoenix, Arizona. Dr. Haddad earned the B.A. (1941) and M.D. (1948) at the American University of Beirut, Lebanon. He is a fellow of the

American College of Surgeons and a diplomate of the American Board of Urology. He was chief editor of the *Annual Report* of the Orient Hospital (1957–1974) and the *Lebanese Medical Journal* (1961–1968) and the author or editor of forty-four books and over eleven hundred articles. He was a member and founder of many societies and has received many honors, including the National Order of the Cedars, the Medal of the Egyptian Medical Association, and the Award of Veterans of Foreign Wars (1983).

SALLY ANN HASTINGS, associate professor of history at Purdue University, works on civic organizations, social welfare, and political women in modern Japan. She earned the B.A. degree in history and English from Tufts University, the M.A. in East Asian studies from Yale University, and the Ph.D. in Japanese history from the University of Chicago. Her publications include *Neighborhood and Nation in Tokyo, 1905–1937* (1995); "The Empress' New Clothes and Japanese Women, 1868–1912" (*Historian*, 1993); and, with Sharon H. Nolte, "The Meiji State's Policy toward Women, 1890–1910," in *Recreating Japanese Women, 1600–1945*, ed. Gail Lee Bernstein (1991). She is working on a book on the first generation of political women in Japan.

CAROL HELMSTADTER, government relations officer of the Ontario Nurses' Association, received the B.A. from Wellesley, the B.Sc.N. from Columbia, and the M.A. in history from Columbia. She is the author of several major articles concerning the history of nursing, including "The Passing of the Night Watch" (*Canadian Bulletin of Medical History*, 1994), and "Doctors and Nurses: Class, Gender, Religion and Professional Expertise in London, 1850–1900" (*Nursing History Review*, 1996). She is working on a book on mid-nineteenth-century nursing reforms in England.

PATRICIA EVRIDGE HILL earned her B.A. in history from Southern Methodist University and her M.A. and Ph.D. in humanities with an emphasis in history from the University of Texas at Dallas. She is currently assistant professor of social science at San Jose State University (in an interdisciplinary social science department). Her recent publications include *Dallas: The Making of a Modern City* (1996), "Invisible Labours: Mill Work and Motherhood in the American South," *Social History of Medicine*, 1996), " 'Go Tell It on the Mountain': Hilla Sheriff and Public Health in the South Carolina Piedmont, 1929–1940," (*American Journal of Public Health*, 1995), "Real Women and True Womanhood: Grassroots Organizing among Dallas Dressmakers in 1935," (*Labor's Heritage*, 1994). She is working on a book-length biography of Hilla Sheriff.

ANN BOWMAN JANNETTA, associate professor of history at the University of Pittsburgh, works on the history of disease, health, and medicine in Japan. Her B.A. is from the University of Pennsylvania; the M.A. and Ph.D. are from the University of Pittsburgh. Publications include *Epidemics and Mortality in*

Early Modern Japan (1987); "Famine Mortality in Nineteenth Century Japan: The Evidence from a Temple Death Register" (*Population Studies*, 1992); and with Samuel H. Preston, "Two Centuries of Mortality Change in Central Japan: The Evidence from a Temple Death Register" (*Population Studies*, 1991). She is working on a book on the history of vaccination in Japan.

ALAN M. KRAUT is professor of history at American University in Washington, D.C., where he teaches immigration and ethnic history, the history of medicine, and southern history. His books include *The Huddled Mass: The Immigrant in American Society, 1880–1921; American Refugee Policy and European Jewry, 1933–1945* (coauthored) and, most recently, *Silent Travelers: Germs, Genes, and the "Immigrant Menace,"* which received the 1995 Theodore Saloutos Prize from the Immigration History Society and the 1995 Phi Alpha Theta Award for the Best Subsequent Book in History. He is currently working on a scholarly biography of Joseph Goldberger.

SUSAN E. LEDERER is associate professor in the Department of Humanities, Pennsylvania State University College of Medicine. She is the author of *Subjected to Science: Human Experimentation in America before the Second World War* (1995) and is completing a history of animal experimentation in twentieth-century America.

SUSAN RIMBY LEIGHOW is an assistant professor of history at Shippensburg University of Pennsylvania. She has published several articles dealing with the history of nursing as well as *"Nurses' Questions/Women's Questions": The Impact of the Demographic Revolution and Feminism on United States' Working Women, 1946–1986* (1996). She received her Ph.D. in history from the University of Pittsburgh.

LOIS N. MAGNER, professor of history at Purdue University, received her Ph.D. from the University of Wisconsin. She teaches courses in the history of medicine and science. Her publications include *A History of Medicine* (1992) and *A History of the Life Sciences* (1994).

DEBORAH KUHN MCGREGOR, assistant professor of history and women's studies, University of Illinois at Springfield (formerly Sangamon State University), earned her Ph.D. in history from the State University of New York at Binghamton. Her publications include *Sexual Surgery and the Origins of Gynecology: J. Marion Sims, His Hospital and His Patients* (1989), and " 'Childbirth-Travells' and 'Spiritual Estates': Anne Hutchinson and Colonial Boston, 1634–1638" (*Caduceus*, (1989). She is researching the history of midwifery in south-central Illinois.

MARCIA MELDRUM is a visiting assistant professor at the Center for Cultural Studies of Science, Technology, and Medicine at the University of California at Los Angeles. She received her Ph.D. in 1994 from the State University of New York at Stony Brook, where her dissertation, '' 'Departures from the Design': The Randomized Clinical Trial in Historical Perspective, 1946–1970,'' won the Distinguished Doctoral Scholar Award. Her most recent publication is "Simple Methods and Determined Contraceptors: The Statistical Evaluation of Fertility Control, 1957–68'' (*Bulletin of the History of Medicine*, 1996).

GENEVIEVE MILLER is associate professor emerita of the history of medicine, Case Western Reserve University School of Medicine, retired director of the Howard Dittrick Museum of Medical History, Cleveland, Ohio, and editor of the *Newsletter* of the American Association for the History of Medicine. She is the author of many books and articles, including *The Adoption of Inoculation for Smallpox in England and France* (1957), *Bibliography of the Writings of Henry E. Sigerist* (1966), and *Letters of Edward Jenner and Other Documents Concerning the Early History of Vaccination* (1983). She earned her A.B. from Goucher College in 1935, the M.A. from Johns Hopkins University in 1939, and the Ph.D. from Cornell University in 1955.

ALAN L. MOORE is completing a degree in history at the Johns Hopkins University. He plans to pursue a doctorate in modern American history. Mr. Moore has served as David P. Adams's senior research assistant on a variety of projects.

T. J. MURRAY is professor of medical humanities at Dalhousie University, Halifax, Nova Scotia, Canada. He has held many administrative roles at this institution, including dean of the medical school, 1985–1992, and head of the Division of Neurology. He and his wife, Janet, have just completed a biography of Sir Charles Tupper, a physician who was a Father of Canadian Confederation, and briefly prime minister of Canada. Dr. Murray was awarded the 1995 Neilson Award of the Hannah Institute for the History of Medicine. He is an officer of the Order of Canada.

SIDNEY OCHS has taught and carried out research on the nervous system— on the cerebral cortex, spinal cord, and peripheral nerves—since his doctoral graduation from the University of Chicago in 1952. He is the author of many research papers, book chapters, the textbook *Elements of Neurophysiology* (1965), and the monograph *Axoplasmic Transport and Its Relation to Other Nerve Functions* (1982). He is professor emeritus of physiology and biophysics in the Department of Physiology and Biophysics at the Indiana University School of Medicine in Indianapolis, where he continues his experimental studies on nerve properties and writes on historical aspects of the nervous system.

JOHN L. PARASCANDOLA is historian for the U.S. Public Health Service. He formerly served as chief of the History of Medicine Division at the National Library of Medicine and as professor of history of pharmacy and history of science at the University of Wisconsin–Madison. His book, on *The Development of American Pharmacology: John J. Abel and the Shaping of a Discipline* (1992), was awarded the George Urdang Medal of the American Institute of the History of Pharmacy.

T.V.N. PERSAUD, M.D., Ph.D., D.Sc., F.R.C.Path. (London) is professor of anatomy at the University of Manitoba. He was chairman of the Department of Anatomy in the Faculties of Medicine and Dentistry from 1977 to 1993 and past president of the Canadian Association of Anatomists (1981–1983). Dr. Persaud's research interests are in the areas of embryology, teratology, and history of medicine.

CYNTHIA DE HAVEN PITCOCK is assistant professor in the history of medicine for the College of Medicine Division of Medical Humanities at the University of Arkansas for Medical Sciences. She studied at Vanderbilt University on a Ford Foundation grant and at Washington University in St. Louis before receiving a Ph.D. in history from the University of Memphis. She teaches the history of medicine to senior medical students. She has published articles in the *American Journal of Obstetrics and Gynecology*, the *Journal of the History of Medicine and Allied Science*, and the *Missouri Historical Review* and has made numerous presentations to clinical faculty at schools of medicine and nursing and at national and international conferences.

JOHN POTTER received his B.A. in history from the University of Massachusetts at Amherst, his M.A. in history from the University of Massachusetts at Boston, and is currently a Ph.D. candidate at Clark University in Worcester, Massachusetts. He is writing his dissertation on the history of child labor regulation in Massachusetts. He has published articles on the history of industrial safety and on industrial hygiene and is the coauthor of an essay on nineteenth-century homeopathic psychiatry, which will be published by the American Psychiatric Association Press as part of a forthcoming collection of essays.

JUAN A. DEL REGATO was awarded the M.D. by the University of Paris. He served as assistant at the Institut Curie, Paris. He was director of the Penrose Cancer Hospital, Colorado Springs, Colorado, from 1949 to 1974. He is a Department of Veterans Affairs Distinguished Physician and Emeritus Professor of Radiology at the University of South Florida. Dr. del Regato was a pioneer in the training of radiation oncologists and a pioneer of radiotherapy research. He has been widely honored for his success in identifying therapeutic radiology as a separate medical specialty.

ANA CECILIA RODRIGUEZ DE ROMO, M.D., University of Mexico. Ph.D., Sorbonne, University of Paris, is professor in the Department of the History and Philosophy of Medicine, Faculty of Medicine, National University of Mexico.

Her publications include "Tallow and the Time Capsule: Claude Bernard's Discovery of the Pancreatic Digestion of Fat" (*History and Philosophy of the Life Sciences*, 1989) and *Epidemia de cólera en 1850* (1994).

CHRISTOPHER J. RUTTY received his Ph.D. from the University of Toronto's Department of History in 1995. His dissertation, " 'Do Something! . . . Do Anything!' Poliomyelitis in Canada, 1927–1962," is being revised for publication. Born in Burlington, Ontario, Rutty possesses a diploma in classical animation from Sheridan College of Applied Arts and Technology, Oakville, Ontario (1981–1984), a combined honors B.A. in history of science and history from the Faculty of Science, University of Western Ontario, London (1985–1989), and an M.A. in history from the same institution (1989–1990). Dr. Rutty has established his own consulting company, Health Heritage Research Services, which specializes in medical history, or health heritage research, consulting and archival services. He is planning further work on the history of Connaught Laboratories, the Ontario March of Dimes, and polio.

JONATHAN SADOWSKY, assistant professor of history at Case Western Reserve University, studies the history of psychiatric institutions in Africa. He received his B.A. from Wesleyan University, his M.A. from Stanford University, and his Ph.D. from Johns Hopkins University. His article, "The Confinements of Isaac O.: 'A Case of Acute Mania' in Colonial Nigeria," appeared in *History of Psychiatry* (1996), and he is completing a monograph on the social history of mental illness in Nigeria.

G. TERRY SHARRER is curator of health sciences at the Smithsonian Institution, where he has worked for more than twenty-five years. He speaks and writes about several agricultural and medical subjects, but his research interests focus on epidemiology and biotechnology. He holds a Ph.D. in history and agricultural economics from the University of Maryland and has authored some three dozen publications.

SHIFRA SHVARTS, professor of health policy and management, Ben Gurion University, Beer Sheva, Israel, earned her B.A. and M.A. in history and geography from the Faculty of Humanities and her Ph.D. from the Faculty of Health Sciences, Ben Gurion University of the Negev, Israel. She is the author of numerous articles on the development of health services and health policy in Israel. She teaches courses in the history of medicine, history of public health, and health policy and health politics in Israel.

LYNNE PAGE SNYDER works as staff historian in the Office of the PHS Historian, Public Health Service, U.S. Department of Health and Human Services. She received her doctorate in the history and sociology of science from the University of Pennsylvania in 1994. She is working on a number of projects about the history of federal environmental health policy.

STEPHEN SOREFF, M.D., is a health systems consultant for the Healthcare Quality Alliance, University of Massachusetts Medical Center, director of quality improvement, HMA Behavioral Health, Inc. in Worcester, Massachusetts, and president of Education Initiatives. His most recent books are *Handbook for the Treatment of the Seriously Mentally Ill* (1995) and, with M. A. McDuffee, *The Documentation Survival Handbook for Psychiatrists and Other Mental Health Professionals: A Clinician's Guide to Charting for Better Care, Certification, Reimbursement, and Risk Management* (1993). His M.D. is from Northwestern University Medical School, Chicago. He is board certified in psychiatry by the American Board of Psychiatry and Neurology.

WILLIAM C. SUMMERS is professor at Yale University, where he teaches both science and history of medicine and science. He has published articles on microbiology, biochemistry, and genetics, as well as on the history of microbiology and the history of medicine in China. He earned the B.S., M.S., M.D., and Ph.D. degrees from the University of Wisconsin between 1961 and 1967. After a year of postdoctoral study at the Massachusetts Institute of Technology, he joined the Yale faculty in 1968.

MICHEL VALENTIN (M.D., Paris, 1939) is an honorary member and former vice president and general secretary of the French Society of the History of Medicine, a laureate of the Institute of France and the Academy of Medicine, and a fellow of the Royal Society of Medicine (London). He is the author of many publications in ergonomics, industrial health, and the history of medicine, including *Work of Men and Forgotten Scholars, History of Ergonomics and Industrial Health* (1978), and biographies of François Broussais (1988) and Louis-René Villermé (1993).

SIGNILD VALLGÅRDA is an assistant professor in the Department of Social Medicine at the University of Copenhagen. She is trained as a historian and doctor of medical science. Her thesis topic was "Hospitals and Hospital Policy in Denmark 1930–1987: A Contribution to the History of the Specialized Danish Hospital Sector" (in Danish, 1992). She is undertaking research into maternal care and perinatal epidemiology in Denmark and Sweden. Her recent publications include "Trends in Perinatal Mortality Rates in Denmark and Sweden, 1915–1990" (*Paediatric and Perinatal Epidemiology*, 1995) and "The Hospitalization of Deliveries: The Change of Place of Birth in Denmark and Sweden from the Late Nineteenth Century to 1970" (*Medical History*, 1996).

EUGENE D. WEINBERG received his Ph.D. degree in microbiology at the University of Chicago in 1950. He has been a faculty member at Indiana University since 1950 and became head of the microbiology section of the Medical Sciences Program in 1963. He was selected for the Indiana University 1995–1996 Distinguished Faculty Research Lecture Award. His research has explored the interactions of microbial and animal cell physiology in determining the outcome of infectious and neoplastic diseases, especially offensive strategies whereby pathogenic microbes and cancer cells obtain iron from their hosts and the defensive measures by which hosts attempt to withhold iron from the invaders. Two of his publications have been designated as Benchmark Papers in Microbiology.

DORA B. WEINER is professor of the medical humanities at the University of California at Los Angeles (UCLA), where she cochairs the UCLA Programs in Medical Classics. Her books include *Raspail: Scientist and Reformer* (1968), *From Parnassus: Essays in Honor of Jacques Barzun* (1976, coedited with William R. Keylor), and *The Citizen-Patient in Revolutionary and Imperial Paris* (1993). She is coeditor of *The World of Dr. Francisco Hernandez* (forthcoming), editor of *Jacques Tenon's Memoirs on Paris Hospitals* (in press), and is preparing a book tentatively entitled *Observe and Heal: Philippe Pinel (1745–1826) and Humane, Comprehensive Public Medical Care in Revolutionary and Imperial Paris.*

ALLEN WEISSE received his undergraduate degree at New York University (1950) and his medical degree from SUNY Downstate Medical Center in Brooklyn (1958). He trained in internal medicine in San Francisco (University of California hospitals) and cardiovascular research at the University of Utah in Salt Lake City. He has been a member of the faculty at the Seton Hall College of Medicine, now the New Jersey Medical School in Newark, for more than thirty years. He has been the head of the echocardiography laboratory at Martland and University Hospital in Newark since 1975. He is the author of many articles and books, including *Medicine: State of the Art* (1984), the award-winning *Conversations in Medicine: The Story of Twentieth Century American Medicine in the Words of Those Who Created It* (1984), *Medical Odysseys: The Different and Sometimes Unexpected Pathways of 20th Century Medical Discoveries* (1991), and *The Man's Guide to Good Health* (1991).

PHILIP K. WILSON, M.A., Ph.D., is an assistant professor of the history of science at Truman State University (formerly Northeast Missouri State University) in Kirksville, Missouri. He studied human biology at the University of Kansas, medical history at the William H. Welch Institute for the History of Medicine at the Johns Hopkins School of Medicine, and received his Ph.D. in the history of medicine from the University of London. He has held postdoctoral positions at the University of Hawaii–Manoa and Yale University School of Medicine. His numerous publications include chapters in *The Popularization of*

Medicine, 1650–1850, Medicine and the Enlightenment, and *The Secret Malady: Venereal Disease in Eighteenth-Century Britain and France.* He edited *Childbirth: Changing Ideas and Practices in Britain and America 1600 to the Present* (forthcoming).

ISBN 0-313-29452-6

HARDCOVER BAR CODE